DATE DUE FOR RETURN

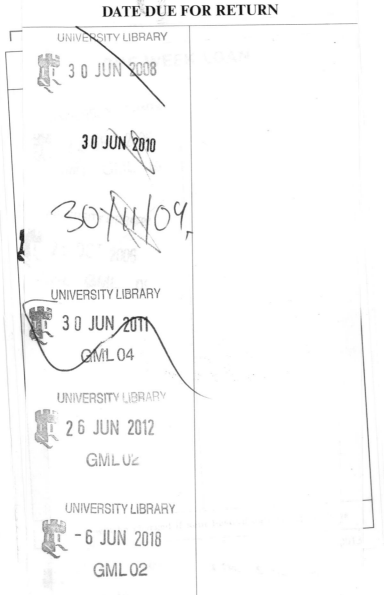
This book may be recalled before the above date.

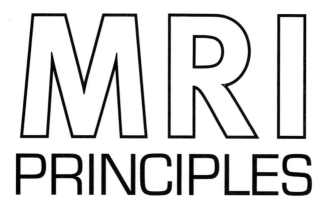

MRI
PRINCIPLES

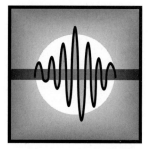

SECOND EDITION

Donald G. Mitchell, M.D.
Professor of Radiology
Director, Magnetic Resonance Imaging
Thomas Jefferson Medical College
Philadelphia, Pennsylvania

Mark S. Cohen, Ph.D.
Professor of Psychiatry, Neurology, Radiology
and Biomedical Physics
Brain Mapping Division
UCLA School of Medicine
Los Angeles, California

SAUNDERS

An Imprint of Elsevier

SAUNDERS
An Imprint of Elsevier Inc.

The Curtis Center
Independence Square West
Philadelphia, Pennsylvania 19106

MRI PRINCIPLES   ISBN 0–7216–0024–7

First Edition 1999.

Library of Congress Cataloging-in-Publication Data

Mitchell, Donald G.
    MRI principles / Donald G. Mitchell, Mark Cohen.—2nd ed.
      p. ; cm.
    ISBN 0–7216–0024–7
    1. Magnetic resonance imaging. I. Cohen, Mark, Ph.D. II. Title.
    [DNLM: 1. Magnetic Resonance Imaging—methods. 2. Mathematics. WN 185 M681m 2004]
    RC78.7.N83M55 2004
    616.07′548—dc22   2003054493

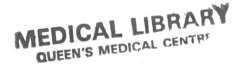

Printed in the United States of America

Last digit is the print number: 9 8 7 6 5 4 3 2 1

To Debbie, Rebecca, and
Liz and to Susan, Danielle,
and David for their love
and support.

Preface

Judging from the sustained book sales and the positive reviews and comments from readers, the first edition of *MRI Principles* appears to have been highly successful. Even Korean and Chinese translations have been published. Four years have passed since the first edition, and the field of magnetic resonance imaging has continued to advance rapidly. Contrast-enhanced MR angiography, functional neuroimaging, and parallel imaging are just a few of the advances that have become part of routine clinical MRI examinations during this period. Because of these developments, we believe that a second edition is in order.

To improve the depth and technical accuracy of *MRI Principles* without reducing its level of clarity for individuals who are not facile in the language of mathematics and physics, the second edition is a collaboration of two individuals with highly complementary backgrounds and interests who have known each other for well over a decade. Mark S. Cohen, Ph.D., has directly helped revise, and add new material to, Chapters 1–12, 16–20, 25, and 26. He has also provided insights that have helped improve the other chapters.

All chapters have been reviewed and revised extensively to keep current with the rapidly advancing state of MR technology. There are several new illustrations, and illustrations seen in the first edition have been modified in most cases to render the annotation and symbols more consistent with the standard conventions used in other publications. We have expanded the description of contrast-enhanced MR angiography and those of advanced neurologic and cardiac applications. We added a final chapter that discusses the logic of protocol construction and optimization, utilizing the principles described earlier in the book.

Despite the almost prosaic quality the examination now has, MRI remains difficult to understand. Whereas x-rays behave more or less like conventional light, the magnetic resonance signal is novel and completely beyond direct human sensation. The very presentation of MR data as images is a distortion, as the signal has nothing to do with light and dark; the organization into spatial maps is superimposed on it, and the primary contrast comes from temporal information. Our experience with MRI has shown that novices must open their minds to several new concepts, none of which can be grasped without understanding the others. Although it can be frustrating, learning to understand MRI can also be delightful, as each time the student integrates a new idea it results in a series of epiphanies about the others.

Although this book was written primarily for clinicians, of necessity it is a physics text. For our readers, however, we assume that the physics material is a means to an end. We have included information that our readers must have to prescribe tailored examinations and to make clinical decisions based on the images, avoiding details for their own sake. During its evolution MRI moved from clinical imaging to new and unexpected terrain; other scientists, including psychologists, psychiatrists, neuroscientists, cardiologists, and oncologists also need to understand how MRI works without being overwhelmed by obscure physics. They too should be able to use the material in this book to get started.

Having been involved personally with MR for most of its history, we offer this observation: The rate of new development has *not* slowed. Researchers are still discovering new physical principles that will expand the already vast array of applications for MRI. In fact, there is a new application to be found in virtually every MR artifact. The field of MR angiography, for example, arose from carefully studying artifacts due to motion; magnetization transfer, diffusion, perfusion, and other techniques have a similar history.

The volume of new material in this second edition, written only a few years after the first, is testimony to the evolution of the field and to the continuing need for practitioners to remain informed and on top of the latest developments.

Acknowledgments

As with the first edition, the second edition of *MRI Principles* has been "usability tested" by several individuals at the Thomas Jefferson University Department of Radiology, Division of MRI. I am particularly grateful to Drs. Christopher Roth, Jaime Checkoff, and Hongyu Shi for their highly insightful comments that helped improve the clarity of the second edition. I am also grateful to David Friedman, M.D., for his helpful comments regarding neurologic applications. Finally, I thank Mark Cohen, for his patience and dedication during the revisions. His contributions have added substantially to the quality and usefulness of this book.

Donald G. Mitchell, M.D.

I could never have gotten this far without the help of literally dozens of mentors in MRI. At the risk of leaving out many, I express my appreciation to Philip Femano, Dennis Atkinson, Wilfried Löffler, Piotr Starewicz, Truman Brown, Richard Rzedzian, Ian Pykett, Michael Rohan, and Robert Weisskoff, each for explaining to me how this particular process of image creation works. I take this opportunity also to thank my co-author, Donald Mitchell, for the chance to work with him on this second edition. I have been brutal about insisting on hundreds of changes to suit my own particular need for accuracy and detail, and he has been tirelessly gracious about accepting them. My hope throughout has been to help improve an already highly successful work.

Mark S. Cohen, Ph.D.

In this book, which is a practical guide rather than a review, we have elected not to reference any original work from the literally thousands of scientists, physicians, physicists and engineers who have contributed to the field known now as Magnetic Resonance Imaging. In so doing, we hope that we have added clarity and compactness to this volume, rather than to diminish the many contributions of our colleagues. Two particular investigators, Paul Lauterbur and Sir Peter Mansfield, received the 2003 Nobel Prize for Medicine for their groundbreaking work on the formation of images from the Nuclear Magnetic Resonance signal. This book is further dedicated to their accumulated work, which brought Magnetic Resonance Imaging from laboratory curiosity to clinical practice.

Contents

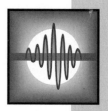

What Is Magnetic Resonance Imaging?

How This Book Is Organized and Why?

Magnetic resonance imaging (MRI) exploded onto the scene of clinical imaging during the mid-1980s. Compared to x-ray-based methods, MRI offers a remarkable combination of safety, spatial and contrast resolution as well as multifaceted sensitivity and specificity: It can be used to create images of startling clarity not only of body tissues but of their chemical constituents, depicting their functional status and providing quantitative measurements of velocity or other physical properties. Furthermore, when used properly, MRI is relatively free of biohazards, making it suitable for use with young children, pregnant women, normal volunteers, and other sensitive populations.

Unfortunately, with all of its power comes an extraordinary level of complexity.

Learning about MRI for the first time can be daunting. Many of the physical principles may be entirely new to the reader, and they are interdependent in such a way that understanding some of these principles requires comfort with many of the others. Our experience has shown that the best way to learn this material is to circle around it; to provide an overview of these topics and their interdependence and then to cover them in more detail. This chapter therefore starts with a brief overview of the fundamentals of MRI. Chapter 2 follows with a deeper view of the process of exciting protons and of using the resulting signals to create images. More detail, and more direct clinical relevance, follow in later chapters.

This book is a guide for the "mathematically illiterate," that is, those not fluent in the language of mathematics. However, it is not a book for the cognitively impaired; we know that readers of this book are not "dummies." Although we systematically avoid using either advanced mathematics or an equation as a proxy for a concept, there are times when a simple formula can help clarify a principle. In those cases, we give you the equations or formulae that amplify the text, and we do our best to summarize those concepts in words. Fortunately, most of the principles of MRI can be cast in terms of familiar material and experience.

What Is Magnetic Resonance?

Magnetic resonance imaging is based on the phenomenon of nuclear magnetic resonance (NMR), that is, the resonance of atomic nuclei. Resonance is defined as increased amplitude of the oscillation of a system exposed to a periodic force, the frequency of which is approximately equal to the system's natural frequency. NMR, in particular, involves measuring signals emitted from atomic nuclei in response to radio waves that have the same natural frequency (resonant frequency) as the nuclei themselves.

Hydrogen is the simplest and most abundant element in the human body. Every water molecule contains two hydrogen atoms; larger biological molecules, such as lipids and proteins, contain many. A hydrogen atom consists of a proton nucleus, carrying a unit positive electrical charge, and a single electron, which has a negative electric charge equal in magnitude to that of the proton (Fig. 1-1). Hydrogen nuclei, which do not contain neutrons, are often referred to simply as *protons*. Most clinical magnetic resonance utilizes protons, but the nuclei of other common atoms, such as sodium, phosphorus, fluorine, lithium, or others, can be used as well for imaging, spectroscopy, or other measurements.

The exact molecular environment where these protons are located has a profound effect on the nature of the MR signals created and thus gives rise to the remarkable power and versatility of clinical MRI and MR spectroscopy. The behavior of biological

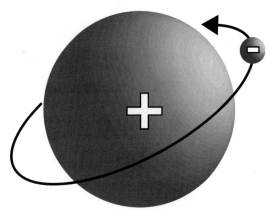

Figure 1-1
A hydrogen atom consists of a large proton, with positive charge (+), and a smaller electron, with negative charge (−).

protons in the presence of a magnetic field is considered in greater detail in Chapter 3.

An overview of the entire process by which images are created from protons is introduced in this chapter. The remaining chapters of the book are devoted to expanding on the various components of this process.

A few physical principles make MRI possible

1. There are fundamental relationships between electricity and magnetism: Moving electrical charges generate a magnetic field, and time-varying magnetic fields create electrical fields that promote the flow of electrical charges (current). The relationship between electricity and magnetism is therefore *reciprocal*.

2. The atomic nuclei of many atoms carry a small *magnetic dipole moment* (that is, they act as small magnets). We deal almost exclusively with protons—the nucleus of the hydrogen atom. (Moment, derived from "momentum," is the tendency of an object to move.)

3. When exposed to magnetic fields, magnets experience an aligning force whereby the "south" pole of one magnet tends to be attracted to the "north" pole of another and repelled by its "south" pole (Fig. 1-2). The term "lower energy"

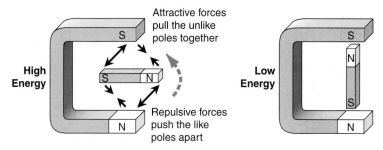

Figure 1-2

Magnets exhibit both an attractive force and an aligning force. When two magnets are brought together, the south pole of one is attracted to the north pole of the other and is repelled by its south pole. Here, the forces interact to make a stable condition, with the north pole of the bar magnet near the south pole of the C-shaped magnet.

describes the more favorable, and therefore more stable, condition when south is aligned with north. As systems move toward equilibrium, they move to lower energy states. At the level of subatomic particles, such as protons, this process is *quantized.* That is, these particles can exist in only a small number of restricted states. Protons can exist only in states that are either "up" (high energy aligned *opposed* to a magnetic field) or "down" (low energy aligned *with* a magnetic field).

4. In addition to their magnetic moment, protons carry "angular momentum." For our purposes we can imagine them as spinning, like tops. Angular momentum is the tendency for a spinning object to continue to spin about the same axis. When force is applied to change the axis of rotation, angular momentum results in *precession*: These objects or particles rotate around such forces.

5. The rate at which an object precesses is proportional to its angular momentum and to the strength of the forces that tend to change it.

To cover this material, we refer at times to mathematical constructs such as vectors, and we explain them as we go. For completeness, we include a few equations, when they add clarity. In the majority of cases, you can ignore these equations without losing hold of the concepts because we rely primarily on description and illustration to reinforce them.

In Chapter 2, we expand on these principles, discussing the nature of protons, magnetic fields, and radio waves and how they are used to construct MR images. First, however, in the remainder of this chapter we review briefly the basic components of the MRI instrument.

MRI Instrument Overview

The MRI instrument includes one or more computers, a radio transmitter, one or more radio transceiver coils and receivers, magnetic field gradient coils, and the main magnet. At the core of all MRI instruments is a homogeneous magnetic field, which is needed to establish longitudinal magnetization of protons within it. Some MRI instruments utilize *permanent* magnets, which contain magnetic materials that directly create magnetic fields. A permanent magnetic field is oriented along an axis that extends between the two poles of the magnet. Usually an MRI system that utilizes a permanent magnet contains a magnetic field that is perpendicular to the scanner table (Fig. 1-3). The configuration of a permanent magnet lends itself particularly well to an "open" configuration.

A magnetic field can also be generated perpendicular to an electric current flowing along a cylindrical coiled wire, as in *resistive* electromagnets (Fig. 1-4). Because the

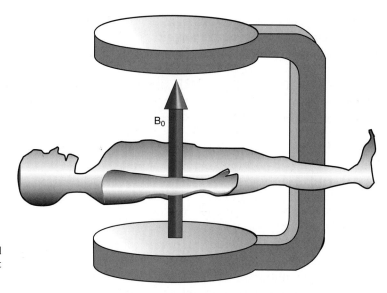

Figure 1-3
Main magnetic field (B_0) oriented along the axis of a permanent magnetic field.

magnetic field is generated within a cylinder, the configuration is typically "closed."

The strength of the magnetic field created by a permanent or resistive magnet is limited to approximately 5000 gauss (10,000 times the strength of the earth's magnetic field), or 0.5 tesla (T). Stronger magnetic fields can be created by *superconducting magnets*, wherein resistance to the flow of electric current can be nearly eliminated by using appropriate materials and a sufficiently low temperature. Although the design issues have been challenging, superconducting technology has now been adapted to produce open MRI units with field strengths of 1.0 T and higher.

Creating MR images depends upon exciting protons within a magnetic field using pulses of radiofrequency (RF) energy, often referred to in this book as radio pulses. Specific portions of the body parts of interest

are excited, and the locations of the signals are determined by creating predictable variations in the magnetic field by applying supplemental magnetic field *gradients*. Because the frequency of the NMR signal depends on the magnetic field, these gradients encode position. This process is expanded upon in Chapter 2 and again in further depth in later chapters.

The timing and strength of magnetic field gradients and radio pulses are controlled through an acquisition computer that uses parameters chosen by the MRI operator. The commands from the computer are sent to gradient and RF amplifiers, which, generate, respectively, gradient and radio pulses. The waveforms for radio pulses are subsequently sent from the RF power amplifier to a radio transmitter that is near or surrounds the patient.

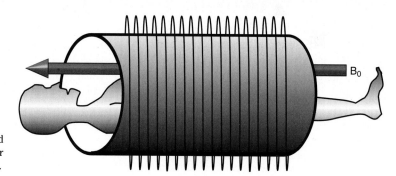

Figure 1-4
Main magnetic field (B_0) oriented along the axis of a resistive or superconducting magnetic bore.

Following excitation of tissue by an RF pulse, a signal is created, the amplitude of which decays rapidly. This initial rapidly decaying signal is called a *free induction decay* (FID). Often, additional RF and gradient pulses are used to create echoes of each signal. The timing of these radio and gradient pulses and their effects on the information content of MR signals are considered in more detail in Chapters 3 and 4. Methods of restoring the MR signal after the FID are discussed in Chapter 6.

The RF pulse is usually transmitted from a "coil." Although the coil can be as simple as a wire loop, a more complex coil configuration is usually used to improve the accuracy or homogeneity (or both) of the RF pulse. In some instances, the same coil is used to send and to receive MR signals. One example of a transmit–receive coil is the large circumferential coil that is built into the bore of most commercial MRI units, typically referred to as the "body coil." Smaller circumferential transmit–receive coils are often used to image smaller structures such as the head or extremities. In other instances, as for imaging superficial structures, a separate *receive-only coil* is used to detect the MR signals that result after excitation by a radio pulse transmitted by the body coil. The signals from the body part of interest are sent from the receiving coil to an RF amplifier, which increases the magnitude of the signals.

Initially, the received signal consists of a continuously varying (analog) waveform that contains signals with a wide range of frequencies, corresponding to the various locations along the imaging gradients. These data do not directly indicate the spatial location of the protons from which they originated. First, the MR signals undergo analog-to-digital conversion (ADC), producing digital data that consist of a set of numbers representing distinct time points along the waves. These data are processed by the MR acquisition computer. In their raw form, the digital data are the "Fourier transform" of the actual MR image. If we consider a two-dimensional picture to be a map of "image space," the corresponding two-dimensional raw data are said to be mapped in "*k-space*" (Fig. 1-5).

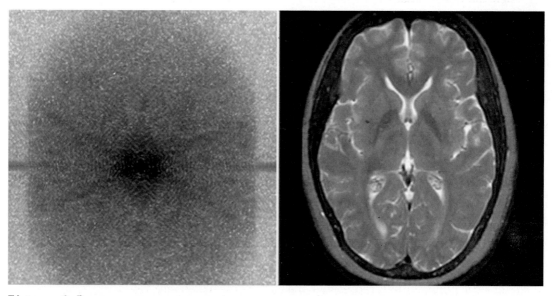

Figure 1-5
k-Space (*left*) is a map of digital data that, when subjected to Fourier transform analysis, generates an image of physical space (*right*). The image at right is a 256 × 192 fast spin echo image with a TR/TEef of 2317/90.

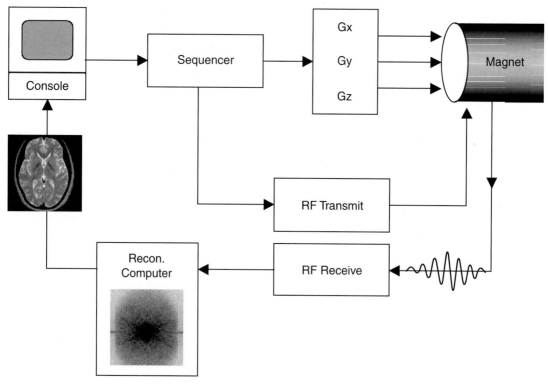

Figure 1-6

General schematic of an MRI instrument. Pulse sequence parameters are sent from the scanner console to the sequencer, a computer component that generates the radiofrequency (RF) transmit and gradient instructions. The resulting signals are received, and analog-to-digital conversion yields raw data that can be displayed as k-space. This is stored and processed by the reconstruction computer, and the resulting pixel data are sent to the scanner console for viewing, printing, or archiving.

Different locations in k-space correspond to differences in spatial frequency—how rapidly the signal intensity varies as we move across an image. Each point in k-space contains data from all portions of an MR image. The centermost point in k-space contains information about the intensity and contrast of the entire image, and the data points at the edges of k-space encode information about the fine details of the image. Figure 1-5 demonstrates an image and its corresponding k-space map. The concept of k-space is discussed and illustrated in greater detail in Chapter 7.

The Fourier transform of k-space yields pixel data that allow construction of a two- or three-dimensional image. Each pixel is assigned a number that represents the MR signal amplitude (intensity) from that spatial location. These pixels form images that are sent to the host computer for display, printing, or further manipulation or analysis. Because the NMR signal intensity depends on the receiver gain and other factors, absolute signal intensity numbers may be meaningless by themselves. The signal intensities of pixels in an image relative to each other, however, are quite useful.

Figure 1-6 describes the basic features of an MRI system as outlined above. The details of MR image creation and how MR parameters can be adjusted to alter the appearance and information content of MR images are addressed throughout the remaining chapters of this book.

▼
Essential Points to Remember

1. Current clinical methods of MR imaging involve the excitation of hydrogen nuclei, which consist of protons.

2. In a magnetic field the most common state of protons is aligned along with the magnetic field.

3. An MRI instrument includes a strong homogeneous magnet which may be superconducting, resistive, or permanent.

4. MR images are created by using radio pulses to excite spinning protons within a magnetic field and then analyzing the resulting signals.

5. The location of excited protons is determined by creating predictable variations in the magnetic field by applying magnetic field gradients.

6. The radio signals are received by the same RF coil that transmitted the exciting radio pulses or by a separate receiver coil matched to the local part of the body.

7. The amplitude, frequency, and phase of MR signals are converted to digital data and are used to create a map of k-space by a process known as the Fourier transform. The Fourier transform of k-space is the final MR image.

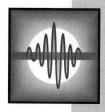

From Protons to Images

The phenomenon of magnetic reso-nance lies at the boundary between quantum and classic physics. Most of quantum physics is outside our direct experience and therefore foreign to us. Fortunately, most of what we need to know about MRI can be cast into the more famil-iar world of our experience, although some consideration of quantum effects can help us understand the basics of MRI. Formal derivation of these quantum effects are well beyond the domain of a book intended to minimize mathematics, so the reader is expected take them at face value.

Atoms and Protons

The formation of atoms into molecules (a.k.a. chemistry) changes their magnetic properties and therefore has substantial effects on the MR signal. This is the funda-mental basis of MR spectroscopy, and we expand on the effect of molecular environ-ments in later chapters as needed. For the present, however, we will think only about atoms in isolation, including the three par-ticles that make up the atoms: electrons, protons, and neutrons. Whereas electrons and protons contain negative and positive electrical charges, respectively, the neutron is uncharged (and is not considered here any further).

Generally, single atoms must have an equal balance of positive and negative charges and thus an equal number of elec-trons and protons. Despite their equal charge, the masses of the proton and elec-tron are vastly different, with the mass of the proton being at least 2000 times larger.

The simplest atom, the hydrogen atom, contains but one proton and one electron. It is also by far the most ubiquitous atom in the universe. Protons carry the properties of both electrical charge and magnetic moment, meaning that when they are exposed to a static magnetic field (one that does not vary), they experience a force that causes them to align with that field.

Longitudinal Relaxation Forces

If magnets are placed into a magnetic field, they experience aligning forces that tend to pull their "south" poles toward the "north" pole of that field. (The convention for labeling north and south poles refers to the magnetic field orientation of the earth.) When the south pole of a magnet is pointing to the north pole of an applied magnetic field (and *vice versa*), its potential energy is low. When north points to north and south to south, the magnets are in a high energy state.

Like other magnets, the individual protons have low and high energy orientations to an applied magnetic field. The laws of thermodynamics dictate that higher energy states are less stable, and that systems tend to change to their lower energy "equilibrium" conditions. Unlike conventional magnets, however, protons can adopt only two states (high and low energy), without any intermediate orientations. It is in this sense that the magnetic orientation is "quantized" (Fig. 2-1).

The transition to the lower energy "relaxed" state releases energy into the surroundings. The amount of energy released is identical to the energy difference between the north-to-north versus the north-to-south conditions. The laws of quantum physics require that this energy be transferred to or from the environment, usually because of a collision or similar interaction with neighboring particles. Because the amount of energy transferred must be *exactly* the difference between high and low energy orientations, spontaneous transitions are infrequent. When the magnetization is far from equilibrium, *most* of these collisions

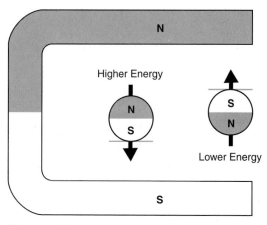

Figure 2-1
Protons can adopt only two states (high and low energy) without any intermediate orientations. Magnetic orientation is therefore "quantized." The preferred low energy state here is indicated with an *arrow* pointing upward, in the direction of the aligning force.

result in proton spins flipping from *high* to *low* energy states.

Over time, as individual protons flip to lower energy orientations, a net excess of spins in the lower energy state accumulates. Each of these protons carries its own magnetic field and interacts with its neighbors. Although the magnetic moment of individual protons is exceedingly small, it is large enough to influence protons close-by. Therefore, not all protons flip to the low energy state with respect to an external field because the magnetic field from their neighbors tends to counteract the external field.

At equilibrium, there is a slight excess of spins in the low energy state to exactly balance all of the forces from both local and external magnetic fields. In this condition, the sample overall is said to be "magnetized" as there is a net difference in the number of spins in the low and high energy states. At this point the sample is in equilibrium, and collisions with particles in the environment are equally likely to flip individual spins to low or high energy states. This net excess of magnetization within the sample (the difference between the number of spins in the high and low energy states) is known as its *longitudinal magnetization* (Fig. 2-2).

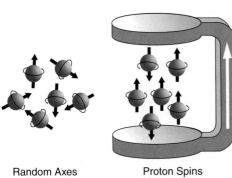 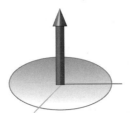

| Random Axes of Rotation | Proton Spins Aligned Along Magnetic Field | Net Magnetic Vector of Protons in Magnetic Field |

Figure 2-2
Proton rotational axis in the absence of a magnetic field (*left*) is random. In the presence of a magnetic field (*middle*), there is a net excess of protons aligned with the direction of the main magnetic field. This produces longitudinal magnetization (*right*).

The approach to equilibrium is initially rapid but slows as the overall system comes close to its balanced state. Figure 2-3 shows total magnetization as a function of time after a sample is placed in a magnetic field.

Even though protons are small and experience a considerable aligning force when placed in a magnetic field, they do not change immediately to their preferred, lower energy state. Instead, as we see in more detail in Chapter 3, it may take some time for a biological tissue, containing a huge number of protons, to reach its lower energy state. The rate at which a material approaches equilibrium is determined by a time constant known as its T1, which is characteristic of the material. The recovery is logarithmic; T1 is the time required for about 63% of the magnetization to recover. The rate of recovery is the inverse of the time, or 1/T1.

Mathematically, the logarithmic curve for recovery of longitudinal magnetization is described by the equation:

$$M_z(t) = M_0(1 - e^{-t/T1})$$

This states that the magnetization along the z direction (by convention, the direction of the external magnetic field is known as z and is usually drawn vertically), known as M_z, is equal to the equilibrium magnetization M_0 times a factor that depends on time (t) and the constant T1. Whereas M_0 is essentially fixed by the strength of the magnetic field, T1 is a characteristic of the sample and describes how rapidly that sample magnetizes.

The approach to equilibrium, along the z axis, is known as *longitudinal* relaxation.

Because the approach to equilibrium requires quantized energy of just the right amount, the overall process can be quite slow. If the collisions are between rapidly moving particles, the energy levels are likely to be too high to cause spin flips. Likewise, if the particles are moving too slowly, the energy levels are too low to cause the state transition.

One factor that strongly influences the motional energy of a system of particles is

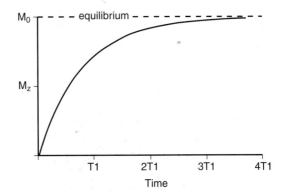

Figure 2-3
Once a sample is placed in a magnetic field, it starts to "magnetize." By convention, the orientation of the external magnetic field is along the z axis, so the magnetization of the sample is called M_z. When first placed in the field, magnetization is relatively rapid but slows as the sample comes close to its final equilibrium, magnetization. Different body tissues magnetize at different rates; on this curve, the characteristic logarithmic magnetization rate for a tissue is the inverse of its T1, which has units of time. After three or four T1 periods, the sample is effectively magnetized fully.

the temperature. Temperature is, in fact, a reflection of the velocities of the molecules that make up a substance. Therefore, the rate at which samples reach magnetic equilibrium depends critically on temperature. Small particles tend to be in more rapid motion than large molecules, so particle size has a strong effect on the rate at which samples magnetize.

The magnetization time, T1, of body tissues varies from a tenth of a second or so for fat, to several seconds for simple fluids such as cerebrospinal fluid (CSF). The T1 also changes in a variety of pathological states and can be manipulated by contrast agents. T1 is a major determinant of contrast in MRI.

To summarize:

■ When placed into a magnetic field, body tissues change gradually from a demagnetized state to a magnetized state.
■ The rate at which a sample magnetizes is determined by its T1.
■ The T1 of body tissues ranges from about 0.1 to 4.0 seconds.
■ T1 depends strongly on the mobility of protons and on their temperature.

Angular Momentum and Precession

Momentum describes the tendency of an object, once moving, to continue moving in the same direction. Stopping a moving object requires applying a force in the direction opposite to its direction of motion; applying a force in any other direction alters its direction of travel but does not stop the motion. Angular momentum is similar: It is the tendency of a spinning object to continue to spin about the same axis of rotation.

Bicycle wheels provide a familiar example of angular momentum. Once the wheels are spinning, their angular momentum tends to keep them rotating. It also keeps the entire bike from falling over, as tilting a spinning wheel to the side amounts to changing the direction of the axis about which the wheel spins and therefore causing a change in its angular momentum.

When a force is applied that would change a spinning object's direction of rotation, its angular momentum opposes the force, causing the object to wobble. Gyroscopes demonstrate this "conservation of angular momentum." Once a gyroscope is spinning, it does not immediately fall over from the force of gravity. Instead, it wobbles about slowly in a circle. This slow circular motion is known as "precession" (Fig. 2-4). The rate of this precession depends not only on the momentum of the object but also on the strength of the force that is trying to change it.

Like bicycle wheels, tops, and gyroscopes, the subatomic protons and electrons of atoms possess angular momentum (Fig. 2-5). The magnitude of this momentum (the proton's magnetic moment) is "quantized"

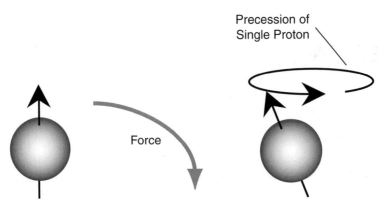

Figure 2-4
When force is applied to change the axis of rotation, angular momentum results in "precession."

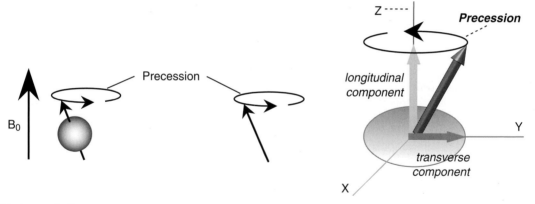

Figure 2-5
Each proton has a small magnetic field and a quantum property called angular momentum, or "spin." Its angular momentum causes it to precess when it is placed in a magnetic field (denoted here as B_0). These diagrams are all equivalent representations. In the *middle* we show only the precession, and on the *right* the precession is separated into its nonspinning longitudinal (along z) component and a transverse component, spinning (precessing) in the xy plane.

(as in quantum physics), meaning that it can only attain certain fixed values. The protons of all hydrogen atoms, for example, have the same angular momentum. When protons are placed in a magnetic field, their intrinsic magnetic moment results in their experiencing an aligning force that gives them a preferred (lower energy) orientation. However, the angular momentum of the protons prevents them from simply aligning their magnetic axis with the external magnetic field. Instead, they spin, or precess, about it. This precession is particularly important, as it gives rise to the signal that is detected to form MR images.

Because all protons have the same mass and angular momentum, they all precess about the external field at the same rate. This relation between the strength of a magnetic field and the rotational rate of the atomic nuclei is of fundamental importance for MRI. It is expressed by the simple formula known as the Larmor relation:

$$f = \gamma B \qquad (1)$$

In this equation, f represents the frequency of rotation (the number of rotations per second), B is the magnetic field strength, and γ is known variously as the "gyromagnetic

ratio," the "magnetogyric ratio," or simply the Larmor constant. For protons, γ is approximately 42.58 millions of cycles per second per tesla of magnetic field (abbreviated as 42.58 MHz/T). The gyromagnetic ratio differs, and is lower, for other atomic nuclei. The Tesla is a unit of magnetic field strength; 1 T is about 20,000 times the strength of the magnetic field of the earth. Magnetic field strength is sometimes measured in "gauss" where 1 T = 10,000 gauss. The simple relation between magnetic field strength and precessional frequency is exploited throughout the MRI process.

The frequency at which the nuclei precess in a given magnetic field is known as their "Larmor frequency." In a magnetic field of 1.0 T, the protons precess at 42.58 MHz. In a 1.5 T field, the precessional frequency is 63 MHz, and so on. Many texts, including this one, sometimes refer to the individual nuclei as "spins," as this is often the single parameter of most interest in magnetic resonance. The term "spin" is also sometimes used as a synonym for the angular momentum of the nucleus.

Figure 2-6 shows the precession of a single proton about a magnetic field applied along the z (vertical) axis. Its travel describes a cone shape oriented about the z axis.

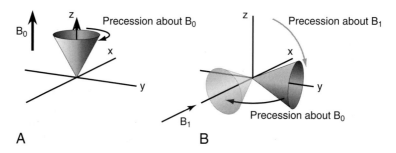

Figure 2-6
At equilibrium, net magnetization is oriented along B_0 (*A*). If we apply a second magnetic field (B_1) at right angles to the static field (B_0), rotating at the Larmor frequency, we can cause the longitudinal magnetization to precess about the B_1 field. If B_1 is of the right magnitude and is applied for just the right amount of time, the sample's longitudinal magnetization rotates by 90°, so it is at right angles to B_0. All of the sample's magnetization is now a rotating field, precessing about B_0 at the Larmor frequency (*B*).

When we look at a collection of such protons, they all precess at the same rate, but at any given time individual protons are likely to be pointing in a random direction. It is easiest to consider the magnetic moments of the individual protons as vectors, where each has a vertical component (directed along z) and a horizontal component that is aligned along the plane made by the x and y axes (the "x-y plane") (Fig. 2-5). The horizontal vector component rotates about the z axis, and stays within the x-y plane.

Nuclear Magnetic Resonance

Suppose we place a sample containing protons (such as a human) in a strong static (stable, not changing) magnetic field, called B_0. After a few seconds, the protons within it reach a low energy state, as described above, aligned along the static field. The protons have now reached equilibrium, with their net magnetization aligned longitudinally (Figs. 2-2 and 2-6A).

Then we apply a second magnetic field, called B_1, which is oriented at right angles to B_0 (aligned along the x axis) and rotating about the z axis at the same rate as the individual protons. Because it is rotating along with the protons, this B_1 field is

experienced, with respect to individual protons, as if it were a *constant* magnetic field at right angles to B_0. To help understand this concept, imagine yourself precessing with a proton (a situation known as the "rotating frame"). Because B_1 is rotating at the same rate as you (the proton), its orientation with respect to you seems to be constant. However, B_1 is just another magnetic field, so you and the other individual protons tend to precess about *it*, as shown in Figure 2-6. Thus the cone of magnetization that describes the orientations of the ensemble of many protons also rotates about B_1.

The rate at which the protons precess about the B_1 field is also governed by the Larmor equation and therefore depends on the magnitude of B_1. The larger the magnitude of the B_1 field, the faster do the protons change the orientation of their precession; moreover, the longer B_1 is left "on," the further the protons rotate. For example, if B_1 has a magnitude of 1 gauss, the protons complete a rotation about B_1 every 1/4258 seconds—about once every 1/4 msec. In just about 1/16th of a millisecond, they have done a one-quarter turn, or 90°. At that time, the cone of magnetization has been rotated from the z axis into the xy plane.

Let us examine this special case in more detail. Each proton's z vector component has now been rotated by 90° (Fig. 2-7). Because initially there were more protons pointed along positive z than along negative z, there

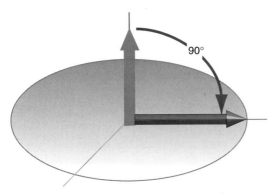

Figure 2-7
A 90° excitation pulse rotates longitudinal magnetization into the transverse plane. In this simplified diagram, net magnetization is represented as vectors (*arrows*).

are now excess protons pointed along one direction in the xy plane. Whereas initially there were more protons in the equilibrium, low energy state, a result of this rotation is that there are now an equal number of protons in the low and high energy states.

Once the spins have flipped by 90°, we can turn off the B_1 field and step away from the rotating frame (that is, relative to the rotating proton) into the stationary frame. From this perspective, we see the net magnetization from the individual spins rotating about the z axis, in the x-y plane, at a rate proportional to the static field strength B_0. The sample is therefore completely demagnetized and far from equilibrium along the longitudinal z axis. It then starts to recover its magnetization at a rate determined by its T1, similar to the original magnetization process when the spins first entered the magnetic field. This recovery of magnetization toward the equilibrium low energy state is referred to as T1 relaxation.

Meanwhile, in the x-y plane, the vectors from all of the individual protons now sum constructively to form a magnetic field rotating at the rate γB_0 the product of the main magnetic field and the gyromagnetic constant of the material. For protons in a 1.5 T magnetic field, for example, this corresponds to a magnetic field rotating in circles

about 63 million times per second. It is this magnetic field, rotating in the transverse plane, that we detect a magnetic resonance signal.

Because the magnetization has been forced out of its equilibrium longitudinal state, the sample is "excited" into a higher energy state. Stated somewhat differently, the B_1 magnetic field rotates the initially longitudinal (along B_0) magnetization into the transverse plane, producing transverse magnetization. A 90° pulse, in particular, rotates all of the magnetization into the transverse plane, eliminating the component along the longitudinal axis; the system thus is said to be "saturated."

This change in the magnetic orientation occurs if the B_1 magnetic field is rotating at precisely the same rate as the individual protons, thereby making the entire process a "resonant" phenomenon—hence the term nuclear magnetic resonance (NMR). If B_1 is made to rotate too slowly or too rapidly, the individual spins wobble back and forth but do not precess smoothly around B_1. In other words, the frequency of the excitation radio pulse must match the natural frequency of the protons, which is determined by the magnetic field in which they are residing.

Radio Waves and Magnetic Fields

Electricity and magnetism are deeply linked forces and concepts. In particular, electrically charged particles, exposed to a time-varying magnetic field, experience a displacement force (electromotive force, or *e.m.f.*). Likewise, an electrical current (the flow of charged particles) creates a magnetic field. The orientations of these fields are interdependent: The magnetic field created by a current encircles the direction of current flow, and the flow of current is at a right angle (orthogonal) to the change in magnetic field (Fig. 2-8). This relationship

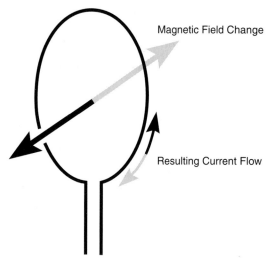

Magnetic Field Change

Resulting Current Flow

Figure 2-8
If a conductor is placed in a time-varying magnetic field, the electromotive force created by the magnetic field causes a current to flow. In this example, the magnetic field oscillates back and forth, as might occur in the presence of rotating nuclear spins and results in a current in the wire loop (antenna), which also oscillates. Typically, this oscillation is at frequencies of several tens of megahertz, corresponding to the Larmor frequency of protons in magnetic fields of several tesla.

is fundamental to MRI, so it is important to become comfortable with it.

The interdependence of electricity and magnetism can be easily verified. For example, if you place an ordinary compass next to a piece of wire and then connect each end of that wire to a battery, the compass aligns itself perpendicular to the direction of current flow.

A static magnetic field does not, by itself, create electricity. However, time-varying magnetic fields cause electrical currents to flow within conductors. Excitation of the sample by NMR, as described above, produces a magnetic field that oscillates at several million times per second, in the *radiofrequency* (RF) range. This time-varying magnetic field creates an e.m.f. that can be detected using standard radio electronics. The strength, or magnitude, of the electrical current depends on factors such as how many protons get together to create it and how rapidly it varies.

What we know of as radio waves are rapidly varying fields of electrical and magnetic force. Like any other source of magnetism, radio waves also affect the orientation of protons. In fact, the rotating field used to induce the magnetic resonance signal is itself simply a pulse of an ordinary radio signal. One should think of magnetic resonance as the interaction of radio and magnetism on the protons. Furthermore, the radio pulse adds energy to the sample (the patient) by moving it away from magnetic equilibrium. As we see in Chapter 3, the strength of the NMR signal depends on how far the sample is from equilibrium. This is a crucial factor for the contrast we see in magnetic resonance images.

Longitudinal magnetization, by the way, cannot be detected readily, principally because in the equilibrium state it is not time-varying, or varies so slowly (as tissues approach equilibrium) that it generates negligible e.m.f. Furthermore, because the e.m.f. is proportional to the magnetic field's rate of change, the NMR signal becomes greater when the sample is placed within the field of stronger magnets (i.e., as the Larmor frequency increases). This is a primary reason that relatively large magnetic fields are used for MRI and why there is often a push in both clinical and research environments to use ever stronger imaging magnets.

Summarizing this material tells us the following.

- A sample containing protons, when placed in a magnetic field B_0, reaches an equilibrium where the magnetic fields of all of the individual protons sum to create a single vector aligned along, and opposed to, the external magnetic field.
- Individual protons precess about the external field at the Larmor rate: 42.58 MHz/T.
- If a second magnetic field (B_1) is applied that rotates about B_0 at the Larmor rate, protons are forced to precess about B_1.
- By adjusting the duration and amplitude of B_1 we can force the protons to flip (rotate) as far as we desire. This brief burst of rotating magnetization is known

as an RF pulse. If the duration is such that the spins flip by 90°, it is called a 90° RF pulse.

- Any magnetization we create in the plane orthogonal to B_0 is time-varying at the Larmor rate and can be detected as the magnetic resonance (MR) signal.

Transverse Relaxation: T2 and Its Friends

Thus far we have discussed how to create a macroscopically detectable signal from the magnetization of body tissues, and we have looked at an important tissue-specific parameter, T_1, which is characteristic for different body tissues. We now look in more detail at the transverse magnetization we created. This transverse magnetization, remember, is the MR signal that is detected to form images.

The magnetization in the x-y plane, known as "transverse" magnetization, is composed of the contributions of myriad individual protons. In a perfectly homogeneous magnetic field, once this MR signal was created it would remain present until longitudinal relaxation had caused the net transverse component to become zero. In fact, however, the rotating signal always decays somewhat more rapidly. This is because the protons can never *all* be in identical magnetic fields. This is due to several factors. First, even if we were able to create a perfectly homogeneous magnet, each of the protons, with its own small magnetic field, slightly perturbs the magnetic field experienced by its neighbor. As a result, the individual protons precess at slightly varying rates and over time begin to point in different directions, so their magnetization in the xy planes eventually cancels. Once the protons are pointing in opposite directions in the transverse plane, the total signal is eliminated completely (Fig. 2-9).

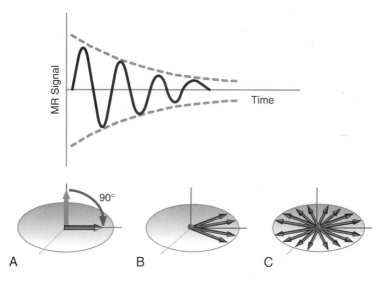

Figure 2-9

The decaying magnetic resonance (MR) signal is represented as an oscillating wave, the magnitude of which is depicted as the space between the *gray dotted lines*. Initially, after a 90° radiofrequency (RF) pulse, the magnetization from all protons in the sample is summed in the transverse plane and precesses together, yielding a large MR signal (*A*). Over time, differences in the local magnetic field cause the spins to precess at slightly different rates and to go out of phase, resulting in a loss of signal (*B*). Ultimately (*C*), the signal goes to near zero when the magnetization from individual spins is canceled by oppositely directed spins. The rapid decay of the signal is depicted at the *top*, the "free induction decay."

The consequence of the spread of proton precessional frequencies is that the MR signal, once created, decays fairly quickly. Figure 2-10 shows the signal decay as a function of time. The graph is described mathematically by the equation

$$M_{xy}(t) = M_0 \, e^{-t/T2}$$

where M_{xy} refers to the transverse magnetization. T2, like T1, is a magnetic relaxation rate. If T2 is short, the MR signal decreases rapidly; if T2 is long, the signal decreases more slowly. Because transverse magnetization can easily be detected as an MR signal, it would be equally accurate to refer to the vertical axis of this graph as the MR signal.

It is extremely difficult to construct imaging magnets whose fields are homogeneous over samples as large as the human body. Although it is now routine to have fields that vary by as little as one part per million over regions as large as the abdomen, it still results in the proton spins varying in frequency by several tens of hertz. Thus the protons in different positions, initially

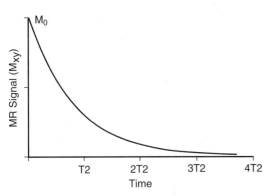

Figure 2-10
After a 90° RF pulse, the proton magnetization is rotated into the transverse (xy) plane. Because the protons start off precessing together (in phase) the signal is strong initially. Over time, however, the differences in the precessional rates of the individual spins causes the total transverse magnetization (and therefore the MR signal) to decay. The decay rate is tissue-specific and is known as T2. The signal decays to near zero after three or four T2 periods.

pointing in the same direction (precessing "in phase") are now pointing in opposite directions within only a few milliseconds, as the faster protons rapidly leave the slower protons behind and the magnetizations go out of phase.

Spatial Localization

Unfortunately, the radio signal does not contain much localization information (although the radio antenna is somewhat more sensitive to nearby signals than to distant ones, a principle that can be exploited to reduce imaging time with advanced methods of imaging, as discussed in Chapter 17). High resolution imaging requires a different, more flexible, means of spatial encoding. In particular, we can take advantage of the proportionality between the magnetic field strength and the proton rotational frequency: If the magnetic field is made to vary predictably with location, the frequency of the MR signal also depend on the location.

The fundamental process used to determine the location of sources of MR signals is the application of supplemental magnetic fields, referred to as *imaging gradients*. In a homogeneous magnetic field, water protons resonate at the same frequency, regardless of location. If we superimpose a second magnetic field on the main magnetic field, we cause a predictable variation in the magnetic field along a predetermined axis. The resulting total magnetic field (the sum of the main and gradient magnetic fields) is highest at one end and lowest at the other; between are intermediate values along the axis of the gradient. Because the resonant frequency of a proton is directly proportional to the magnetic field that contains it, the magnetic field gradient produces a predictable variation in resonant frequency along this axis. Thus application of the magnetic field gradient causes protons at one end of the gradient to spin slower and protons at the other end to spin faster (Fig. 2-11). By detecting the

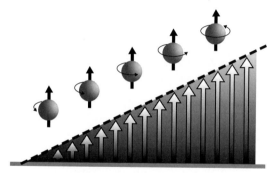

Figure 2-11
Magnetic field gradient applied in addition to the homogeneous main magnetic field. The magnetic field increases to the right along the axis of this gradient, increasing the resonant frequencies of the affected protons.

frequency of the signal, we can determine its position.

Magnetic field gradients are usually produced by gradient coils within the bore of the main magnet. Magnetic field gradients are applied in three orthogonal axes, at different times, allowing three-dimensional localization of the signals' origins. The application of these gradients and the methods by which the signals are used to construct images are discussed in more detail in Chapter 6.

By calculating the strength of the MR signal at each frequency, we create an image showing the signal strength at each location. The mathematics that allows us to calculate the signal frequency is known as the Fourier transform (Fig. 2-12),

a topic of advanced mathematics. In this book, we cover some of the results of Fourier mathematics, as we need them to understand MR image formation, but we do not need to do the calculations or to consider them in any detail.

Magnetic resonance induction, image contrast, and image formation are highly interdependent. We see in later chapters that part of the process of spatial localization involves restricting magnetic resonance induction to a localized region in space, such as by slice-select gradients. Furthermore, the timing of the sequence of radiofrequency (RF) and gradient pulses determines the contrast in the images, which also depends on the tissue relaxation times T1 and T2. One reason MRI can be a challenge to understand is that understanding image contrasts requires some understanding of spatial localization and vice versa.

The MRI process is basically as follows.

1. Magnetize the region of interest.
2. Use a radio signal to alter its magnetization.
3. Collect a resultant radio signal from the patient. The timing of the signal generation and data collection determines the image contrast.
4. Distort the magnetic field so the signal frequency is a function of position.
5. Repeat the process as often as necessary to acquire sufficient data to construct the desired images.
6. Analyze the signal frequencies emitted from the region of interest to form the image.

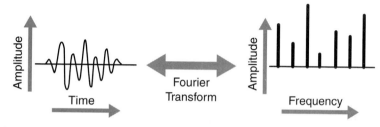

Figure 2-12
Fourier transform analysis involves converting the frequency data in a complex wave into a map of amplitudes for each frequency.

▼
Essential Points to Remember

1. Moving electrical charges generate a magnetic field, and time-varying magnetic fields create electrical fields that promote the flow of electrical charges (current). The relationship between electricity and magnetism is therefore reciprocal.

2. In the presence of a magnetic field, protons spin at a frequency that is directly proportional to the strength of that magnetic field.

3. The net magnetization of protons at equilibrium is called *longitudinal magnetization*, which is oriented in the same direction as the magnetic field of the imaging magnet.

4. When excited by a radio pulse of identical frequency, the magnetization of spinning protons is rotated toward the transverse plane. The strength and duration of this excitation radio pulse determine how far this magnetization is rotated.

5. A radio pulse that rotates the magnetization of spinning protons by 90° is referred to as a *90° pulse*. A 90° pulse converts **all** *longitudinal magnetization* to *transverse magnetization*.

6. Equilibrium (longitudinal) magnetization cannot be measured easily. Magnetization must be rotated into the transverse axis for it to be detected.

7. The rate at which a tissue becomes magnetized is determined by its T1, which depends on the mobility of its protons.

8. The MR signal, derived from transverse magnetization, decays at a rate determined by the T2 of the tissue.

9. The location of MR signals is determined by applying magnetic field gradients, which cause the resonant frequency of protons to vary predictably along the axis of the magnetic field.

Chapter 3

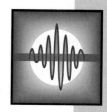

Proton Environments and T1 Relaxation

A ll other factors being equal, a higher density of mobile protons results in a stronger magnetic resonance (MR) signal and brighter pixels on MR images. This dependence of contrast on density also applies to radiography and scintigraphy. However, there are other mechanisms for MR tissue contrast that often are more important which relate to the local environment of protons. That is, the signal arising from a given proton varies according to its position within a molecule and its relationship to other molecules. Much of the tissue contrast in MR images is based on the different rates between tissues of magnetization and demagnetization.

In Chapter 2 we outlined the importance of the longitudinal and transverse relaxation rates, T1 and T2. This chapter and the next focus on developing a deeper understanding of the relationship of T1 and T2 to the physical environment created by human tissue and physiology. In this chapter, we concentrate

on water, the principal source of most signals used for MR imaging. The rate at which water magnetizes (or re-magnetizes after magnetic resonance induction) in a given body tissue is tissue-dependent, and these differences in magnetization rates can be exploited to create MR image contrast. This chapter concerns some of the physical factors that determine T1 and relates them to the strength of the magnetic field and to some specific aspects of the timing of the magnetic resonance process.

Water

The structure of water in biological tissues is surprisingly rich. To understand tissue contrast on MR images, however, a simplified two-compartment model is generally sufficient. These two water compartments

21

are referred to commonly as *free water* and *bound water*.

Free water consists of water molecules in solution that are not in immediate proximity to macromolecules such as proteins, phospholipids, or DNA. Free water moves rapidly and is highly *disorganized* at the local level (although forces such as van der Waals attraction give water bulk organization). Bound water, on the other hand, is close enough to macromolecules for its motion to be restricted. The restriction of the motion of bound water is principally through hydrogen bonding, which occurs when the highly polar water molecule is near charged molecules, such as those that appear on the surface of living cells or within intracellular organelles. Bound and free water are illustrated in Figure 3-1.

The relative amounts of free and bound water within tissues vary greatly throughout the body. Soft tissues with abundant intracellular organelles, such as brain, pancreas, and liver, have a large intracellular surface area. The proportion of bound water in these tissues therefore is large. In contrast, there is a large proportion of free water in urine and cerebrospinal fluid (CSF), as well as within cysts, follicles, and glands. Water in these locations thus appears different from water in solid tissues in the MR images (Fig. 3-2).

T1 Relaxation (Recovery)

As discussed in the Chapter 2, exposure to a radio pulse with a frequency that matches a proton's precessional frequency induces magnetic resonance, rotating the equilibrium

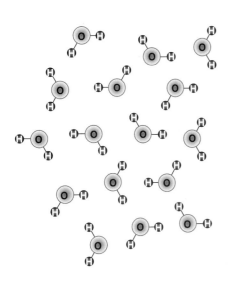
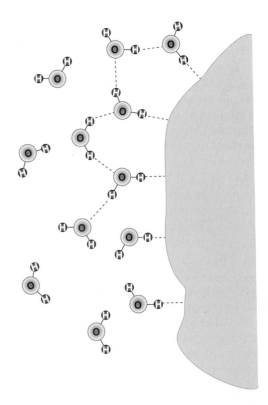

Figure 3-1
Biological water can be considered to be in one of two compartments: free water (*left*) or bound water (*right*), which is closely associated with macromolecules. Dotted lines indicate van der Waals attraction.

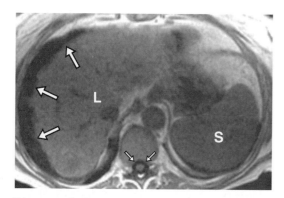

Figure 3-2
Axial T1-weighted image of the abdomen depicts free water in ascites (*large arrows*) and cerebrospinal fluid (CSF) (*short arrows*) as having low signal intensity owing to the long T1 relaxation time of free water. Some of the water in solid tissues such as spleen (S) and liver (L) is bound, causing higher signal intensity. The T1 of liver is shorter than that of spleen, so liver has higher signal intensity.

longitudinal magnetization into the transverse plane. Following magnetic resonance induction, the longitudinal magnetization recovers (Fig. 3-3).

This recovery of longitudinal magnetization requires an exchange of energy (chiefly motional energy) between the protons and their environment. Because the energy exchange is quantized, longitudinal relaxation

is most efficient when there are frequent interactions (such as collisions) between the protons and their environment at specific energy levels. This relationship, between the physical chemistry of molecules and the T1 magnetization rate is one of the main reasons MRI is so useful in clinical practice: It offers a sensitive window into the microstructure of body tissues.

When a patient is placed initially in a magnetic field, or following a 90° pulse, the net alignment of protons is in a high energy state far from equilibrium. At this time most interactions between the protons and their environment result in transitions to a lower energy state. Therefore the approach to the equilibrium magnetization state is initially rapid (Fig. 3-4). Over time, however, the magnetic forces on the protons become more balanced, and individual protons become equally likely to change to their higher or lower energy states. At this point the entire system is at equilibrium because the net magnetization no longer changes.

Figure 3-5 shows, for three body tissues, the initially rapid change in M_z, which slows as it approaches the final equilibrium value of M_0. In Figure 3-5, M_z is equal to the difference in the number of low energy and high energy protons. The magnetization curves depict $M_z(t)$, magnetization as a function of time; time is indicated on the

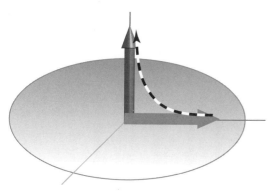

Figure 3-3
T1 relaxation (recovery) converts transverse magnetization back to longitudinal magnetization, its equilibrium state. The loss of transverse magnetization (shown horizontally) occurs independently at the rate, T2.

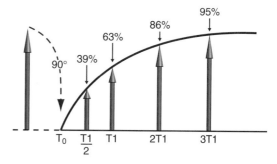

Figure 3-4
T1 relaxation following a 90° excitation pulse, which creates transverse magnetization at T_0. The curve indicates the logarithmic recovery of longitudinal magnetization at T1/2, T1, 2T1, and 3T1.

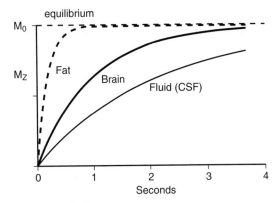

Figure 3-5
T1 recovery curves for three tissues with different T1 values: fat has the shortest T1, cerebrospinal fluid (CSF) has the longest, and brain is intermediate. For all three, recovery is initially rapid, slowing as equilibrium is approached.

horizontal axis in seconds. The *shapes* of the magnetization curves are essentially identical for all body tissues, but the time axis may vary greatly.

Imagine that it is possible to acquire an MR image about 1 second after a subject is placed in the imager. In that case, his or her body fat would be almost fully magnetized because of its short T1. However, the brain, with a much longer T1, would be perhaps 40% less magnetized, and the CSF would be only 30% magnetized. If the signal intensity in the final image is made proportional to the magnetization, the signal from fat is much stronger than that from brain or CSF. Although it is not practical to excite tissue within a second of a patient's entry into the magnet bore, differences in tissues' T1 relaxation rates are indeed used to generate contrast in MR images by applying radiofrequency (RF) excitation pulses that repeatedly saturate the magnetization (described below under "Repetition Time and Contrast"). Figure 3-6 similarly shows recovery curves for two different tissues, indicating recovery of magnetization at the T1 for each of the two tissues.

What accounts for this large difference in magnetization rates? The energy of the molecules' motion is proportional to their velocity, and small molecules generally move more, and faster, than larger ones. Much of the motional energy of the tiny free water molecule is too fast to facilitate relaxation; thus, free water recovers its magnetic equilibrium ("magnetizes") slowly, with a T1 of a few seconds. Conversely, the coordinating effect of macromolecules on the structure of water slows its motion and lowers its average energy. In many cases this decreases T1, so the water near such organizing molecules (bound water) magnetizes more rapidly.

Figure 3-6
T1 relaxation for solid tissue (*gray*) and free water (*black*). In this example, recovery to 63% of equilibrium longitudinal magnetization requires four times as much time for free water as for solid tissue. Therefore T1 relaxation is four times as long for free water as for solid tissue.

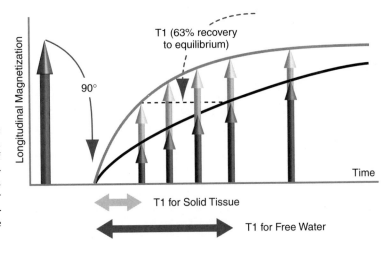

Body Tissues

The upper limit for biological T1 relaxation times is that of pure free water, approximately 3 seconds. The T1 relaxation times of CSF and urine, which contain some electrolytes but few large molecules, are between 2 and 3 seconds. In contrast, the motion of fatty acid protons within adipose tissue is restricted, increasing the efficiency of T1 relaxation and causing adipose tissue to have a T1 shorter than that of most other biological tissues. The T1 of adipose tissue is approximately 100 to 150 msec, depending on the magnetic field strength.

Protons in macromolecules such as protein do not produce an MR signal on currently used pulse sequences (because, as amplified in Chapter 4, their transverse magnetization decays so rapidly that no signals are detected by most current clinical MR techniques). However, such molecules restrict the motion of nearby water and thus shorten its T1 relaxation time. Fluids with high protein content, such as mucus and synovial fluid, have a shorter T1 than do less viscous fluids.

Most normal cellular soft tissues have a large intracellular surface area, which results in a large proportion of bound water. Cellular tissues thus tend to have much shorter T1 relaxation times than do fluids such as urine and CSF (Fig. 3-5).

For many benign and malignant disease processes, at the cellular level the intracellular constituents become relatively disorganized. Together with the edema that often accompanies disease, this increases the relative fraction (ratio) of free/bound water, prolonging the T1.

Field Strength

The difference in energy between high and low energy states generally increases with field strength, whereas the motional energies of the water molecules do not. Field strength therefore has a relatively complex relationship with the T1 relaxation rates (Fig. 3-7): T1 increases for some tissues and decreases for others as the magnetic field strength increases.

For the range of field strengths in clinical use, some generalizations are helpful. Most nonfatty soft tissues have a longer T1 at high field strength. The increased T1 of adipose tissue is less pronounced, and there is no significant change in free water. Therefore T1 contrast between most soft tissues, and between free and bound water, is stronger at low field strength. The contrast between soft tissue and fat is greater at high field strength.

Magnetic field strength is also a major determinant of MR *signal* strength. For this reason, MR images obtained with comparable parameters are usually noisier at

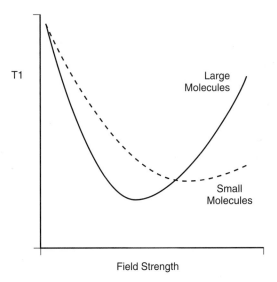

Figure 3-7
The relationship of T1 to field strength is typically U-shaped, depending on molecular size. At lower fields, the relaxation times of large molecules tend to be less than those of small molecules. At high field strengths, the difference between low and high energy states increases so the increase in T1 is less for small molecules.

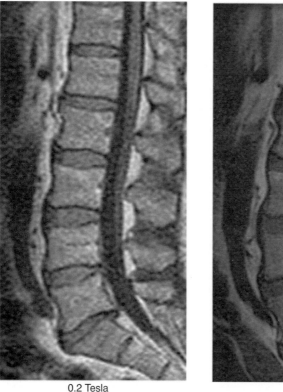
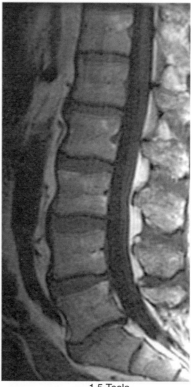

0.2 Tesla   1.5 Tesla

Figure 3-8
Comparison of T1-weighted spin echo images of the lumbar spine of one subject obtained with similar parameters at 0.2 T (*left*) and 1.5 T (*right*). The image obtained at 0.2 T is noisier but has greater contrast between the CSF and the spinal cord or intervertebral discs. However, the contrast between cellular and fatty marrow in the vertebral bodies is greater at 1.5 T. (Courtesy of Lawrence Tannenbaum, M.D. and Edison Imaging, Edison, NJ.)

low field strength (Fig. 3-8). Field strength is discussed in greater depth in Chapter 12.

Repetition Time and Contrast

We indicated in Chapter 2 that, following an RF pulse of proper amplitude and duration, equilibrium longitudinal magnetization (M_0) is converted to the MR signal. Thus the maximum strength of the MR signal is equal to M_0, the magnitude of the longitudinal magnetization that existed prior to the RF pulse. Here, we examine the effects on the MR signal of a series of 90° RF pulses.

For this example we assume that there is no transverse magnetization at the time of the RF pulses. Following each 90° pulse *all* of the longitudinal magnetization is rotated into the transverse plane. Along the longitudinal axis (z axis), the sample is in the same state as before it entered the magnetic field, with no net longitudinal magnetization. Because it is far from equilibrium, the longitudinal magnetization grows rapidly, as shown in Figures 3-4 through 3-6.

In the transverse plane, the magnetization immediately after each 90° pulse is as large as the prior longitudinal magnetization. Owing to transverse relaxation processes (described in Chapter 2 and in more detail in Chapter 4) the signal decays quickly. After a short time (TR), we apply a second 90° RF pulse.

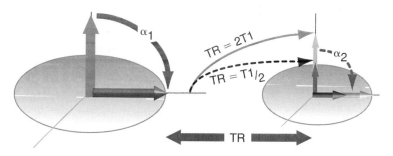

Figure 3-9

Effect of T1 differences in two tissues on the amount of transverse magnetization created. The initial 90° excitation pulse (α_1) rotates all longitudinal magnetization into the transverse plane. T1 for the tissue indicated by the *dark arrow* is four times as long as it is for that indicated by the *light arrow*. The repetition time (TR) is therefore half the T1 for dark and twice that for light. Different amounts of transverse magnetization are thus created by the next 90° excitation pulse (α_2) for each of the two tissues, directly reflecting the different amounts of longitudinal magnetization that had recovered. Thus the differences in T1 between the two tissues produce different amounts of transverse magnetization and different intensities on the resulting image (T1 contrast).

Figures 3-9 and 4-5 shows this process for two different tissues. One, shown with dotted lines, has a long T1, thereby recovering longitudinal magnetization slowly. The other, indicated with solid lines, has a shorter T1. Because both tissues start at equilibrium, the signal strength following the first RF pulse is equal to M_0 for both tissues. After a short interval, the longitudinal magnetization of the tissue with the longer T1 (slower recovery) is less than that of the tissue with the shorter T1. The MR signal thus created in the transverse plane (M_{xy}) by the next excitation pulse is less for the tissue with a long T1. The resulting image shows tissues with a long T1 as darker than tissues with a short T1; the contrast in the image is thus *T1-weighted*.

With each successive 90° pulse the longitudinal magnetization is returned to zero. If the repetition time, TR, between pulses is constant, the longitudinal recovery during each interval is identical, so the signal *contrast*—the intensity difference between tissues with different T1s—is established and steady.

This discussion shows the fundamental relationship between TR (the RF pulse repetition rate) and T1 contrast. T1 contrast is minimized when TR is extremely long, as this allows recovery of longitudinal magnetization for all tissues. As the TR is

reduced, the T1 contrast increases up to a point. When TR is extremely short, however, the signal from all tissues is reduced so much that little usable signal, and therefore little contrast, remains. Figure 3-10 shows this effect. Figures 3-11 and 3-12 further illustrate the interrelationship between TR and T1 contrast.

When a flip angle different than 90° is used, some longitudinal magnetization remains after the RF pulse. In this case it takes more than one RF pulse for the system to reach a steady state. As MR systems are not perfect, even when a 90° pulse is programmed the actual flip angle within the body tissues may be somewhat more or somewhat less. Commercial imaging systems usually include a series of three or more preparatory pulses (dummy pulses) prior to data collection to ensure that a steady state is reached.

Flip Angle

As explained in Chapter 1, during the time the RF pulse is turned on, the magnetization rotates steadily at a rate determined by the strength of the pulse. If the pulse is turned

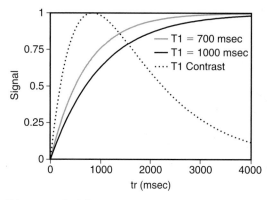

Figure 3-10

Contrast between two tissues as a function of TR. Two tissues are represented: one with a T1 of 700 msec (*dashed curve*), and the other with a T1 of 1000 msec (*solid thin line curve*). The difference in signal intensity (contrast) between these two tissues is indicated with the *heavier solid line curve*. Note that the contrast is small with an extremely long TR when the signal from both tissues is near maximal, and with a short TR when the signal from both tissues is near zero. The vertical scale for contrast and signal are not the same.

on for a shorter time, the resulting flip angle is reduced. If the flip angle is less than 90°, part of the magnetization is rotated into the transverse plane (creating a signal), and part remains along the longitudinal axis. When at least some of the longitudinal magnetization remains, the return to equilibrium requires less time. Under these circumstances, shorter TRs can be used while still maintaining an adequate signal.

Figure 3-13 shows this effect. On the left, a relatively large flip angle rotates most of the magnetization into the transverse plane, leaving a small fraction of the longitudinal magnetization. By comparison, the right panel shows the effects of a smaller flip angle, which disturbs the longitudinal magnetization very little while still producing substantial transverse magnetization and MR signal. Figure 3-14 further illustrates the effect of reducing the flip angle on longitudinal and transverse magnetizations.

With a small flip angle, recovery to equilibrium takes less time, so that even with a short TR the next RF pulse creates a large signal. The effect of flip angle reduction on the strength of the resulting MR signal depends on a balance between the amount

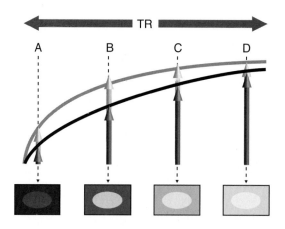

Figure 3-11

T1 relaxation curves of two tissues show contrast based on four repetition time (TR) values (A–D). The *curve* and *arrows* in light gray indicate a tissue with short T1, while the darker shade indicates long T1. If the TR is too short (A), the contrast may be subtle owing to low signal intensity of both tissues. With more moderate TR (B), the contrast may be depicted optimally. As TR increases, the magnetization of the tissue with a long T1 continues to recover, and contrast may become increasingly subtle, as for conditions C and D.

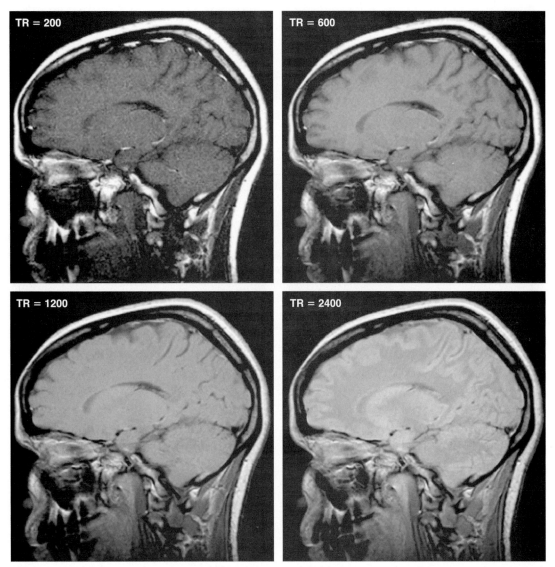

Figure 3-12

Effect on tissue contrast of varying the repetition time (TR). Sagittal fast spin echo images of the brain with a TE of 15 msec and variable TR. With TRs of 200 and 600 msec, there is substantial T1 contrast between gray and white matter and CSF, but the overall signal intensity is higher with a TR of 600 msec. As the TR increases to 1200 and 2400 msec, T1 contrast diminishes.

of transverse magnetization created and the amount of longitudinal magnetization saturated by the excitation radio pulse, as shown in Figure 3-15. A flip angle of 90° creates the most transverse magnetization, which *by itself* results in the *highest* signal intensity on the eventual MR images. However, a 90° pulse also saturates longitudinal magnetization most completely, which *by itself*, results in the *lowest* signal intensity on the eventual MR images when TR's of less than several times T1 are used.

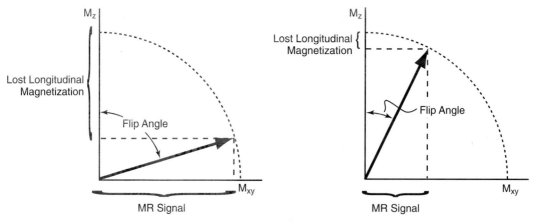

Figure 3-13

Effect of the flip angle on the MR signal. *Left.* A relatively large flip angle rotates most of the longitudinal magnetization (M_z) into the transverse plane, leaving a small amount in place. *Right.* By comparison, a small flip angle little disturbs the longitudinal magnetization but still produces substantial transverse magnetization (M_{xy}) and MR signal. With the small flip angle, recovery to equilibrium takes little time, so the next radiofrequency (RF) pulse creates a large signal. The effect of flip angle reduction on the strength of the resulting MR signal depends on a balance between the amount of transverse magnetization created and the amount of longitudinal magnetization saturated by the excitation radio pulse.

Conversely, flip angles smaller than 90° create less transverse magnetization, but they also saturate less of the longitudinal magnetization.

The advantage of small flip angles is most pronounced in tissues with a long T1. With a low flip angle, even if the TR is short, the longitudinal magnetization recovers in a short time. Because smaller flip angles allow substantial recovery of longitudinal magnetization even of tissues with a long T1, they reduce the influence of T1 on the resultant signal and therefore tend to reduce T1 contrast. Depending on the imaging need, this can be desirable or undesirable. Most importantly, small flip angles allow one to use short TRs while still retaining adequate signal and, when desired, minimal T1 contrast. This is the basis of a variety of imaging methods, including the original FLASH (*f*ast *l*ow *a*ngle *sh*ot) acquisition.

In most commonly used MR acquisition modes, multiple RF excitation/data collection cycles are needed to form a single image. As such, the total imaging time is determined by the TR, and there is great

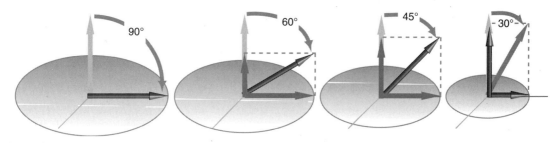

Figure 3-14

Excitation pulses of 90°, 60°, 45°, and 30°, rotating different amounts of longitudinal magnetization into the transverse plane. With a reduced excitation flip angle, such as 30°, less transverse magnetization is created and more longitudinal magnetization remains.

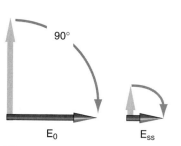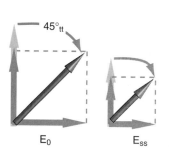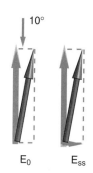

Figure 3-15

Comparison of the amount of transverse magnetization created at steady state by 90°, 45°, and 10° at a given short repetition time (TR) for a tissue with a given T1. Although the amount of transverse magnetization created by the initial excitation pulse (E_0) is greatest for the 90° excitation pulse, most magnetization remains saturated at the time of each excitation pulse during the steady state (E_{ss}). With 45° excitation pulses, T1 relaxation is more complete at the same TR, as less longitudinal magnetization is saturated with each excitation pulse. Thus more transverse magnetization is created during the steady state by 45° pulses than by 90° pulses. Although there is nearly complete T1 recovery between excitation pulses with 10° pulses, little transverse magnetization is created by each excitation pulse. For the tissue and TR in this example, the optimal excitation angle (Ernst angle) is closer to 45° than to 90° or 10°.

incentive to reduce the TR as much as is practical. Often this results in a TR that is much shorter than the tissue T1. In such situations, the flip angle can be lowered to maintain adequate signal strength.

For a tissue with any given T1 and TR, there is an optimum flip angle, known as the *Ernst angle*, that yields the maximum

MR signal. The Ernst angle can be computed using the following formula.

$$\text{Ernst angle} = \text{arc } \cos(e^{-TR/T1})$$

The Ernst angle is plotted as a function of TR/T1 in Figure 3-16. When the TR is relatively long compared to T1 (left panel) the

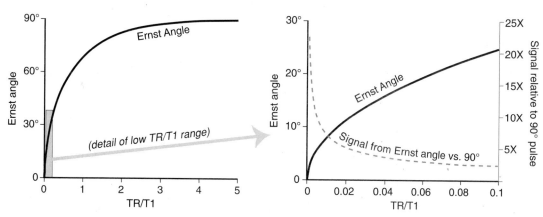

Figure 3-16

Ernst angle for various combinations of TR and T1. The *solid black curve* shows the Ernst angle (the flip angle yielding the maximum MR signal) as a function of the TR/T1 ratio. *Left.* Wide range of TR values relative to tissue T1. *Right.* Enlarged view of the region of the *gray curve* on the left, where the TR is 10% or less of the tissue T1. As the TR becomes shorter compared to T1, the Ernst angle becomes progressively smaller. The signal resulting from excitation at the Ernst angle relative to the signal from a 90° excitation is shown by the *gray dashed line*. As the TR becomes progressively shorter, an RF pulse at the Ernst angle is increasingly advantageous relative to a 90° pulse for creating a stronger MR signal.

effect of the flip angle is less important. When the TR is very short, however (right panel), the optimal flip angle can be extremely small. Under such conditions the signal may be several times higher with small (in contrast to large) flip angles. As the TR becomes longer, however, small flip angles become less advantageous. Figure 3-17 shows the combined effects of the TR and the flip angle.

In most imaging situations we are not necessarily interested in maximizing the signal intensity of a specific tissue but, rather, in maximizing the contrast between

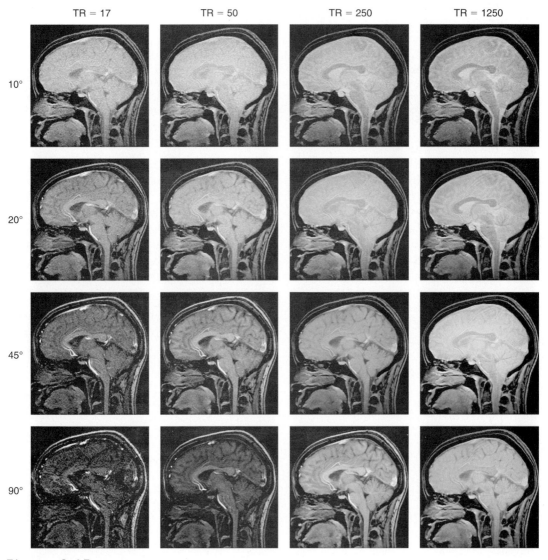

Figure 3-17

Effect on tissue contrast of varying the repetition time (TR) and flip angle. Sagittal spoiled gradient echo images of the brain using variable TR and flip angles. With a short TR and high flip angle (*bottom left*), the overall signal intensity is low. With a long TR and low flip angle (*top right*), the signal intensity is higher but there is little T1 contrast. The best balance between adequate signal intensity and T1 contrast is achieved with TR–flip angle combinations of 17/20°, 50/45°, or 250/90°.

two or more tissues. For T1-weighted images (whose contrast depends strongly on differences in T1), it is important for the tissue with a long T1 to have low signal intensity. Therefore the optimal flip angle for depicting this contrast must be higher than its Ernst angle. T1 contrast at the chosen TR is optimal at or higher than the Ernst angle for the tissue with the shorter T1. In other circumstances—for example when acquiring images that emphasize T2 contrast (T2-weighted images)—T1 contrast must be minimized. In these cases a flip angle smaller than the Ernst angle is appropriate to reduce T1 contrast. T1 contrast, TR, and the flip angle should be considered together because in many cases changes in one should be accompanied by changes in the other. Ernst angles are smaller for tissues with a long T1. Smaller flip angles should be chosen when using short TRs, especially for tissues with a long T1 relaxation time.

▼
Essential Points to Remember

1. Water in biological tissues can be considered as being divided into free and bound compartments. The mobility of the bound water molecules, which are associated with cellular macromolecules, is lower than that of free water.

2. When samples are placed in a magnet, they do not reach their magnetized, equilibrium state immediately. Instead, they must exchange energy through random interactions with their environment.

3. The bound and free water molecules reach magnetic equilibrium at different rates because of the differences in their motional energy.

4. T1 relaxation rates differ greatly among body tissues.

5. Magnetic field strength has a complex relationship with tissue T1 times, increasing the T1 for some and reducing it for others. However, at clinical field strengths, T1 increases with field for most body tissues.

6. If images are acquired with a series of RF pulses (the typical case), TR, the time between successive RF pulses, determines the T1 weighting in the image signal; tissues with a long T1 appear less intense than those with a short T1, especially when the TR is short compared to T1.

7. When flip angles of less than 90° are used, T1 contrast can be reduced, and a shorter TR may be used without increasing T1 weighting.

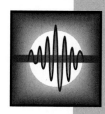

Transverse Magnetization and T2 Contrast

Immediately following induction by a radiofrequency (RF) pulse, the magnetic resonance (MR) signal starts to decay through a process broadly called "transverse relaxation." The many factors that control this transverse relaxation rate are the primary subject of this chapter. We also explore MR methods to control and measure transverse relaxation.

Free Induction Decay

Chapter 1 introduced the notion that the MR signal, once created, is transient because its amplitude depends on the individual spins precessing together in phase. The process of forming the signal is called *magnetic resonance induction*, and the loss of signal intensity over time is called the *"free induction decay"* (FID). Figure 4-1 shows how the FID might appear, for example, on an oscilloscope screen.

The shape of the amplitude of this curve, that is, how fast it decays, is described by the equation:

$$\text{Signal intensity (SI)} = \text{M}(t)e^{-t/\text{T2}},$$

where $\text{M}(t)$ is the starting magnetization (e.g., the transverse magnetization just after a 90° pulse). The parameter T2 determines how rapidly the signal decays. If T2 is small, the signal decays rapidly; in other words, signal decay takes a short time ("short" T2). A large T2 means that the signal decays slowly ("long" T2). The actual observed decay rate depends on many factors, all of which tend to shorten the duration of the FID. Generally, these factors are described as special varieties of T2, such as T2* and T2′. The term T2 is reserved for describing the decay rate that is intrinsic to the tissue or sample.

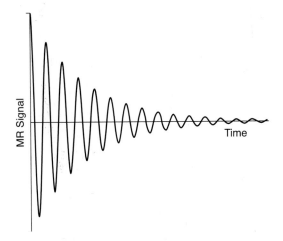

Figure 4-1
Example of the appearance of the free induction decay (FID) on an oscilloscope screen.

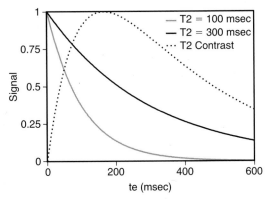

Figure 4-2
Following a single radiofrequency (RF) pulse, the signal intensity and contrast of two tissues are shown as their signals decay. The *dotted line* indicates a T2 of 300 msec and the *solid line* a T2 of 100 msec. After about 150 msec, the signal from the tissue with the longer T2 is about 2.5 times greater.

The T2 of body tissues varies over a broad range, from less than a few milliseconds for bone to more than a second (1000 msec) for simple fluids such as bulk water. Figure 4-2 shows the signal intensities and contrast following a single RF pulse in two different tissues as their signals decay. Note that the tissue shown with a dotted line has a T2 of 300 msec, whereas the other has a T2 of 100 msec. After about 150 msec the signal from the tissue with the longer T2 is about 2.5 times greater.

To form an MR image, several milliseconds usually must pass between the end of the RF excitation pulse and collection of the MR signal. This time, called TE, is often referred to the *echo time*. Although most currently used MRI techniques involve sampling an "echo" of the original FID, some methods (e.g., projection reconstruction) utilize the original FID. Therefore, TE might be more accurately considered the *time after excitation*. The horizontal axis in Figure 4-2 therefore is labeled TE, as it represents the strength of the MR signal as a function of the time between RF excitation and MR data collection.

The decay of transverse magnetization during the TE period reduces the signal intensity on the resulting image. This reduced signal intensity is especially significant for tissues with short T2 relaxation times. Images with a TE such that the signal intensity is influenced primarily by T2 differences between tissues are referred to as *T2-weighted images*. Images with TEs much shorter than the T2s of the tissues of interest have little T2 weighting, so the image contrast is determined principally by other factors. Images with TEs comparable to, or slightly longer than, the T2s of the tissues of interest are considered to have substantial T2 weighting. Images with TEs much longer than the T2s of the tissues of interest may exhibit so much decay of transverse magnetization from all tissues that they are of little clinical use. Figures 4-2, 4-3, and 4-4 show the relationship between the signal-to-noise ratio (SNR) and contrast as the TE increases.

Figure 4-5 depicts the combined effects of T1 recovery and T2 decay on tissue contrast. Although neither the repetition time (TR) nor the excitation flip angle directly affect T2 contrast, they are important determinants of T1 contrast, as discussed in Chapter 3. For an image to be T2-weighted, it is generally beneficial to minimize T1 contrast,

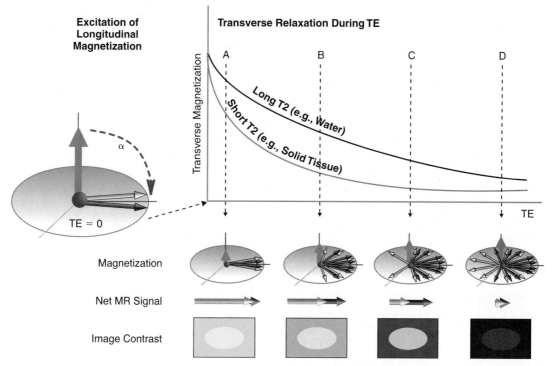

Figure 4-3
T2 relaxation curves of two tissues show contrast based on four TE values. The T2 decay of solid tissue (*gray curve*) is faster than that of free water (*black curve*). If the TE is too short (A), the signal-to-noise ratio (SNR) is high but contrast may be poor owing to insufficient decay of transverse magnetization from either tissue. With more moderate TE (B and C), the contrast may be optimal. As the TE increases further, transverse magnetization of the tissue with a long TE continues to decay, and contrast may become increasingly subtle (D). *Vertical gray arrows* indicate longitudinal magnetization, which recovers more slowly than transverse magnetization decays.

as a strong component of T1 contrast tends to obscure T2 contrast. Therefore, T2-weighted images usually have a long TR, a low excitation flip angle, or both.

For optimal T2 contrast between two tissues, it is desirable for most of the signal intensity of the tissue with the shorter T2 to have decayed. Conversely, it is essential for ample signal intensity from the tissue with the longer T2 to remain. Thus, to depict T2 contrast between two tissues, an optimal TE balances sufficient decay of transverse magnetization from one tissue against sufficient remaining transverse magnetization from the other. In other words, the difference in signal between two tissues (contrast) is zero at a TE of zero (when both signals are maximal) and falls to zero as TE becomes very long (when the signals from both tissues are minimal). The contrast peaks at a TE between the T2s of the two tissues.

Non–T2 Causes of Transverse Magnetization Decay

Each tissue has a characteristic T2 relaxation time that is not directly dependent on magnetic field strength. The T2 relaxation time is approximately equal to the time at which the signal has decayed by two-thirds due to properties intrinsic to the tissue. However, the actual rate of signal decay, depending on the

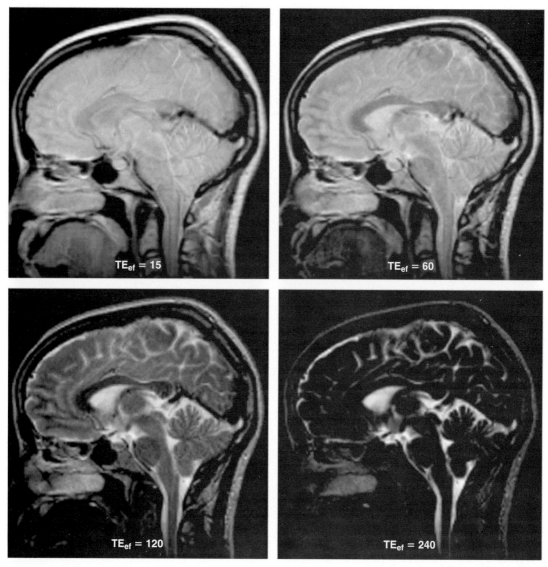

Figure 4-4

Varying the TE affects tissue contrast. Sagittal fast spin echo images of the brain with increasing effective TE (TE_{ef}) show minimal T2 contrast at 15 msec. T2 contrast increases up to 120 msec. With an effective TE of 240 msec, there is good T2 contrast between brain and cerebrospinal fluid (CSF), but the signal intensity of "non–CSF" tissues is too low for adequate contrast.

pulse sequence, is often more rapid than predicted based on T2 (Fig. 4-6). This actual observed transverse relaxation time, referred to as T2* (pronounced T2 star), is affected by additional factors, including magnetic field heterogeneity, motion, and chemical shift. T2*, in contrast to T2, is reduced substantially for many tissues at high magnetic field strength.

When transverse magnetization is first created by excitation of longitudinal magnetization, the spins in the transverse plane are coherent; that is, they precess in phase with one another. Anything that

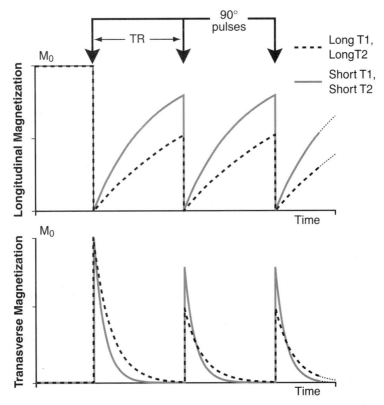

Figure 4-5

Top. Simultaneous changes in longitudinal magnetization. *Bottom.* Dependence of the amount of transverse magnetization on T1 and T2 for two tissues. The tissue shown with *dotted lines* has a longer T1 and T2 than the tissue shown with *solid lines*. The transverse magnetization (signal) following the first radiofrequency (RF) pulse has a strength of M_0 for both tissues. After the second RF pulse, the longitudinal magnetization of the tissue with the longer T1 (*dotted lines*) is less than that of the tissue with the shorter T1. The MR signal created in the transverse plane is therefore less. With each successive 90° pulse the longitudinal magnetization is returned to zero. The longitudinal recovery therefore is the same during each interval, so the signal *contrast*—the difference in the intensity of the tissues with different T1 values—is established and steady.

causes spins to precess at different rates leads to dephasing, which causes the combined transverse magnetization to decay (Fig. 4-7).

Intrinsic Sources of Transverse Relaxation

When the longitudinal magnetization of a material has reached its equilibrium, there can be no transverse magnetization. Therefore, the T1 relaxation time places an upper limit on T2. Beyond that, there are many reasons for the loss of phase coherence. Like other nuclei, protons cause small local perturbations in the magnetic field by orienting in their high or low energy states. When the relationship between these and nearby protons is fixed (as in large molecules that contain many protons), the magnetic perturbations produced by each proton slightly affect the field experienced by the others, causing the overall field to be less homogeneous. The T2 of such tissues is then shortened. In fact, almost any mechanism that holds protons in a relatively fixed relation to a magnetic field perturbation reduces the T2.

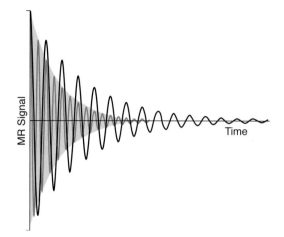

Figure 4-6

T2 relaxation is depicted as the decaying *black oscillating wave*. Decay from T2*, depicted by the *gray oscillation*, is faster.

By contrast, when protons are free to move about rapidly, as in fluids such as water, the field experienced by all protons, on average, becomes essentially identical. The T2 of simple water therefore can be extremely long—more than a second for distilled water. When the fluid contains dissolved materials or is viscous, the field within it becomes less homogeneous and the T2 is consequently reduced. The measured T2 of cells, especially dense cells, is much shorter than that of free water; neoplastic cells, in contrast, generally have a longer T2 owing in part to their relative lack of internal structure (Figs. 4-8 and 4-9). On the extreme end, in the immediate vicinity of blood clots the decaying hemoglobin exposes the neighboring water to iron atoms that perturb the magnetic field strongly, causing the T2 to become very short. All of these factors make T2 variations a remarkably sensitive indicator of different tissue types and an excellent marker for disease.

Heterogeneous Magnetic Field and Susceptibility

When a tissue is placed in a magnetic field that is not homogeneous, the precessional frequencies vary from location to location: Remember that the precessional frequency is directly proportional to the magnetic field strength. Protons exposed to strong local magnetic fields precess faster than those in weak magnetic fields (Fig. 4-10). This causes dephasing and accelerated decay of transverse magnetization during the TE, resulting in areas of signal loss and distortion.

Every effort is made to construct homogeneous magnets for use in MRI units. Supplemental magnetic field coils, referred to as *shim gradients*, are adjusted to correct for minor heterogeneities of the main magnetic field. Today's modern imagers can achieve fields that are uniform to within a fraction of one part per million over areas the size of the human torso.

Magnetic susceptibility is a measure of the relative magnetic field strength in a material expressed as a fraction of the magnetic field in which it is contained. This varies because tissues induce additional magnetization once they themselves are magnetized.

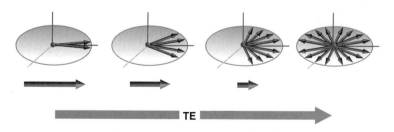

Figure 4-7

Progressive loss of coherent transverse magnetization during the interval between the creation of transverse magnetization by the excitation pulse and measurement of the signal at the echo time (TE). The *horizontal arrows* below the circles indicate decreasing net transverse magnetization.

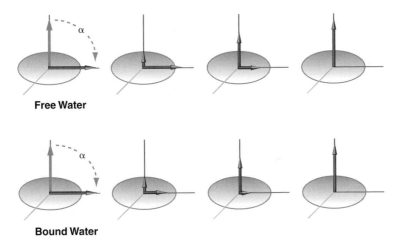

Figure 4-8
T1 and T2 relaxation for free and bound water. *Top.* For free water, T2 is nearly equal to T1. Thus transverse magnetization decays at a rate comparable to the rate at which longitudinal magnetization recovers. *Bottom.* For bound water, T2 is shorter than T1. Thus transverse magnetization decays faster than longitudinal magnetization recovers.

The induced magnetization is proportional to the square of the main magnetic field.

Even if shimming is perfect, the magnetic field is disturbed once a patient lies within it. This is largely because of differences in magnetic susceptibility between the patient's tissues relative to each other and relative to air or other materials.

Most body tissues are slightly *diamagnetic*, meaning that the field within them is a few parts per million weaker than the magnetic field applied to them. The paired electrons in these materials cause slight dispersion of local magnetic forces, thereby weakening the magnetic field in their proximity. The magnetic properties of other substances are generally considered relative to those of water, which has an extremely weak diamagnetism (nearly zero).

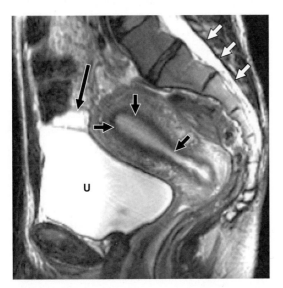

Figure 4-9
Sagittal T2-weighted image of the pelvis depicts free water in urine (U), endometrial glands (*short black arrows*), bowel lumen (*long black arrow*), and CSF (*white arrows*) as having high signal intensity owing to the long T2 relaxation time of free water. Solid tissues such as uterine myometrium and skeletal muscle have shorter relaxation times and therefore lower signal intensity on this image.

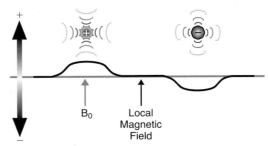

Figure 4-10
Effects on the local magnetic field relative to the main magnetic field (B$_0$) of positive (+, *left*) and negative (−, *right*) susceptibility. A superparamagnetic focus, such as a particle of iron, has positive susceptibility, increasing the local magnetic field in its vicinity. An air bubble or focus of calcium has negative susceptibility, decreasing the local magnetic field in its vicinity.

Paramagnetic materials, which have unpaired electrons, concentrate local magnetic forces, thereby increasing the local magnetic field. The T1 and T2 relaxation of water protons is enhanced by proximity to paramagnetic materials; the relaxation times of water protons are reduced by nearby paramagnetic substances. Examples of T1 and T2 relaxation enhancement by paramagnetic materials include the effect of MRI contrast materials and signal alterations of tissues secondary to the presence of iron.

Superparamagnetic materials contain particles with strong positive susceptibility—stronger than that of paramagnetic materials. *Ferromagnetic* materials contain larger solid or crystalline aggregates of molecules with unpaired electrons that interact with each other across multiple associated magnetic domains. Ferromagnetic materials have "magnetic memory," so a lingering magnetic field is created after exposure to an external magnetic field.

Overall, the effect of magnetic field heterogeneities is to reduce the T2*. This is because spins in a heterogeneous magnetic field precess at a variety of frequencies, causing the signal to dephase and therefore to decay rapidly. If the signal decay due to such heterogeneities is faster than the T2 of the tissue on its own, the intrinsic tissue T2 has little effect on the signal. The transverse relaxation component due to local heterogeneities of the magnetic field is sometimes given the label T2′ (pronounced T2 prime).

There are a few areas in the body in which it is notoriously difficult to achieve a homogeneous magnetic field. They include the air-filled sinuses of the head, the interior spaces of the lung, and of course any place in the body containing foreign metallic objects (Fig. 4-11). If signal loss from a heterogeneous magnetic field is not corrected through the use of refocusing pulses (described later in the chapter), the areas of signal loss become larger and more severe with longer TE (Fig. 4-12). The susceptibility effect, and thus the sensitivity to superparamagnetic substances, increases with the second power of the magnetic field

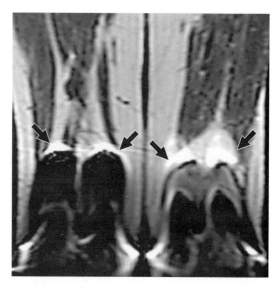

Figure 4-11
Coronal T1-weighted spin echo image of the lower thighs of a patient with bilateral metallic knee prostheses. *Arrows* indicate distortion due to susceptibility differences between stainless steel and body tissue.

strength (Fig. 4-13). For example, the sensitivity to superparamagnetic materials at 1.5 T is nine times higher than that at 0.5 T.

Some artifacts from air–tissue interfaces can be reduced by placing water or materials with similar susceptibility (e.g., fluorocarbons) adjacent to the patient, displacing the air away from the patient's skin. Other air–tissue interfaces, such as those in cranial sinuses, airways, lung, and bowel, cannot be eliminated. Bone also has negative susceptibility, and bone–tissue interfaces are present throughout the body. With some MRI systems, patient-induced magnetic field heterogeneity is minimized by applying additional shimming while the patient lies within the magnetic field and before imaging begins, though this can correct only for gross effects, not for local field heterogeneities.

The effects of paramagnetic and superparamagnetic materials on MR images are completely unlike those of any material on images produced by any other modality. For instance, dense materials such as iodine and calcium prevent photons from reaching a radiographic detector or film and thus

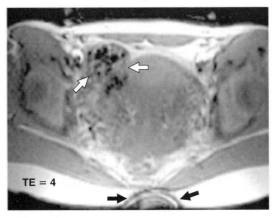 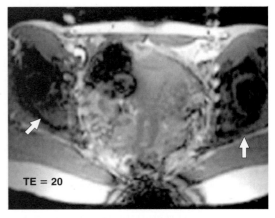

Figure 4-12
Effect of increasing TE on susceptibility effects. Spoiled gradient echo images were obtained at 1.5 T. *Left.* With a TE of 4 msec, air and stool are visible in the sigmoid colon (*white arrows*). Artifact due to metal is noted posteriorly (*black arrows*). *Right.* Increasing the TE to 20 msec intensifies these susceptibility artifacts and susceptibility-induced signal intensity loss from bone trabeculae in the acetabula (*white arrows*).

have direct effects on the final radiographic image. Similarly, radioactive materials emit photons that are detected directly and displayed on scintigraphic images. In contrast, paramagnetic and superparamagnetic materials are not detected directly; all current clinical MR images are derived from signals produced by protons. A compound containing paramagnetic materials is not depicted on an MR image unless that

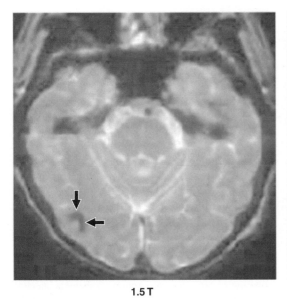 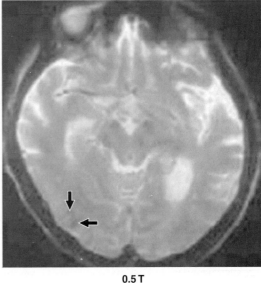

Figure 4-13
T2-weighted spin echo images of the brain show a small hemorrhagic infarction (*arrows*) with low signal intensity that is due to the susceptibility effects of the iron in hemosiderin. The lesion is better visualized at 1.5 T than at 0.5 T owing to the greater susceptibility at higher magnetic field strength. Both images are at the level of the hemorrhage, but other anatomy is different because of different patient positioning. (Courtesy of W.G. Bradley.)

compound also contains mobile protons, and their effects are greatest on water protons.

The alteration of tissue relaxation times by magnetic materials depends on the concentration of these magnetic materials and their microscopic interactions with water protons. For example, a paramagnetic substance may have little effect on a tissue if it is shielded from close contact with tissue water. Similarly, a superparamagnetic material has greater effect on a tissue if it is distributed heterogeneously, producing more pronounced variation in the local magnetic fields. Thus, the concentration and microscopic distribution of magnetic materials are important determinants of the resulting signal intensity on MR images (Fig. 4-14).

Chemical Shift

The chemical shift between water and CH_2 protons is discussed in Chapter 5. Briefly, the resonant frequency of protons varies slightly based on their molecular environment, particularly at high magnetic fields, where the absolute frequency differences are large. Heterogeneous chemical shift, such as in tissues that contain both lipid and water, can contribute to signal loss that depends on the TE.

■ Refocusing Radio Pulses and the Spin Echo

There are some applications in which decay of transverse magnetization from heterogeneous susceptibility, heterogeneous chemical shift, or both is acceptable or even desirable. In most cases, however, T2* is dominated by factors of little clinical interest, such as imperfections in the basic magnetic field or less than perfect shimming, both of which

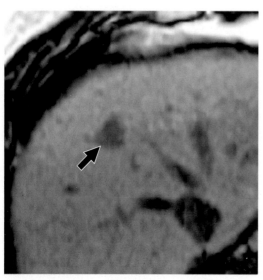
Baseline

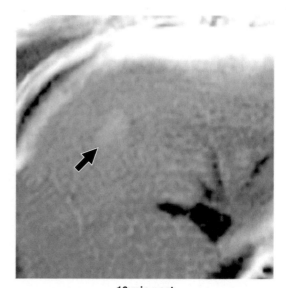
10 min post

Figure 4-14

Hepatic cavernous hemangioma (*arrows*) on T1-weighted images before and 10 minutes after intravenous injection of iron oxide particulate contrast material. The paramagnetic effects of the contrast agent vary depending on its distribution. After 10 minutes, many particles have been taken up heterogeneously by reticuloendothelial cells, decreasing the hepatic signal intensity because of heterogeneous magnetic susceptibility. Intravascular distribution within the hemangioma is more homogeneous, decreasing the susceptibility-induced signal loss. Additionally, the intravascular particles are in closer approximation to water, increasing the paramagnetic enhancement of T1 recovery and, in turn, increasing the signal intensity of the hemangioma.

cause signal losses. Fortunately, signal cancellation from a heterogeneous magnetic field and that due to phase opposition from chemical shift, can be eliminated through the use of the "spin echo," a clever method developed in 1950 by Erwin Hahn.

The spin echo is easiest to visualize when a 90° radiofrequency (RF) pulse is followed a short time later by a 180° pulse at one half of the TE, as in Figure 4-15. The spins, oriented initially along the longitudinal axis, are first rotated into the transverse plane by a 90° RF pulse (Fig. 4-15, 1). At this time they are in phase. Over time, the spins in lower magnetic fields, which precess more slowly, fall behind the faster moving spins, and the magnetization begins to dephase (Fig. 4-15, 2) until ultimately there is no net transverse magnetization or MR signal. At this point (Fig. 4-15, 3), a 180° pulse is applied, rotating all of the spins about the same axis. The result is that the faster moving spins are now placed *behind* (i.e., with a phase *lag* relative to) the slower moving spins. Because their position in the magnetic field was not changed by the RF pulses, the faster moving spins continue to precess

more rapidly, and after a short time the magnetizations from all of the spins rephase to form the spin echo (Fig. 4-15, 4). Specifically, if a period τ elapses between the 90° and 180° pulses, after another identical period τ the signal reforms as a spin echo (2τ following the 90° pulse).

The net effect of the spin echo is that the dephasing due to magnetic field inhomogeneity is reversed completely so long as the spins do not move during this period. If the signal collection is timed to coincide with the spin echo, the contrast in the final image depends on T2 but not on T2*.

Consider a tissue that contains tiny foci of iron, such as those that may be present in hemosiderin following hemorrhage. These iron foci have positive susceptibility and therefore increase the magnetic field in their immediate proximity. The protons nearest the iron precess faster than other protons. Thus, shortly after creation of transverse magnetization by the excitation radio pulse, protons near the iron gain phase relative to other protons. At a time halfway between the excitation pulse and the desired echo peak, a 180° refocusing

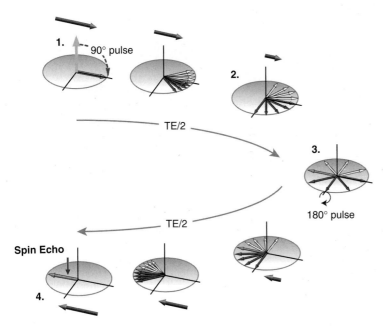

Figure 4-15
Effect of a 180° refocusing pulse, which reverses the phase accumulation of spins at the midpoint of the TE. When first created, transverse magnetization is completely coherent (1). Spins that precess at relatively high frequency (*light arrows*) gain phase relative to other spins (*dark arrows*), causing phase dispersion (2). During the second half of the TE, after being rotated 180° in the transverse plane by the refocusing pulse (3), the spins represented by *light arrows* are behind in phase but continue to precess faster. At the TE, all spins are back in phase (4).

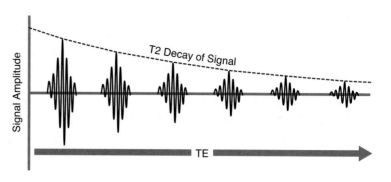

Figure 4-16
Exponential decay of MR signal due to T2 relaxation, sampled after each of many refocused echoes. The signal strength of each echo is weaker as the echo time (TE) increases.

pulse is applied, which rotates all spins in the transverse plane, reversing the phases of these protons relative to each other. The protons near the focus of iron still precess faster than other protons, but their phase is now behind. As time passes, the rapidly precessing protons near the iron focus regain this phase, "catching up" at the TE, forming the spin echo.

Refocusing pulses also correct dephasing between tissues having different chemical shifts, such as between adipose tissue and water. A 180° pulse, applied halfway between the excitation pulse and the signal collection, reverses the relative phases of water and lipid protons, so that water protons are placed behind in phase relative to lipid protons. During the second half of the TE period, the phase of the water protons approaches the phase of the protons, so net magnetization reaches a peak at the spin echo.

Once the spins are again in phase, the entire process of echo formation can be repeated simply by following with another 180° pulse whose timing is selected to form a second echo at another desired TE. The signal strength resulting from numerous refocused echoes decaying according to a tissue's T2 is shown in Figure 4-16.

The spin echo is easiest to understand graphically, and has the largest amplitude, when it is formed by a combination of 90° and 180° pulses. However, spin echoes form with most sequences that include repeated RF pulses, always at twice the time between the pulses. The use of echo-forming (or *refocusing*) pulses of less than 180° is common in modern equipment, as it can reduce the amount of RF power needed to form spin echoes, with little loss of signal. ·

▼
Essential Points to Remember

1. Once created by nuclear magnetic resonance induction, the MR signal decays rapidly as a result of many factors that cause the individual proton spins to dephase relative to one another.

2. The observed decay rate, T2*, is always faster than the tissue's intrinsic T2 owing to factors that include local heterogeneities of the magnetic field that cause the precessional rates of the individual spins to differ. T2* is always shorter than T2.

3. The interval between creation of transverse magnetization and its measurement is the TE. Because the T2s of body tissues vary, TE can be used to adjust tissue contrast.

4. For depiction of T2 differences between tissues (T2 contrast), there is an optimal TE that is long enough to allow sufficient decay of transverse magnetization of short-T2 tissues but short enough to minimize decay of transverse magnetization of long-T2 tissues.

5. When protons in a tissue precess at the same frequency, transverse magnetization decays at a rate determined by the tissue's T2 relaxation time. When protons in a tissue precess at a range of frequencies, transverse magnetization of the tissue decays faster than its T2 relaxation time predicts.

6. Protons precess at different frequencies when they are bound to different atoms. This change in frequency is called *chemical shift*. Tissues that contain more than one chemical shift have a signal amplitude that cycles up and down at different TE values as the different magnetizations cycle into and out of phase with respect to each other.

7. When two or more RF pulses are used in succession, a spin echo is formed. Its amplitude does not depend on the magnetic field homogeneity.

Chapter **5**

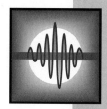

Chemical Shift

E ven in a perfectly homogeneous magnetic field, not all protons resonate at the same frequency. The motion of a proton in a magnetic field is affected by its local molecular environment, changing its resonance frequency. This is referred to as *chemical shift*.

Chemical shift, which defines the resonant frequency of protons, is largely *independent of relaxation time,* which defines the time it takes protons to magnetize. For example, free and bound water have the same resonant frequency and therefore the same chemical shift, whereas their relaxation times are quite different. Similarly, adipose tissue and some forms of hemorrhage may have similar T1 relaxation times, whereas their chemical shifts are different.

Lipid and Water Resonance

There is a single resonant frequency for protons in water at a given magnetic field strength, whereas protons in other molecules (e.g., silicone, lactate, various fatty acids) resonate at slightly different frequencies. In other words, the protons in these various molecules have slightly different chemical shifts. In fact, protons at different sites in a given complex molecule [e.g., methylene (CH_2) and methyl (CH_3) protons in triglycerides] may have different chemical shifts. Protons in some components of adipose tissue, such as unsaturated olefinic acids ($-CH=CH-$) actually have resonant

49

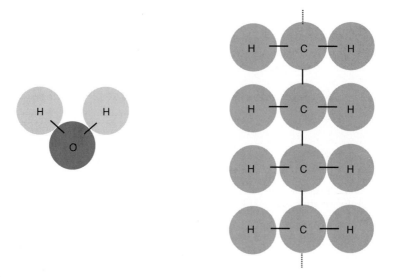

Figure 5-1
Electron sharing across covalent bonds, such as between oxygen and hydrogen, is unequal. The dense electron cloud surrounding the oxygen nucleus, which holds the electron cloud tightly, is depicted as a dark shade of gray. As a result of the unequal sharing, the magnetic shielding created by the electrons about the proton nucleus is less in water (*left*) than in the hydrocarbon chains that occur in lipids (*right*). The carbon nuclei hold the electron cloud less tightly than do oxygen nuclei, so the electron clouds surrounding the hydrocarbon protons are depicted as darker than those surrounding water protons. These water protons therefore have a slightly higher magnetic resonance (MR) frequency than do the hydrocarbon protons.

frequencies closer to that of water than to the resonant frequencies of most other lipid protons.

The most important chemical shift in most magnetic resonance (MR) imaging applications is that between water protons and CH_2 protons in long-chain fatty acids (e.g., triglyceride) in adipose tissue (Fig. 5-1). The chemical shift of water relative to CH_2 is caused by water's strongly electronegative oxygen atom, which displaces the electron cloud away from the hydrogen protons. The chemical shift between protons in different magnetic environments is proportional to the overall magnetic field in which they lie. That is, the higher the frequency at which the protons precess, the larger the chemical shift. Therefore, the magnitude of chemical shifts is expressed relative to their precessional frequency, in parts per million (ppm). For example, the chemical shift between water and

methylene protons is approximately 3.5 ppm (Fig. 5-2).

The actual value of this chemical shift, in hertz, is directly proportional to the main magnetic field, so the chemical shift between water and lipid is larger at high magnetic field strength. The magnitude of the chemical shift is determined by multiplying the precessional frequency, expressed in hertz, by the relative magnitude of the shift, expressed in parts per million. At 1.5 T, for example, protons precess at 63.9 MHz; multiplying this by 3.5 ppm yields 224 Hz, the chemical shift between water and CH_2 protons at 1.5 T. At 0.5 T protons precess at 21.3 MHz, so the chemical shift between water and CH_2 protons is 74.5 Hz.

Chemically nonselective excitation pulses have a bandwidth (frequency range) large enough that water and lipid are both excited. Chemical shift techniques that

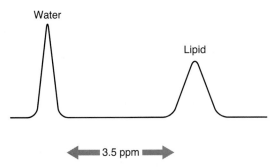

Figure 5-2

The difference in resonant frequency between water (*left*) and lipid (*right*) protons is approximately 3.5 ppm, or 3.5 Hz/MHz. There are several lipid resonances, so the composite peak for lipids is broader than the simple peak for water.

involve selective excitation or saturation of either water or CH_2 protons utilize radio pulses with a range of frequencies narrow enough that only one of these groups of protons is affected.

Theoretically, chemical shift magnetic resonance imaging (MRI) techniques are possible at any field strength, although they are technically difficult at low field strengths owing to the smaller absolute differences between the resonant frequencies of lipid and water protons and the lower signal-to-noise ratio (SNR) realized at reduced magnetic field strength.

Heterogeneous Chemical Shift

Tissues that contain protons bound to a variety of atoms, such as adipose tissue, have heterogeneous chemical shifts. The MR signal from adipose tissue is dominated by saturated CH_2 protons in the triglycerides, although protons from unsaturated fatty acids and water in blood vessels and connective tissue also provide some signal. Once magnetized, the protons of water and

CH_2 precess at different frequencies. If the heterogeneous chemical shift in adipose tissue is not corrected for, such as by use of a 180° refocusing pulse, the different precessional rates of protons result in periodic dephasing and rephasing of transverse magnetization. The magnitude of these uncorrected phase differences depends on the time that elapses between the creation of transverse magnetization and its measurement (i.e., the TE).

Because water protons precess faster than CH_2 protons in adipose tissue, they gain in phase. When first created, the transverse magnetizations of water and CH_2 protons are in phase with respect to each other, but the phase gain of water relative to CH_2 protons increases with time until the phases are maximally opposed with respect to each other (i.e., 180°). At this time, destructive interference between these two populations with opposite phases reduces the net transverse magnetization and results in lowered signal intensity (Fig. 5-3). As TE increases beyond the time of the 180° opposed phase, the phase of water proton magnetization continues to gain with respect to that of CH_2 protons, so the phase difference between them reaches 360° (which is equivalent to 0°). At this time, water and CH_2 proton magnetizations are once more in phase (Fig. 5-4).

As the TE increases, transverse magnetization varies owing to the combined effects of cyclic dephasing from chemical shift heterogeneity and the exponential decay from a heterogeneous magnetic field (T2* decay). Figure 5-5 depicts these combined effects. T2* decay is represented as an exponential decay curve drawn along the peaks of a graph depicting cyclic variations of signal intensity as the TE increases. This curve represents signal loss due to the combined effects of T2* and chemical shift heterogeneity. An example of this oscillation of signal intensity with increasing TE is shown in Figure 5-6.

The signal intensity oscillations that result from chemical shift differences between water and CH_2 protons form the

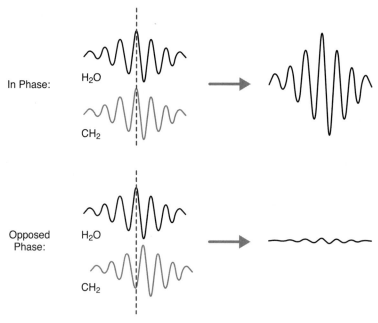

Figure 5-3
Summation of two in-phase waves (*top*) and cancellation of two opposed-phase waves (*bottom*).

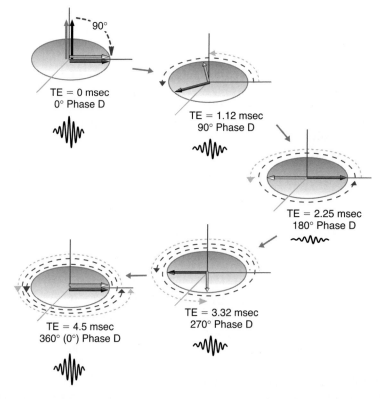

Figure 5-4
Phase differences between water and lipid with changing TE. In this example, the TEs are appropriate for a field strength of 1.5 T. At a TE of 2.25 msec, water (*black arrows*) and lipid (*gray arrows*) magnetizations are 180° out of phase with respect to each other, leading to maximal phase cancellation. At TEs of 0 and 4.5 msec, water and lipid magnetizations are in phase with respect to each other, leading to maximal summation of the signal.

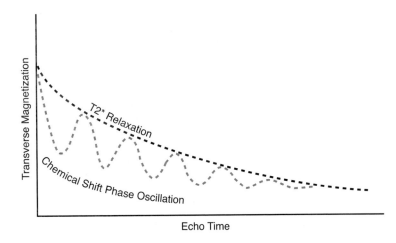

Figure 5-5
Decay of transverse magnetization due to T2* relaxation, corresponding to the peaks of decay of transverse magnetization of a tissue with heterogeneous chemical shift. The *gray curve* represents the combined effects of T2* decay and superimposed oscillations due to chemical shift heterogeneity.

basis for a simple yet powerful tool for characterizing some tissues on MR images. By a simple comparison between gradient echo images with two different TEs where these protons are, in-phase or opposed-, tissues that contain lipid and water can be identified with extremely high accuracy (Fig. 5-7). This technique can be used successfully at a variety of field strengths, although the TEs that yield opposed-phase and in-phase images will differ (Fig. 5-8). In particular, the time difference between in-phase and opposed-phase TEs is directly proportional to the field strength. For example, this time difference is about 2.2 msec at 1.5 T and 11.0 msec at 0.3 T (Fig. 5-8).

Spectroscopy

The magnitudes of the proton chemical shifts vary systematically with the chemical bond (i.e., with the *electronegativity* of the atom to which they are bonded). In addition, there are small magnetic interactions among nearby protons, called "J-coupling," that alter the frequencies slightly. These effects are quantitative: The strength of the proton signal at any frequency is proportional to the number of similar protons, and the changes in frequency for each of the various atomic bonds is reasonably well known. When the MR signal from a complex molecule is analyzed carefully for its energy at each frequency (i.e., its "spectrum"), it is possible to calculate the relative number of protons that appear in each of the chemical bonds. Such an analysis can give specific information as to the chemicals contained in a solution or even the intact human body. In fact, it constitutes a form of nondestructive chemical analysis.

The study and analysis of a spectrum of signals is known as spectroscopy, and magnetic resonance spectroscopy (MRS) is a specific variant. A spectroscopic signal contains information about characteristic changes in the chemical composition of diseased tissues.

Protons are not the only source of MR signals. For example, by analyzing the spectrum from the phosphorus atom, it is possible to look at the ratios of adenosine tri-, di-, and monophosphates (ATP, ADP, AMP), the primary energy transfer molecules in biological systems. Similarly, changes in the chemical shift can be used

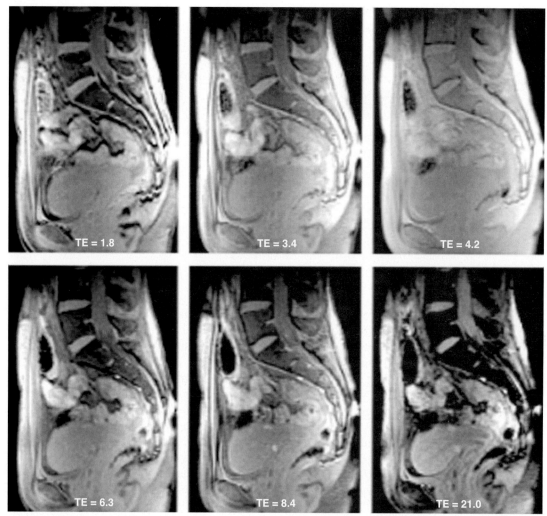

Figure 5-6

Sagittal gradient echo images of the pelvis and lower lumber spine with increasing TE show a combination of T2* and chemical shift effects. At a TE of 1.8 msec the phases of lipid and water proton magnetizations are nearly 180° opposed; at 4.2 msec they are nearly in phase. Thus, the signal intensity of bone marrow increases through this range of TEs. At 8.4 and 21.0 msec lipid and water proton magnetizations are also approximately in phase, but the heterogeneous magnetic susceptibility of trabecular bone causes a short T2* and therefore rapidly decreasing signal intensity as the TE increases.

to measure crucial biological values, such as tissue pH.

Although MRS is not new, there are many complexities in the acquisition and analysis of spectral data, so it has been relatively slow to gain acceptance. With rare exceptions, at the time of this writing analysis of MRS data is the domain of physicists with highly specific expertise. As the field advances, however, MRS is likely to have a growing impact on clinical medicine and decision making.

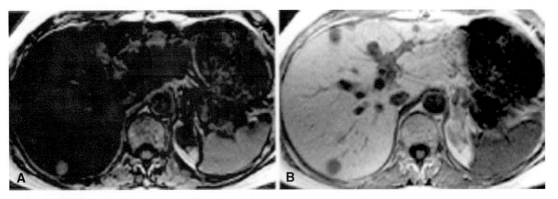

Figure 5-7
Gradient echo images obtained at 1.5 T that are identical in all aspects except for the TE. These images can be used to identify tissues that contain lipid and water. (*A*) With the TE at 2.3 msec, the phases of CH_2 and water protons are 180° out of phase relative to each other. (*B*) With the TE at 4.6 msec, they are now in-phase. Liver parenchyma, which contains water and lipid, therefore has reduced signal intensity relative to other tissues in *A*, including the focal liver metastases.

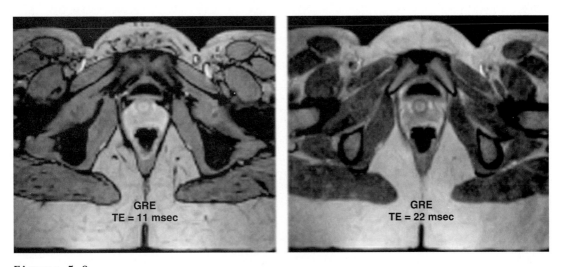

Figure 5-8
Axial gradient echo images of the pelvis at 0.3 T. CH_2 and water protons are out of phase at a TE of 11 msec (*left*) and in-phase at a TE of 22 msec. These values are five times as long as corresponding values at 1.5 T.

▼ Essential Points to Remember

1. The precessional frequency of protons varies, depending on their position within a molecule. The difference between two such frequencies is called *chemical shift*.

2. Protons in water, silicone, and lipid have different chemical shifts.

3. Chemical shift differences are independent of differences in relaxation times.

4. Chemical shift frequency differences are greater at higher magnetic field strengths.

Chapter **6**

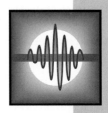

Spatial Localization: Magnetic Field Gradients

Thus far we have looked at the magnetic resonance (MR) properties of tissues without considering how signals from different locations are resolved and depicted in their correct positions. To move beyond analysis of bulk tissue properties toward creation of useful diagnostic images, a reliable method for locating the source of MR signals is needed. This is not a simple process, as the MR signal on its own does not yield adequate positional information to form an image. By analogy, when we listen to a radio we cannot determine from which direction the radio station is broadcasting. Although the distance from various components of a complex receiver coil can be used to provide some spatial information (see Parallel Imaging, Chapter 17), a variety of clever techniques in combination is needed to resolve this complex collection of radio signals in three dimensions, producing useful MR images.

The fundamental principle used to determine the location of MR signal sources is the application of supplemental magnetic field gradients, referred to as *imaging gradients*. In a homogeneous magnetic field without applied imaging gradients, protons with identical chemical shift precess at the same frequency regardless of location. If we superimpose a spatially-varying magnetic field on a homogeneous main magnetic field, we cause a predictable variation along a predetermined axis. When the supplemental field is set up to decrease gradually from one end of the magnet to the other, the resulting total magnetic field (the sum of the main and "gradient" magnetic fields) is strong at one end, weak at the other end, and intermediate between those points. Because the precessional frequency of a proton is proportional to the magnetic field to which it is exposed, the magnetic field gradient produces a systematic variation in frequency along this axis. Thus, the presence of the gradient causes protons at one end of the magnet to precess slower, and those at the other end to precess faster, relative to protons between these two extremes.

Slice Selection

If we transmit an excitation radio pulse into a tissue when a magnetic field gradient is present, not all tissue is excited. The excitation radio pulse excites only tissues that precess at the appropriate frequency, corresponding to a particular position along the axis of the imaging gradient. Thus, only a limited "slice" is excited. An imaging gradient applied during exposure to an excitation or refocusing radio pulse is referred to as a *slice-select gradient*. Appropriately oriented slice-select gradients can be used to excite protons selectively in an axial plane (Fig. 6-1), a coronal plane (Fig. 6-2), or a sagittal plane.

Two or more slice-select gradients can be applied simultaneously to excite protons selectively in any arbitrary slice orientation (Fig. 6-3).

Notation

To help understand the timing with which magnetic field gradients are turned on and off, we introduce a simple, commonly-used, annotation. This and other elements of pulse sequence annotation are used throughout the remainder of this book. We use conventions typical within the MR community.

A flat line, in "neutral" position, indicates that the imaging gradient is turned off. When the imaging gradient is turned on, the level of the line changes to above neutral for positive polarity or below neutral for negative polarity. Figure 6-4 shows the annotation for slice-select gradients applied during the 90° and 180° radio pulses of a standard spin

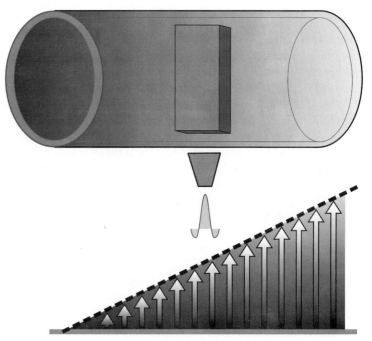

Figure 6-1
Slice-select gradient. *Top.* Magnet bore and the transverse slice in it that is selectively excited by the radiofrequency (RF) pulse. *Bottom.* Magnetic field gradient that alters the main magnetic field: in this example along the axis of the magnet bore. The magnetic field at one end of the magnet bore is thus weaker than at the other end. The transmitted radio pulse has a frequency that was chosen to match the frequency of the desired image slice, resulting in an axial image.

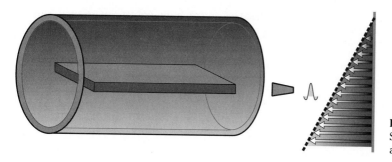

Figure 6-2
Slice-select gradient used to generate a coronal image slice.

echo pulse sequence. Note that for the 90° excitation radiofrequency (RF) pulse, the gradient is initially applied with positive polarity, but this is reversed after the RF pulse. As explained later in the chapter (page 61), the polarity is reversed so the effects of the gradient on the phase of transverse magnetization is balanced.

Frequency Encoding

In the absence of imaging gradients, all protons in an imaging plane precess at identical frequencies (except for small variations resulting from magnetic field heterogeneity and differences in chemical shift). If an imaging gradient is applied along one axis of an image plane while the MR signal is being measured, variations in signal frequency are created along that gradient axis. The frequency of the MR signals measured during readout is high at one end of the gradient axis and low at the other end. This provides an opportunity, within a previously selected slice, to localize the source of MR signals in one dimension. This process of encoding the spatial location of protons based on their positions along a gradient applied during their measurement is called

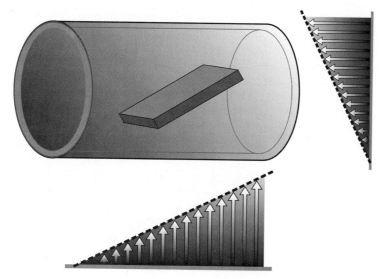

Figure 6-3
Simultaneous application of two slice-select gradients generates an oblique slice.

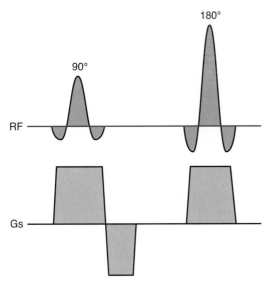

Figure 6-4
Slice-select gradients (Gs) applied for 90° excitation and 180° refocusing radio pulses. The polarity (direction of strong versus weak) of each gradient is indicated by its position above or below the neutral line. RF, radiofrequency.

frequency encoding; a gradient applied to encode the signal frequency during readout is called a "frequency-encoding," or "readout," gradient.

The process of in-plane frequency encoding is based on principles similar to those of slice selection, as both involve spatial localization based on resonant frequency. There are also important differences. Slices are *selected* by applying an imaging gradient during radio *excitation*. After the slice is excited a signal is measured, which is then encoded to create an image. Spatial information in one axis of the image, the frequency-encoding axis, is determined based on the frequency of spins. In other words, frequency is *encoded* by applying an imaging gradient during the *measurement* of MR signals. The signals themselves are a result of the excitation, which affected only the desired slice because of slice selection. A conceptually similar method, referred to as *phase encoding* (described later in the chapter), is used for the third axis.

Chemical Shift Misregistration Artifact

The sources of MR signals are mapped along the axis of the frequency-encoding gradient based on their frequencies during readout. The assumption inherent in this method is that any difference in frequency between spins is caused by a difference in location along the frequency-encoding gradient. Any additional cause of differences in resonant frequency produces frequency-encoding errors. One salient example of such a frequency-encoding error is signal misregistration secondary to chemical shift differences, producing chemical shift misregistration artifact.

At any given site along the frequency-encoding axis, all water protons precess at the same frequency. Methylene (CH_2) protons in lipids precess at a lower frequency, however (see Chapter 5). Thus, these lipid signals are represented on the resulting MR image at a site different from water signals from the same region. In particular, lipid signals are misregistered toward the low end of the frequency-encoding axis relative to water signals arising from the same location. A typical MR image consists of superimposed water and lipid images that are aligned imperfectly.

As an example, consider an image obtained at 1.5 T using a 32-kHz sampling bandwidth (the range of frequencies sampled is 32 kHz) and 256 frequency-encoding pixels. Dividing the range of frequencies sampled by the number of pixels shows us that each pixel represents a 125 Hz band. Because the chemical shift between water and CH_2 is 224 Hz, the chemical shift here is equivalent to approximately 2 pixels. In this image, consider that a "water object" such as a kidney is surrounded by lipid (adipose tissue). The water image of the kidney shifts toward the high end of the frequency-encoding axis relative to the fat image from adipose tissue. At the high end of the axis, water signals from kidney are misregistered so they are mapped overlapped onto the same location as perinephric fat signals. The signals of water and fat are added together here, producing a high signal intensity interface at the high end of the frequency-encoding axis. At the low end of the frequency-encoding axis, signals from renal water are shifted away from adjacent fat, leaving a void (i.e., no signal). This is shown in Figure 6-5, and an example of chemical shift artifact at the edges of a kidney is shown in Figure 6-6.

Gradient Dephasing and Rephasing

Slice-Select Gradient Rephasing

To select the appropriate image slice, the slice-select gradient determines that only a slice of tissue with a certain range of frequencies along this axis is excited. Next, for spatial localization along one axis of this slice, a frequency-encoding gradient is applied while the MR signals are measured. During application of each of these imaging gradients, protons spin at nonuniform frequencies; therefore, the gradients rapidly destroy the phase coherence of spins. This gradient dephasing causes a potential problem because it is essential that the MR signals have maximum phase coherence to generate enough signal to produce images.

During slice selection, when the radiofrequency (RF) pulse and slice-select gradients are applied simultaneously, the spins dephase from this gradient effect. To compensate for this dephasing, the slice-select gradient is reapplied in the reverse-direction orientation (swapping ends of the magnet that are at relatively high and low field strengths) to bring the spins in the excited slice back into phase. The initial application of the slice-select gradient is sometimes called the *dephasing lobe* of the slice-select gradient because it dephases the resonating spins. The repeated but reversed application

of the slice-select gradient is referred to as the *rephasing lobe*.

The dephasing and rephasing lobes of the slice-select gradient, and the accompanying phase changes of the transverse magnetization, are shown in Figure 6-7. Only the transverse component of the magnetization is subject to dephasing, however, and it develops slowly over the course of the RF pulse application. The product of the amplitude and duration of the rephasing lobe (its "area") is determined to be just enough to compensate for the dephasing that occurs during application of the RF pulse; the area of the rephasing lobe is roughly 60% of that used during excitation when a 90° pulse is in operation. In Figure 6-7 the amplitudes of the dephasing and rephasing lobes are identical, whereas the duration of the rephasing lobe is less than that of the dephasing lobe. Alternatively, the rephasing lobe could have the same duration and about half the amplitude. A rephasing lobe is not needed after a 180° refocusing pulse; the portion of the gradient lobe after the 180° pulse corrects the phase changes caused before the 180° pulse, as the 180° pulse had reversed the phase of the transverse magnetization.

Frequency-Encoding Gradient Rephasing

For in-plane frequency encoding, the challenge is to measure MR signals that have a wide range of frequencies (so position can be encoded based on these frequency differences), although MR signals such as these do not remain coherent. For conventional image reconstructions, it is essential that we sample a moment in time when all of the spins are in phase, in addition to the time points when the signal is altered by the spin dephasing. With most current imaging methods this is accomplished by applying a dephasing lobe of the frequency-encoding gradient prior to measuring the MR signals, which in turn occurs during application of the rephasing lobe.

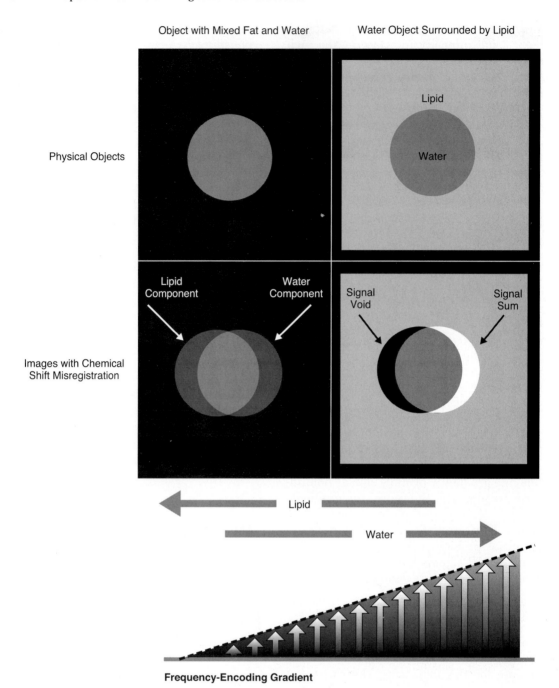

Figure 6-5

Chemical shift misregistration artifact. *Left.* Smearing of a round object that contains a mixture of lipid and water. *Right.* Typical artifact that results at the edges of "water objects" such as kidneys that are surrounded by adipose tissue. Relative to surrounding lipid, the round water-containing object is mapped toward the right, producing a crescent-shaped set of high signal intensity pixels to the right, which represents signals from both lipid and water. The crescentic signal void to the left reflects an absence of the signal mapped to this region.

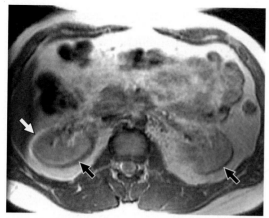

Figure 6-6
Chemical shift misregistration artifact. Water in the kidneys is misregistered along the frequency axis toward the right relative to adipose tissue. This causes black signal voids at the kidneys' left margins (*black arrows*) and white summation lines at their right margins (*white arrow*).

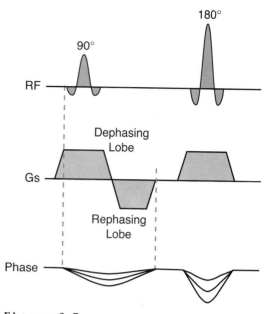

Figure 6-7
Phase of transverse magnetization during application of the dephasing and rephasing lobes of a slice-select gradient (Gs). Once transverse magnetization is created by the 90° pulse, the continued presence of the dephasing lobe of the gradient causes phase dispersion. It can be reversed by application of the rephasing lobe. All spins are in phase when the effects of the dephasing and rephasing lobes are balanced. The 180° refocusing pulse reverses the phase of the transverse magnetization, so continued application of Gs causes rephasing. RF, radiofrequency.

During application of an imaging gradient's dephasing lobe, protons at one end of the gradient precess faster and thus gain in phase relative to precessing protons at the other end. When the frequency-encoding gradient's dephasing lobe is turned off, the frequencies of the spins in the image slice become identical once more (except for differences due to magnetic field heterogeneity and chemical shift differences). The phase differences created by the gradient persist, however; they remain out of phase with each other, neither gaining nor losing phase. Then, near the echo time (TE), the frequency-encoding gradient's rephasing lobe is applied. Spins that have gained phase now precess more slowly and thus lose phase relative to spins at the opposite end of the gradient. As with the slice-select gradient, the dephasing and rephasing lobes of the frequency-encoding gradient have opposite polarities, but the products of their strength and duration are set up to ensure that the spins come back into phase at the desired moment. This produces a "gradient" echo that peaks at the time TE, allowing efficient measurement while controlling

contrast. The timing of the dephasing and rephasing lobes with respect to the echo is shown in Figures 6-8 and 6-9.

Gradient Echoes and Spin Echoes

As described above, applying two frequency-encoding gradient lobes with opposite polarities creates an echo. Because this echo is created by reapplication of a magnetic gradient, it is referred to as a *gradient echo*. If a refocusing radio pulse (usually about 180°) is applied during the interval between these two frequency-encoding gradient lobes, the echo obtained is called a *spin echo*. The spin echo occurs at a time following the

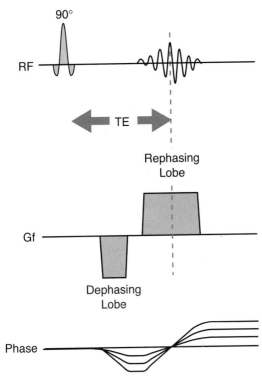

Figure 6-8
Effects on phase coherence of the dephasing and rephasing lobes of a frequency-encoding gradient (Gf) and the signal that results at the echo time. RF, radiofrequency.

180° pulse that is equal to the time between the 90° and 180° pulses. Usually, the gradient echo and spin echoes are made to coincide, as this results in image contrast that most accurately represents the spin echo.

Application of a 180° refocusing pulse compensates for frequency variations due to magnetic field and chemical shift heterogeneity. Variations due to magnetic field heterogeneity include those imposed by main magnetic field imperfections and heterogeneous susceptibility (see Non–T2 Causes of Transverse Magnetization Decay, Chapter 4). In contrast, reapplication of an imaging gradient compensates only for itself (Fig. 6-10). If there is no 180° refocusing pulse, a gradient echo is formed by reapplying the frequency-encoding gradient

with *reversed* polarity, compensating for its dephasing lobe. If a 180° refocusing pulse is applied, the phase differences between spins are reversed. In this situation, applying a rephasing lobe that has the same polarity as the dephasing lobe (Fig. 6-11) creates an echo.

When a second RF pulse (a 180° pulse is typically used for this purpose) follows the RF excitation, it refocuses the transverse magnetization and results in the formation of a *spin echo*. Regardless of whether a refocusing pulse is applied, an MR echo is created by applying dephasing and rephasing lobes of the frequency-encoding gradient; this echo could therefore be considered a gradient echo. In most cases the gradient echo and spin echo are made to coincide, in which case the echo is generally referred to as a spin echo. If there is no refocusing pulse, the echo is referred to as a gradient echo.

When the gradient echo and spin echo occur at the same moment, the signals from fat and water components are in phase at the center of the gradient echo. As the image contrast overall is dominated by the signal at the center of the gradient echo (see Chapter 7) (the center of k-space), the signals from fat and water in any given voxel are additive.

If, on the other hand, the gradient echo is offset in time from the spin echo, it is possible to construct images wherein the transverse magnetization from fat and water components of the signal are out of phase with one another and therefore interfere destructively, causing voxels that contain both fat and water to have a reduced signal (Fig. 6-12). Classifying the contrast as "spin echo" or "gradient echo" in these images is ambiguous. Likewise, the label for the TE is potentially ambiguous, although the time of the gradient echo is generally used.

Phase Encoding

Thus far we have discussed spatial localization using frequency differences that depend

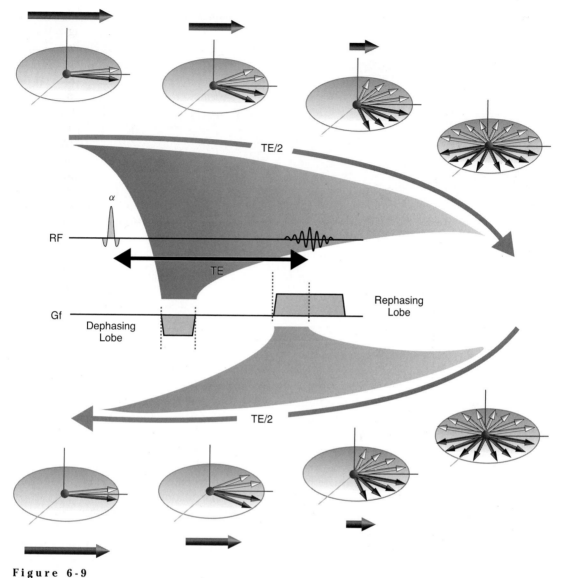

Figure 6-9
Gradient echo technique shows phase dispersion and refocusing caused by, respectively, the dephasing and rephasing lobes of the frequency-encoding gradient (Gf). The dephasing lobe causes some protons *(dark arrows)* to precess faster than others *(light arrows)*. The rephasing lobe, with opposite polarity, causes the spins that have lost phase to precess faster, so their phase "catches up," forming a gradient echo at the echo time (TE). RF, radiofrequency; α, excitation pulse.

on position along the axis of a magnetic field gradient. This includes selective excitation to choose an image slice, and frequency encoding, which is used to encode one axis within an image. The second in-plane axis of the image is localized by *phase encoding,* which involves mapping the location of the sources of MR signals based on differences among their phases at readout. Because many individuals find phase encoding particularly difficult to understand, we explain it in two ways, first discussing the sequence of events

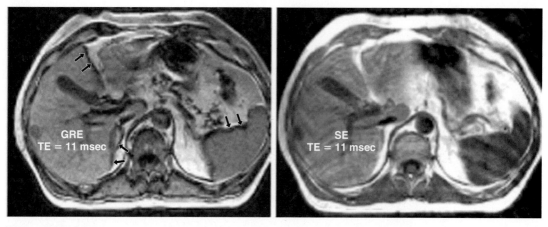

Figure 6-10
Images with TE = 11 msec, obtained at 0.3 T using the gradient echo (*left*) and spin echo (*right*) techniques. *Arrows at left* indicate chemical shift cancellation artifact at fat–water interfaces, as CH_2 and water proton magnetizations have opposite phases at 11 msec. At *right*, even though the TE is identical, the 180° refocusing pulse has corrected for these differences, so there are no cancellation edge artifacts.

that occur and then focusing on the similarity of the actual encoding process.

The phase-encoding gradient is established by applying a single brief magnetic field pulse perpendicular to the axes of slice-selection and frequency encoding. This brief gradient pulse causes precessional frequencies to vary momentarily along this axis. Once the phase-encoding gradient pulse has ended, the precessional frequencies are once again uniform, but the phase changes persist. The signal acquired during echo readout therefore contains phase differences caused by the phase-encoding gradient.

The phase-encoding gradient must be applied repeatedly at different strengths to locate the sources of MR signals along the phase-encoding axis. Frequency encoding, by contrast, maps all points along the frequency-encoding axis based on information contained in each signal. Although each signal contains data from throughout the entire two-dimensional image slice, data from multiple signals are needed to solve for the signal location by two-dimensional Fourier transformation (2D-FT).

Although the specific events involved in phase encoding differ in some respects from what happens during frequency encoding,

the actual encoding processes in each are essentially identical. We therefore explore their similarities.

Whenever a gradient is applied, spins in different locations along it precess at different frequencies, causing modulation (fluctuation) of the MR signal. This modulation takes place because the signals from these individual spins go in and out of phase with one another, causing either constructive or destructive interference. When the signal is sampled during continuous application of the gradient, the signal is said to be "frequency"-encoded. If sampling is performed *after* the gradient has been applied, however, the signal is said to be "phase"-encoded. In practice, they are the same.

This is perhaps easier to see if you consider the sampling process itself. As discussed in Chapter 1, the MR instrument captures the signal as a series of digital samples. Figure 6-13A shows sampling in the presence of a gradient. The arrows in the circles represent the direction of the transverse magnetization, which changes with time as the spins precess in the magnetic field. This is shown for two locations along the gradient, precessing at different rates. The observed signal (dashed lines) is

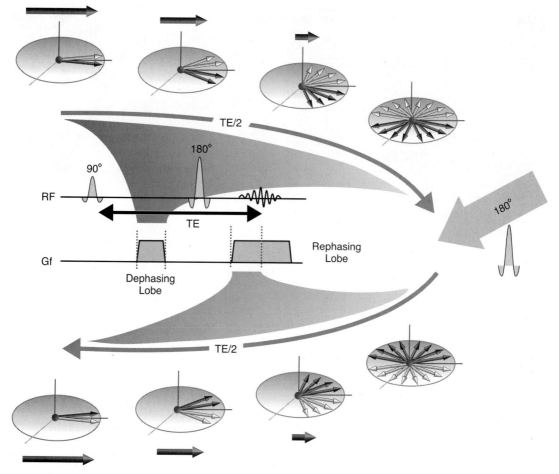

Figure 6-11

Spin echo technique, showing refocusing of transverse magnetization by a 180° radio pulse, which occurs at the middle of the echo time (TE) (compare Fig. 6-9). The 180° pulse corrects for differences in precessional frequency that are due to a heterogeneous chemical shift and a heterogeneous magnetic field. During the first half of the TE, some protons *(dark arrows)* resonate faster than others *(light arrows)*. The 180° pulse reverses the phases of the fast and slow spins. During the second half of the TE, the frequency-encoding gradient (Gf) is reapplied using the same polarity. The phase of the fast spins "catches up" to the phase of the slow spins, forming a spin echo at the TE. RF, radiofrequency.

the sum of the components for the two locations shown.

In this simple example, the signal is modulated between sample points by the effects of the gradient, which causes periodic dephasing and rephasing of the magnetization from the two locations. Initially they are in phase, and the combined signal from the two is large. As time progresses, the phase shift between the two results in their signal sum decreasing until they point in opposite directions (180° out of phase), and the signal cancels completely. Thereafter the signal increases again, periodically increasing and decreasing in amplitude.

The farther these two spins are from each other, the more their frequencies differ owing to the greater differences in their local magnetic fields brought about by the gradient. Consequently, they go in and out of phase with one another more quickly. Because the strength of the combined signal

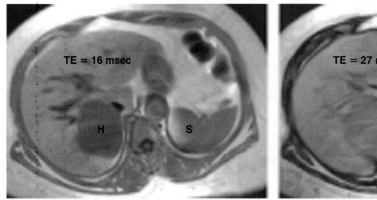
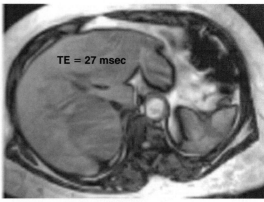

Figure 6-12
Complete (*left*) and incomplete (*right*) refocusing. There is a single excitation pulse followed at 8 msec by a 180° refocusing pulse and echo sampling at 16 msec. Then, 11 msec later, a second rephasing gradient lobe forms a second echo, at 27 msec. Therefore, this second echo is 11 msec removed from spin echo refocusing, which occurred at 16 msec. For these images, obtained at 0.3 T, 11 msec is the appropriate time for 180° opposite phase between CH_2 and water protons. Note that the hemangioma (H) and spleen (S) are much less intense than the liver on the in-phase image (*left*) but nearly isointense in the opposed-phase image (*right*) because of fatty infiltration of the liver.

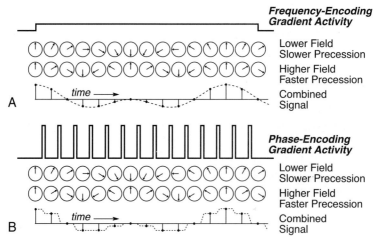

Figure 6-13
Signal modulation due to phase changes during frequency encoding (*A*) and phase encoding (*B*). The *arrows in circles* represent the direction of the transverse magnetization, which changes with time as the spins precess in the magnetic field. This is shown for two locations along the gradient (low and high fields), precessing at different rates (slow and fast precession). The observed signal (*dashed lines*) is the sum of the components for the two locations shown. Because the strength of the combined signal from all of the protons in a sample depends on the relative phases of the individual spins, we can say that the MR data have been encoded by phase. In *A* the frequency-encoding gradient is applied continually, whereas in *B* the phase-encoding gradient is applied discontinuously as a series of brief pulses. Each pulse has an area equal to that of the continuous gradient between samples and therefore has the same effect on the proton spins.

from all of the protons in a sample depends on the relative phases of the individual spins, we can say that the MR data have been encoded by phase.

Consider an alternative version (Fig. 6-13B). Here, the gradient is applied discontinuously as a series of brief pulses. Each pulse has an area (the product of time and duration) equal to that of the continuous gradient between samples and therefore has the same effect on the proton spins.

The effect on the relative phases of the spins in different positions would be the same whether the gradient pulses are repeated rapidly or separated greatly in time. In fact, this is the means by which the third image dimension is encoded in standard imaging sequences. With conventional MR image encoding, the slice-select and readout encoding are complete for each excitation, whereas the third dimension is encoded by a series of gradient pulses of varying duration, amplitude, or both that differ from one excitation to the next. As suggested in Figure 6-13, the effect of phase encoding is essentially identical to that of frequency encoding.

Strong phase-encoding gradients accentuate differences between two structures that are near each other; thus, they are useful for resolving fine detail. However, the resulting large differences in phase cause these signals to have lower-amplitude MR signals than do signals produced with weaker phase-encoding gradients (Fig. 6-14). The number of phase-encoding gradient strengths directly determines the number of locations mapped along the phase-encoding axis, thereby determining the spatial resolution in this axis and affecting the image acquisition time.

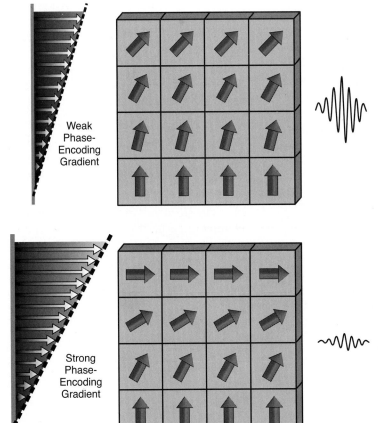

Figure 6-14
Effect of phase-encoding gradient strength on spatial resolution and echo amplitude. Weak phase-encoding gradients cause mild dephasing across the phase-encoding axis and thus give rise to strong echoes. Strong phase-encoding gradients accentuate differences between nearby points and thus help to resolve fine detail; however, the increased phase differences across the image secondary to the stronger phase-encoding gradients cause dephasing of these echoes. Thus, the echoes obtained using stronger phase-encoding gradients have lower amplitude and contribute less overall signal to the image.

The slice-select and frequency-encoding gradients include dephasing and rephasing lobes to ensure that the phases of MR signals are coherent while being sampled. There is no rephasing lobe along the phase axis before the MR signal is measured, as a rephasing lobe would eliminate phase differences and thus prevent phase encoding. In some pulse sequences, *rewinding* gradient pulses with identical amplitude and reversed polarity relative to the phase-encoding gradient pulses are applied to eliminate the phase differences *after* signal collection and prior to the next excitation pulse. This sustains the transverse magnetization across TR intervals.

▼
Essential Points to Remember

1. Applying a magnetic field gradient along any axis causes the precessional frequency of protons to depend on their position along this axis.

2. Image slices are excited selectively by applying a slice-select gradient during application of radio pulses so the frequency of the radio pulse corresponds to the frequency of protons in the desired image slice but not to protons outside this slice.

3. The position of protons along one axis in an MR image can be determined by obtaining the MR data during application of a frequency-encoding gradient.

4. Because CH_2 protons precess at a frequency different from that of water protons, signals from these lipid protons are misregistered relative to signals from water protons in the MR image along the frequency-encoding gradient. This is called *chemical shift misregistration artifact.*

5. The timing and polarity of magnetic field gradients often is indicated using a line, with the deflections above and below baseline indicating application of a magnetic field gradient with, respectively, positive and negative polarity.

6. Application of a magnetic field gradient dephases the MR signal. Reapplication of a comparable gradient with reversed polarity rephases the MR signal, restoring phase coherence.

7. To produce a coherent signal during frequency encoding, it is necessary first to apply a dephasing lobe of the frequency-encoding gradient. The rephasing lobe of the frequency-encoding gradient forms an echo. This echo provides the signal that is measured to create the MR image.

8. A 180° refocusing pulse applied between the dephasing and rephasing lobes of the frequency-encoding gradient reverses the phases of all transverse magnetization. Frequency differences therefore cause dephasing during the first half of the TE and rephasing during the second half of the TE. The 180° refocusing pulse therefore corrects for heterogeneous chemical shift and magnetic field.

9. If a 180° refocusing pulse is applied, the two lobes of the frequency-encoding gradient must have the same polarity to form an echo. This echo is called a *spin echo.*

10. The third axis of an image is encoded by applying a brief phase-encoding pulse to change the phase of signals along this axis. The phase-encoding gradient must be repeated for the generation of each echo, each time with slightly different area.

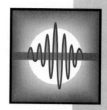

k-Space: A Graphic Guide

In k-space no one can hear you scream.
Bruce R. Rosen, M.D., Ph.D.

The concept of *k-space* is a formalism created to provide a convenient, often graphic explanation for some of the important points about Fourier transform image reconstruction. Physicists refer to k-space frequently when discussing the properties of magnetic resonance (MR) images. Although its derivation requires complex integral calculus, it is usually possible to gain an intuitive understanding of k-space without resorting to higher mathematics. This book is written for those who wish to understand magnetic resonance imaging (MRI) without being confronted with equations. Gaining comfort with the concept of k-space helps make this possible.

From this chapter you should come to an understanding of the interaction of feature-encoding and contrast, some of the tradeoffs associated with MRI between acquisition time and spatial resolution, an improved understanding of artifacts, and useful insight into the designs of advanced spatial encoding

approaches that are discussed later in this book, such as echo-planar imaging, spiral acquisition, and fast spin echo.

What is k-Space?

The MR signal is encoded spatially as it is collected. Remember that in a typical pulse sequence the data are sampled in the presence of a gradient, which causes the spins to precess at a velocity that depends on their position in space (see Chapter 6). A mathematical manipulation, the "Fourier transform," is able to convert such data to a map of the signal intensity as a function of frequency, that is, an *image*. If we were to make a two-dimensional map of the raw signal for a single slice prior to the Fourier transform, the plane on which these data lie would be in "k-space," rather than in conventional image space.

The intensities of the signal at each point in k-space contain information about both contrast and location, but the location information is transformed and distorted. Specifically, k-space is a description of the natural arrangement of the MR raw data.

Some Basic Properties of k-Space

In the absence of gradient spatial encoding, MR data are, by definition, at the center of k-space. More precisely, we are at the location (0,0) in k-space: In a two-dimensional image there are two k-space axes, $k_{readout}$ and k_{phase} (in other places, you may see k_x used for $k_{readout}$ and k_y used for k_{phase}). This point is also known as the "origin." Slice selection is a somewhat special case and is *not* usually best treated in k-space. After selective excitation but before phase- or frequency-encoding by the gradients, the data in the two-dimensional excited slice are all at the k-space origin. The signal has no spatial information at that moment because without the effects of the gradients the spins at all points in the magnet precess at the same frequency (neglecting small effects such as chemical shift and T2).

When gradients are applied to the signal, its intensity evolves as the spins in differing locations go in and out of phase relative to one another. The overall signal therefore contains some spatial information, as it is specifically the difference in the phase as a function of position that has caused the signal modulation. The effective position in k-space is determined by the product of the gyromagnetic ratio, the gradient strength, and the time for which the gradient is left on. Because the gradients are expressed in units of tesla per meter (how much the field strength differs as a function of distance), and the gyromagnetic ratio (γ) is expressed as hertz per tesla (1 Hz = 1 cycle/second = 360°/second), we can determine that the units of k-space are cycles per meter.

Tesla/meter × hertz/Tesla × seconds
   = Tesla/meter × cycles/second/Tesla
      × seconds
   = ~~Tesla~~/meter × cycles/~~second~~/~~Tesla~~
      × ~~seconds~~
   = cycles/meter

The position in k-space, which is therefore expressed in phase per distance, tells us how much the phase between two spins differs as a function of the distance between them after a gradient has been applied. Note also that the position in k-space is the *area* of the gradient waveform (multiplied by γ), as discussed in Chapter 6.

If there were there only *two* spins in the sample, as shown in Figure 6-3, the difference in the signal strength between the center of k-space [k = (0,0)] and a later point in time would be enough to show the locations of both spins. In reality, of course, the distribution of samples placed in the instrument are usually much more complex, and it is necessary to make many more measurements. Generally, one data sample must be collected per pixel. However, each data sample consists of "real" and "imaginary" data, which are symmetrical. Therefore, in practice we need to collect only about half as many samples as there are pixels in the image.

Imaging gradients are set up such that the magnetic field increases with the distance from the center of the MRI device. Thus, the farther spins are from one another, the larger is the frequency difference between them and the greater is the phase difference that accumulates as the gradients are left on. As we move from k = (0,0) to higher magnitudes of k, the signal incorporates larger phase differences. The higher the value of k, the smaller is the distance that can be resolved as separate pixels. In this way, we can see that the amount of spatial encoding—the position of the signal in k-space—determines the *resolution*, or *pixel size*, of the final image. In other words, the distance from the center of k-space determines the spatial resolution of the image.

In k-space each sample point is represented as a complex number (including a "real" and an "imaginary" part), with a position in k-space equal to the product of the gradient amplitude and duration for a specific gradient. In the typical example of a two-dimensional image slice, k-space is expressed in $k_{readout}$ and k_{phase}, which are the gradient areas for the readout and phase-encoding gradients, respectively. The points in k-space do not directly express location; instead, they indicate the amount of spatial encoding that has taken place at that point. More generally, the k-space axes may be labeled by their *functional* assignments $k_{readout}$ and k_{phase} or, for three-dimensional data acquisitions, k_{slice}.

k-Space Trajectories

Importantly, the position in k-space does *not* depend explicitly on time: the data can be placed in k-space in any order, and many MRI pulse sequences differ greatly with regard to the order in which the spatial data are encoded. The data collection order creates a path, or *trajectory,* through k-space. Some examples of k-encoding schemes include echo-planar, rapid acquisition with relaxation enhancement (RARE), and spiral scanning. The encoding scheme used for the most current techniques in clinical practice, as laid out in Chapter 6, is represented in k-space in Figure 7-1.

At the top, Figure 7-1 shows the typical pulse sequence diagram for three TRs of a two-dimensional "gradient echo" imaging sequence [a sequence that has no radiofrequency (RF) refocusing]. Below it is shown the corresponding arrangement of the sample points in two-dimensional k-space. The bold italic letters show the location in k-space at the time indicated in the sequence diagram, and the italic numbers show the sample points in k-space corresponding to the time points in the sequence diagram.

Following the first RF excitation, the data are at the k-space origin (Fig. 7-1, A); the negative pulse along the phase-encoding

gradient creates a negative displacement in the k_{phase} axis equal to the area of that gradient pulse, moving to the location in k-space indicated as B in Figure 7-1. The negative pulse in the readout gradient causes a similar displacement in the negative $k_{readout}$ direction (Fig. 7-1, C). At this point, the readout gradient is applied with the opposite polarity, and data collection is initiated. Each of the successive data samples, 1 through 8, have a different amount of $k_{readout}$ encoding as the gradient is left on for a slightly longer time until the readout gradient has moved the k-space location to D in Figure 7-1.

In this imaging sequence, after each data acquisition the RF pulse scrambles the phases of the spins and thereby removes any effective spatial encoding. As a result, the data return to the k-space origin (Fig. 7-1, A) following each RF pulse. This time a slightly briefer negative pulse of the phase-encoding gradient displaces the data along k_{phase} by an amount equal to its area (Fig. 7-1, E). A negative pulse of the readout gradient moves the position in k-space to the left (Fig. 7-1, F), and acquisition continues for data points 9 through 16. After the third RF excitation, the phase-encoding gradient is left on for an even shorter time, and the position in k_{phase} is displaced downward (Fig. 7-1, H). In a complete imaging sequence, this process continues until enough points are acquired to fill out a two-dimensional grid in k-space.

What we have described is the filling of k-space in two dimensions after magnetization has been created by excitation of a given image slice. For three-dimensional Fourier techniques, a volume is excited and then spatially encoded in three dimensions. For the latter acquisition techniques (discussed in Chapter 8), k-space is filled in three dimensions.

Echo-Planar Imaging

To help understand the value of k-space thinking, we look at an entirely different

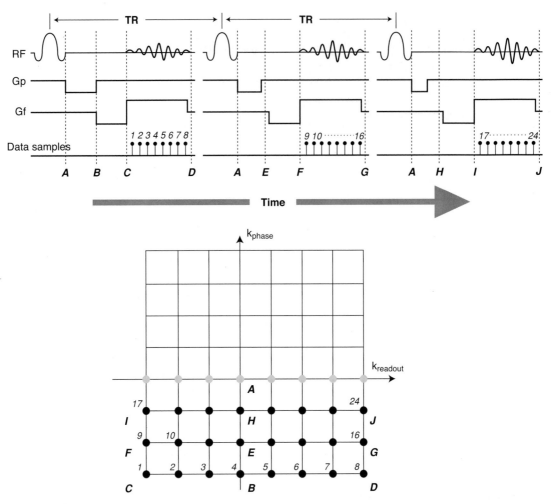

Figure 7-1

Encoding k-space of a typical two-dimensional (2D) "gradient echo" imaging sequence. Below it is shown the corresponding arrangement of the sample points in 2D k-space. *Letters in bold italic* show the location in k-space, and *numbers in italic* show corresponding sample points in k-space. Following the first radiofrequency (RF) excitation, the data are at the k-space origin (A). A negative phase-encoding gradient pulse moves encoding to B. A negative readout gradient causes a similar displacement, to C. A readout gradient is reapplied with opposite polarity, and data samples 1–8 are collected as the k-space location moves to D. After each data acquisition the RF pulse removes the spatial encoding, returning data to A. Following the second RF pulse a slightly briefer negative phase-encoding gradient pulse moves the data to E, a negative readout gradient moves the position in k-space to F, and data points 9–16 are acquired. Similar events occur after the third RF excitation.

imaging sequence. Echo-planar imaging (EPI) was devised to improve the speed of MR data collection. With single-shot EPI, only a single RF excitation is needed to form a complete two-dimensional image. In a single-shot EPI sequence, the complete two-dimensional

k-space grid is therefore sampled following each RF pulse. Figure 7-2 shows the timing diagram (top) and k-space traversal (bottom) for such an EPI acquisition. As in Figure 7-1, the data start at the origin of k-space (Fig. 7-2, A) following RF excitation. With EPI,

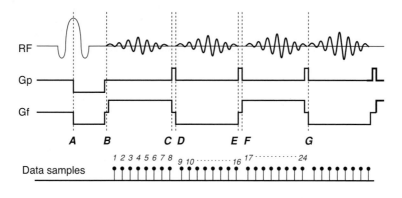

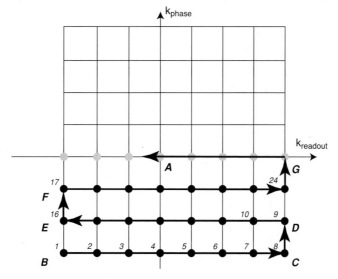

Figure 7-2

Timing diagram (*top*) and k-space traversal (*bottom*) for an echo-planar imaging (EPI) acquisition. As in Figure 7-1, the data start at the k-space origin (A) following RF excitation. Negative readout and phase-encoding gradient pulses applied simultaneously displace the position in k-space (B). The readout gradient is then switched between positive and negative values, and the phase-encoding gradient is pulsed briefly after each reversal. In k-space this causes traversal in a "raster" pattern, as shown by the *heavy arrows*.

negative pulses are applied simultaneously along the readout and phase-encoding axes sufficient to displace the position in k-space all the way to the lower left (Fig. 7-2, B). Following this, the readout gradient is switched between positive and negative values, and the phase-encoding gradient is pulsed briefly after each sign reversal. In k-space this results in a simple, orderly traversal in a so-called "raster" pattern, as shown by the heavy arrows.

Spatial Resolution and Contrast

The largest image features, which vary the least over the span of the image, are said to have the *lowest* "spatial frequency"; smaller image features have a *high* spatial frequency. Remember that the dimensions of k-space are in cycles per meter (i.e., spatial frequency). In fact, the center of k-space encodes information about the largest features in the image, whereas the edges of k-space encode information essentially about the smallest features. (Actually, information about the small features is dispersed in k-space, whereas that from large features is principally limited to the points near the origin.) In other words, the centermost point in k-space (lowest frequency) contains information about the intensity and contrast of the entire image, whereas data points at the edges of k-space (high frequency) encode information about features the size of single

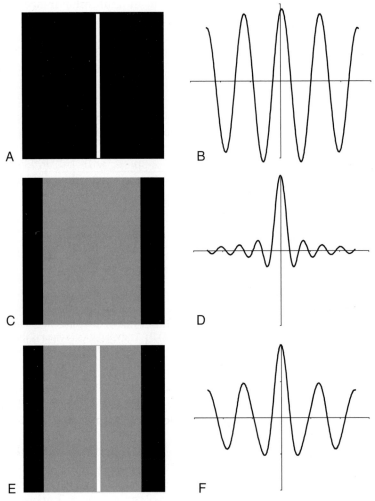

Figure 7-3

Relationship between k-space location and spatial frequency. (A) Image of a vertical bar near the center of the field of view. (B) Its k-space data at the center horizontal line across $k_{phase} = 0$ appear like a sinusoid of nearly constant intensity because all the spins in that object are at approximately the same location in the readout (horizontal axis) and therefore precess at the same frequency. (C) Image of a large object. During signal readout the spins along the readout precess at a variety of frequencies. At the k-space origin, where there is no net gradient effect, all the spins are in phase and the signal is maximal. As the spin phases evolve, moving away from the center of k-space, the signal dephases and rephases. (D) The k-space data for this object has most of its signal in the center of the k-space, where the spins are in phase. (E) Image of the two objects together. (F) Corresponding k-space data.

pixels (picture elements, or dots on the computer screen), providing fine detail of the image. Remember that k-space does not correspond directly to physical space, and a line along the frequency-encoding axis of k-space does not correspond directly to the frequency-encoding axis of the final MR image. Rather, the left and right extremes of the frequency-encoding axis in k-space correspond to the fine detail in this axis, not the left and right portions of the MR image.

Figure 7-3 shows the relation between k-space location and spatial frequency. Imagine a simple object, a vertical bar, near the center of the field of view (Fig. 7-3A). Its k-space data (at the center horizontal line across $k_{phase} = 0$) appear like a sinusoid of nearly constant intensity (Fig. 7-3B). This reflects the fact that all the spins in that object are at approximately the same location in the readout (horizontal) axis and therefore precess at the same frequency. If the object were moved to the left or right, the frequency of this sinusoid in k-space would change. Figure 7-3C shows an image of a large object that nearly fills the field of view. During signal readout the spins along the readout (horizontal) gradient precess at a variety of frequencies. At the k-space origin, where there is no net gradient effect, all of the spins are in phase and the signal is at its maximum. As the spin phases evolve, moving away from the center of k-space, the signal dephases and rephases. The k-space data for this object (Fig. 7-3D) has almost all of its signal in the center of k-space, where the spins are in phase, with little signal elsewhere. In this sense, the edges of k-space can be said to carry *only* information about image detail, and the origin of k-space contains *most* of the information about large image features. Figure 7-3E and F shows an image of the two objects together, along with the corresponding k-space data.

To resolve the fine detail in an image, data corresponding to the periphery of k-space are needed. However, because the position in k-space is the product of the gradient amplitude and time, more time or more gradient power is required. During the time that the gradient is being used for spatial encoding, the MR signal strength evolves as a result of factors such as T1 and T2 relaxation. Generally, any factor that causes the MR signal strength to change during encoding causes deterioration of the resulting image (typically as blurring). If the total time spent on the signal readout is long compared to T2* (the combined transverse relaxation rate), the image becomes blurred. This effect is prominent in multiecho images with long echo trains, few shots, or both, or in images with "low bandwidth" (see Chapter 9), which have long sampling times near physically complex tissue interfaces with a short T2 or T2*.

It is worthwhile to note that k-space is not divided neatly into gross-contrast portions and fine-detail portions. The relative contributions to contrast and detail change gradually between the center and periphery of k-space, with the intermediate portions of k-space providing substantial contributions to both.

Spatial Resolution and Field of View

Diagrams of k-space are helpful for describing the effects of pulse sequence changes on image resolution and field of view (FOV). The depiction of resolution and FOV in k-space, however, is the inverse of their depiction as pixel data in physical MR images. Echoes acquired with strong phase-encoding gradients, providing information about fine detail, are represented at the edges of k-space. Therefore, increasing the spatial resolution of an image involves obtaining data farther from the center of k-space. In other words, increased spatial resolution is represented as increased *area* of k-space. In the physical MR image, however, increasing the spatial resolution of an image means obtaining more pixels per square centimeter of tissue.

To emphasize relative contributions to the image of the center and periphery of k-space,

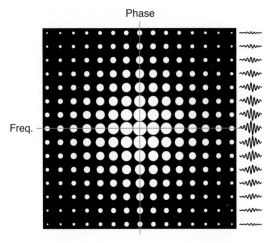

Figure 7-4
A k-space map for a square field of view image with a 15 × 15 matrix. The horizontal axis indicates frequency encoding and the vertical axis phase encoding. The *large dots* at the center of the matrix represent data at the center of k-space. The *small dots* at the periphery of the matrix determine the fine detail of the image. Echoes that correspond to the center of k-space have greater amplitude.

we present a graphic representation of k-space that depicts the center of k-space as large points and the periphery of k-space as finer points (Fig. 7-4). Figure 7-5 shows an image of k-space and its corresponding MR image.

The distance between points in k-space is not affected by changing the spatial resolution of the physical image. As an example, the effect of a 50% reduction of the image matrix shown in Figures 7-4 and 7-5 without changing the FOV is shown in Figures 7-6 and 7-7. An even greater reduction in image matrix is shown in Figure 7-8. Decreased image matrix is represented as k-space of decreased size.

Note that Figures 7-7 and 7-8 show increasing blurring as more of the data from the periphery of k-space are eliminated. Figures 7-9 and 7-10 show the k-space maps and corresponding images reconstructed solely from the periphery of k-space. These images

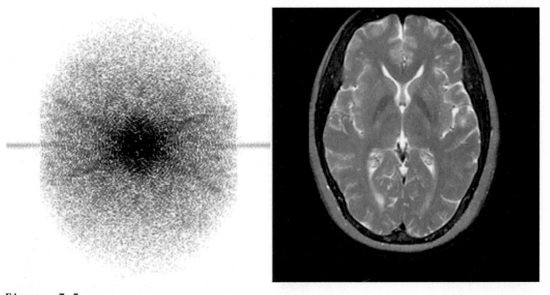

Figure 7-5
Left. A k-space map of digital data acquired from an axial T2-weighted fast spin echo pulse sequence with a 256 × 192 matrix interpolated to a 256 × 256 map of k-space. *Right.* Image that results from Fourier transform analysis.

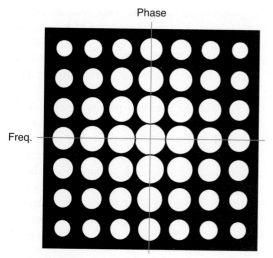

Figure 7-6
k-Space for an image with a field of view identical to that of Figure 7-1 but with lower spatial resolution (i.e., 7 × 7 matrix). The points at the periphery of k-space, which account for the fine detail in Figure 7-2, have not been acquired in this example.

represent the edge information that was absent in Figures 7-7 and 7-8, respectively, without the image contrast from the center of k-space that was present in these images.

Increasing the image FOV involves obtaining additional pixels at the periphery of the physical image. If spatial resolution is not changed, these pixels are of the same size; thus, no additional data are obtained farther from the center of k-space. A larger physical FOV is represented in k-space by decreasing the distance between the points of k-space. In other words, to increase the FOV of the physical image, k-space is filled more densely. For decreased physical FOV, k-space is filled less densely. A 50% reduction in FOV relative to Figures 7-4 and 7-5, without changing the pixel size, is shown in Figures 7-11 and 7-12.

In summary, the representations of image resolution and FOV are inversely related for

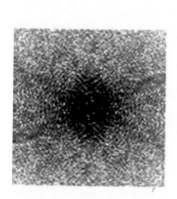
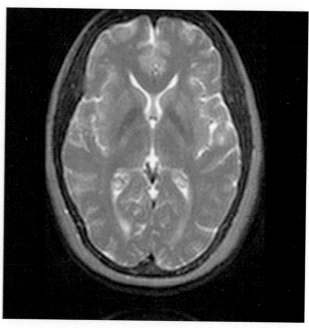

Figure 7-7
The central 128 × 128 points of k-space from Figure 7-2 (*left*) were used to construct the 128 × 128 image at the *right*.

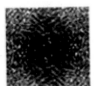

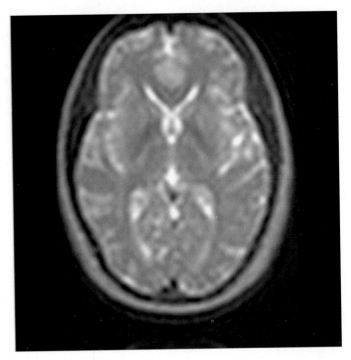

Figure 7-8
The central 64×64 points of k-space from Figure 7-2 (*left*) were used to construct the 64×64 image at the *right*.

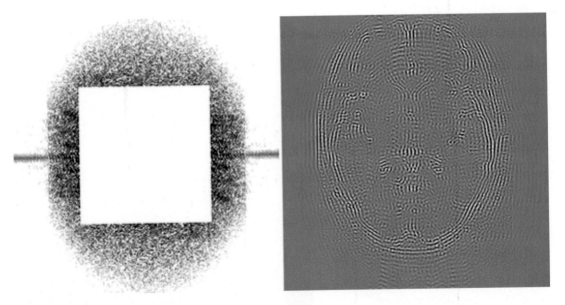

Figure 7-9
The central 128×128 points of k-space from Figure 7-2 (*left*) were eliminated. The remainder of the k-space was used to construct the image at the *right*, which consists entirely of fine detail—and no image contrast.

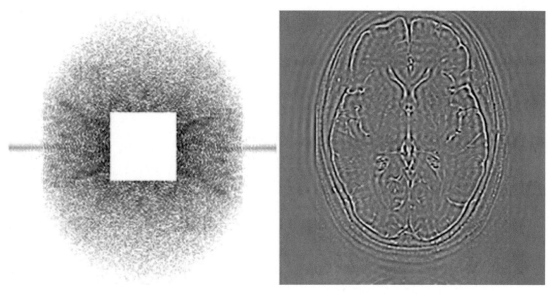

Figure 7-10
The central 64 × 64 points of k-space from Figure 7-2 (*left*) were eliminated. The remainder of the k-space was used to construct the image at the *right*, which consists principally of fine detail—and minimal image contrast.

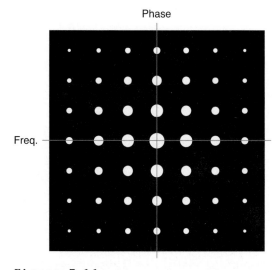

Figure 7-11
A k-space map for a square field of view (FOV) image with identical resolution but dimensions half those seen in Figure 7-1. The k-space is sampled as far toward the periphery, as in Figure 7-1, so spatial resolution is not changed. There is more space between points of k-space, however, so the FOV is reduced.

physical image space, in contrast to k-space. A larger map of k-space indicates high spatial resolution, whereas a map of k-space with points spaced more closely indicates a large FOV.

Zero-Filling of k-Space: Fourier Interpolation

Data corresponding to the periphery of k-space are needed to resolve the fine detail in an image. There are times when generation of additional image pixels is desired but not at the expense of additional image acquisition time. In such situations it is possible to fill in k-space with zeros. If zeros are added at the edges of k-space, the resulting image has a larger matrix composed of more small pixels. However, because the finer

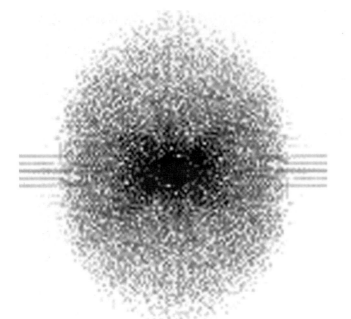

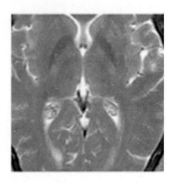

Figure 7-12

The k-space map (*left*) is filled less densely than the map in Figure 7-2, generating an image (*right*) with an FOV half that seen in Figure 7-2 but with identical spatial resolution.

image matrix was generated without benefit of any additional information, there is some blurring between pixels. This is analogous to more conventional forms of pixel interpolation, where new pixels are calculated based on a calculation of nearby pixels.

Interpolation cannot add real information, but poor or inaccurate interpolation can degrade it. In most cases, interpolation by zero filling results in a much more accurate approximation than does pixel-based interpolation based on the image rather than the raw data.

Earlier approaches to MR imaging used radial k-space trajectories (as do certain current experimental methods, in order to achieve special requirements such as extremely short TE—see Chapter 17). In such acquisitions, where only a circular area of k-space is sampled, the more accurate presentation of the image would be on a circular field of view, as any pixels outside of this area would have been formed by

extrapolation of the raw data. All portions of k-space contribute to the final image, however, though the mapping is not point-to-point. Figure 7-13 shows how the outer corners of k-space add meaningfully to the final image. In this, we demonstrate how zero-filling the corners, rather than including the real data that belongs there, results in noticable error and artifact. The figure demonstrates also how data from a limited region of k-space may grossly affect the final images.

▼
Essential Points to Remember

1. K-space is a matrix of raw digitized MRI data prior to Fourier transform analysis. The Fourier transform of k-space is the image.

2. All points in k-space contain data from all locations in an MR image.

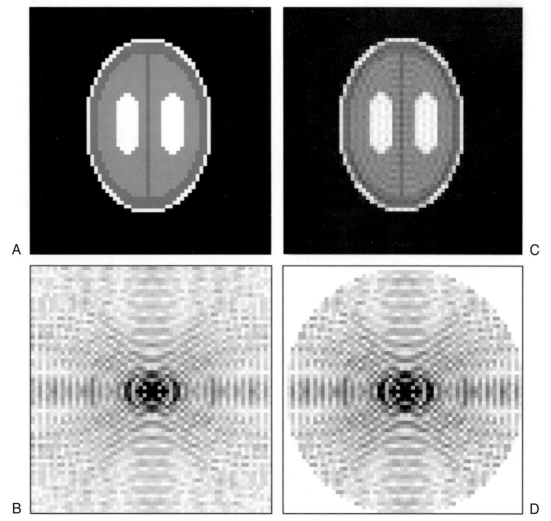

Figure 7-13
Contribution of the corners of k-space to the final image. It is tempting to assume that if k-space is covered to a distance from the origin equivalent to a pre-established pixel resolution (e.g., to 1 mm pixels), that one need only acquire data to a fixed radial distance. In fact, all portions of k-space impact on the final image. *A* shows a reference image, and *B*, below, shows its k-space data. Keeping only a circular portion of k-space around the origin, and zero-filling the corners (*D*) results in a degraded image (*C*) with significant artifact.

3. Points near the center of k-space provide most of the MR image signal intensity and so determine gross tissue contrast throughout the image.

4. Points at the periphery of k-space provide fine edge detail throughout the image, but these points have little effect on image contrast.

5. Adding zeros to the periphery of k-space results in the reconstruction of a larger number of small pixels but generally does not increase spatial resolution.

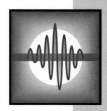

Image Acquisition: Pulse Sequences

Most of our discussion in the first seven chapters addressed the sequence of events involved in the generation of one line of k-space data in a typical magnetic resonance (MR) pulse sequence. These events are typically repeated several times, keeping all factors constant except for the value of the phase-encoding gradient. The time between repetitions is the repetition time (TR), defined earlier during our discussion of T1 relaxation. Within certain constraints, the user can choose the TR. The various techniques for acquiring MR images differ in how slice selection and phase encoding are changed for successive excitations and how the radiofrequency (RF) pulses are used to create transverse magnetization (signal). Combinations of the characteristics and timing of the radio pulses and magnetic field gradients are referred to as *pulse sequences*. Classification and analysis of pulse sequences are greatly facilitated by the use of a standard set of pulse sequence annotations, as discussed below.

Basic Pulse Sequence Annotation

Further discussion of imaging gradients, particularly their timing in relation to other events inherent in generating and measuring MR signals, is facilitated by using a simple form of annotation that describes the timing and configuration of MR pulse sequence events. A pulse sequence is often diagrammed by a set of horizontally oriented lines. The horizontal axis indicates time, the scale of which is identical for all lines in a given example. Each line describes a sequence of radio pulses, image gradients, or magnetic resonance imaging (MRI) signals.

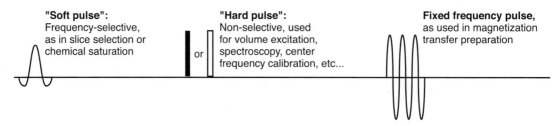

"Soft pulse":
Frequency-selective, as in slice selection or chemical saturation

or

"Hard pulse":
Non-selective, used for volume excitation, spectroscopy, center frequency calibration, etc...

Fixed frequency pulse,
as used in magnetization transfer preparation

Figure 8-1

The notation used for radiofrequency (RF) pulse waveforms varies according to the "type" of RF pulse. A "soft" pulse is a frequency-selective RF pulse such as might be used for slice selection of chemical shift selective excitation. A "hard pulse" is not frequency-selective and is used typically to excite the entire imaging volume simultaneously. Long frequency-selective pulses are used in some cases (e.g., for magnetization preparation).

We began using this annotation in Chapter 6 and continue it throughout the rest of this book. Below, we review the conventions we use.

The top line, abbreviated RF, describes the radiofrequency (radio) pulses. The MR signal, or echo, may also be indicated on this line, although sometimes it is depicted separately on the bottom line. The maximum amplitude of the MR signal corresponds to the time of greatest phase coherence, as determined by the timing of the refocusing lobe of the frequency-encoding gradient. The time between the excitation pulse and the peak of the MR signal defines the echo time (TE). The oscillations of the wave diminish toward the "tails" of the echo both before and after the echo peak.

Slice-selective or frequency-selective RF pulses commonly are represented as a waveform, and a solid vertical bar is often used to indicate a nonselective radio pulse (Fig. 8-1). The height of the waveform or bar indicates the degree of rotation imparted to the affected magnetization. The purpose of the radio pulse is often shown below the bar. In many cases the effective flip angle is indicated next to the pulse. When the flip angle is variable or user-selectable, it is frequently given a variable name, such as α, for an excitation pulse. In Figure 8-2, note that the 180° refocusing pulse is twice as high as the 90° excitation pulse.

The next three lines indicate the timing, amplitude, and polarity of the slice-select (Gs), frequency-encoding (Gf), and phase-encoding (Gp) gradients (Fig. 8-3). A flat line, in "neutral" position, indicates that the imaging gradient is turned off. When the imaging gradient is turned on, the level of the line changes to above neutral for positive polarity or below neutral for negative polarity. The absolute meaning of the polarity is arbitrary, indicating only which end of the gradient is at a higher magnetic field. The identity of the particular gradient illustrated (e.g., slice selection or frequency encoding) is normally shown to its left. Gs and Gf

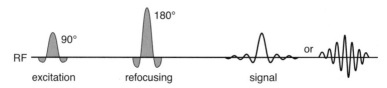

RF

90° excitation

180° refocusing

signal

or

Figure 8-2

Two RF pulses, as might be used to form a spin echo. The flip angle is noted next to each, and the relative sizes suggest the difference in effective flip angle. Two alternative symbols are used to represent the MR signal.

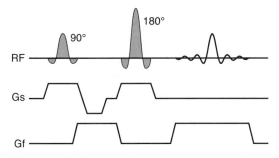

Figure 8-3
Three horizontal lines indicate the timing of the excitation and refocusing pulses, the MR signal, and the slice-select and frequency-encoding gradients.

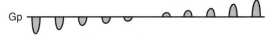

Figure 8-4
Annotation for multiple phase-encoding gradient (Gp) pulses, each occurring after a different excitation. In this example, 11 Gp pulses were applied, beginning with the strongest negative pulses and ending with the strongest positive pulses; the middle pulse has an amplitude of 0.

are indicated in Figure 8-3, showing their timing relative to the RF pulses and data readout.

Some use the abbreviation Gr for *readout gradient* to refer to the frequency-encoding gradient; and some use an alternative "xyz" notation, referring to the slice-select gradient as Gz, the frequency-encoding gradient as Gx, and the phase-encoding gradient as Gy. Although this notation is popular, we do not favor it because these axes may be confused with the physical axes of the magnet bore. If, for example, one mentions the *z axis,* does it indicate the long axis of the magnet bore or the axis of the slice selection? It is only for axial imaging that these axes are identical.

The phase-encoding gradient is indicated as gradient pulses with a series of amplitudes. Sometimes a short, curved line, rather than a rectangular shape, is used for frequency-encoding and slice-select gradients. Repeating the curved line with a different height farther along the time scale (Fig. 8-4) can indicate the variable amplitude of the phase-encoding gradient throughout multiple repetitions. Alternatively, phase-encoding gradient pulses of varying amplitudes within successive repetitions are superimposed, as in Figure 8-5. Figure 8-6 describes the timing of radio pulses and imaging gradients relative to the production of a signal for a standard spin echo pulse sequence. In this and many other examples,

shading is used to highlight the area within each gradient lobe.

Single-Slice Acquisitions

Some pulse sequences involve creating one MR image at a time. The acquisition time for these single-slice techniques is directly proportional to their TRs. When a single image is created using one repetition for each value of the phase-encoding gradient, the acquisition time is simply the number of phase-encoding values multiplied by the TR. Therefore, single-slice acquisitions usually have short TRs, typically 50 msec or less. If a short TR is acceptable or desirable, single-slice acquisitions may be appropriate. The TR, phase-encoding pulses, and echo amplitudes for single-slice acquisition are illustrated in Figure 8-7. Acquisition of one slice does not begin until acquisition of the previous slice is complete.

For some applications a short image acquisition time is paramount. Here, the TR is chosen as the minimum interval achievable within the constraints of the pulse sequence and MRI hardware. In these situations, the TR is limited by the echo time (TE) and the time required to apply the radio pulses and imaging gradients plus any delays between them that may be necessary. For such rapid techniques, minimizing the TR, and thus the acquisition time, usually requires use of the shortest possible TE and most rapid switching of imaging gradients. (As seen later, in Chapter 14, some modern pulse sequences allow the effective TE to exceed the TR.)

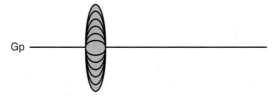

Figure 8-5
Condensed annotation for multiple phase-encoding gradient (Gp) pulses.

Two-Dimensional Multislice Acquisitions

A long TR is desirable for many applications. One example is an image that should show fluid as high signal intensity. Because simple fluid typically has a long T1 relaxation time, increasing the TR allows more time for magnetization to recover, increasing its signal intensity. For images with a long TR, single-slice acquisition techniques may be unacceptably inefficient, as the time between measuring the echo and the next excitation radio pulse (the difference between the TE and the TR) is "dead time." Rather than wasting the time between the TE and the next excitation pulse, another slice can be excited during that interval. Additional slices are excited by reapplying, for each, an excitation pulse of slightly different frequency that causes resonance at the frequency corresponding to a different location along the slice-select gradient.

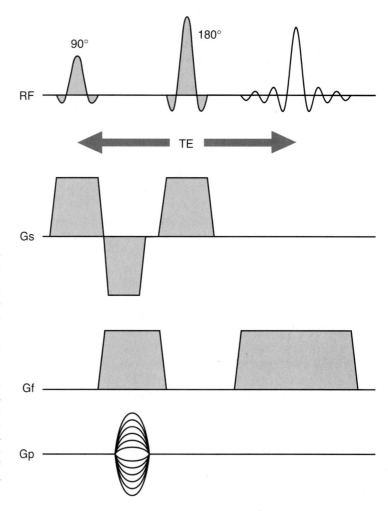

Figure 8-6
Pulse sequence annotation for a conventional spin echo pulse sequence. The first line (RF) describes the sequence of radio pulses (90° and 180°) followed by the signal that occurs at a time (TE) after the 90° pulse. The next two lines (Gs and Gf) describe the timing of the slice-select and frequency-encoding gradients, respectively. Deflection above the baseline indicates positive polarity; deflection below the baseline indicates negative polarity. The shading of these gradients highlights their area. The final line (Gp) indicates multiple pulses of varying strengths of the phase-encoding gradient.

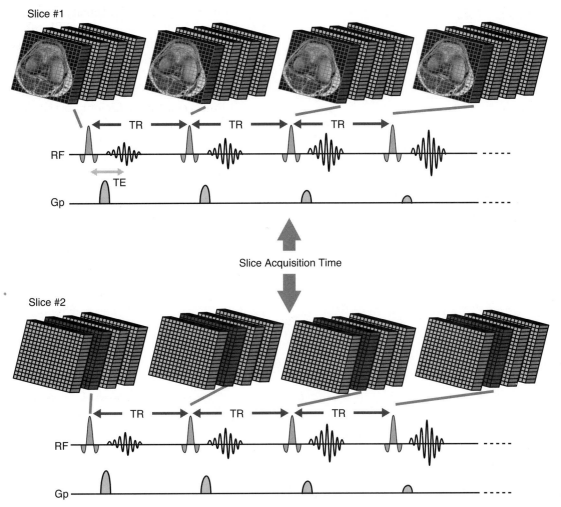

Figure 8-7

Sequence of radiofrequency (RF) and phase-encoding gradient (Gp) events involved in imaging a stack of slices using single-slice acquisition. A given slice is excited repeatedly, varying the strength of the phase-encoding gradient. As the phase-encoding gradient strength decreases, the magnitude of the echo increases. After enough echoes have been obtained to complete the acquisition of a given slice, the process is repeated for a different slice.

A second image slice is thereby excited, followed by measuring the echo from this second slice at its TE. If time permits, additional slices can be thus excited in an "interleaved" manner during each TR, followed each time by measuring the resulting echo. Typically, the slices are not excited in sequential order (i.e., slices 1, 2, 3 ...) but in such a way as to maximize the time elapsing *between* excitation of adjacent slices to reduce the effects of cross-talk (see Cross-Talk, page 90). Figure 8-8 illustrates four slices being excited during each TR.

As an example, let us assume that, for Figure 8-8, the TR is 40 msec and the TE 5 msec. Slice 1 is first excited by a radio pulse during application of the slice-select gradient, and an echo is sampled whose peak occurs 5 msec after the excitation radio pulse. Next, the slice-select gradient is reapplied along with an excitation pulse that has a slightly different frequency, matching the frequency of slice 3. In practice, an excitation

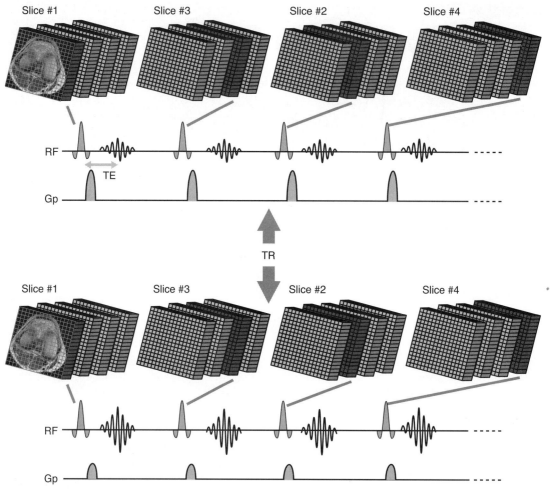

Figure 8-8

Sequence of radiofrequency (RF) and phase-encoding gradient (Gp) events involved in imaging a stack of slices using multislice acquisition. Each slice is excited using a given phase-encoding gradient strength. After each slice has been excited once, all slices are excited a second time using a different phase-encoding gradient strength.

pulse cannot occur immediately after the echo peak because time is required to finish sampling the echo and to apply additional (spoiling and crushing) gradients to reduce artifacts. In this example, let us assume a delay of 5 msec between each echo peak and the next excitation pulse. Thus, slice 3 is excited 10 msec after slice 1. Next in order, the frequency of the excitation pulse is changed so slices 2 and 4 are excited, generating their respective echoes 5 msec after each excitation pulse. Finally, at the TR, 40 msec after the initial excitation pulse,

the value of the phase-encoding gradient is changed and slice 1 experiences its second excitation pulse. Figure 8-9 compares images acquired using single-slice and multi-slice gradient echo techniques.

Cross-Talk

Because the slice profiles for excitation are imperfect, one consequence of multislice acquisitions is the inadvertent excitation of tissue outside the intended image slice.

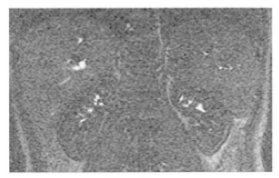
Single-slice TR = 7 msec

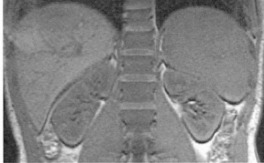
Multislice; TR = 100 msec

Figure 8-9
Coronal gradient echo images of the abdomen acquired using single-slice (*left*) and multislice (*right*) techniques with 90° excitation flip angles. With the multislice technique, a longer repetition time (TR) is possible without a longer acquisition time for the stack of images. The use of a longer TR results in an improved signal-to-noise ratio.

This is referred to as cross-excitation, or "cross-talk." It can reduce longitudinal magnetization and thus decrease signal intensity in the resulting image. In other words, cross-talk can decrease the time between exposures of a slice to excitation radio pulses, thereby reducing the effective TR because the time between excitations of protons at the slice surfaces is shorter than the specified TR (Fig. 8-10). Such cross-talk may also result in the unintended collection of signal from slices other than the one of interest.

Cross-talk generally results in a reduced signal-to-noise ratio (SNR), particularly for tissues with long T1 relaxation times because they recover more slowly from cross-excitation. Cross-talk is especially likely when the gaps between image slices of a multislice acquisition are too small relative to the precision of the excitation radio pulses or when slices are contiguous.

Cross-talk can be reduced by improving the precision of the slice profile of the excitation radio pulses. This may require increased radio energy, increased time, or both, and is not usually an operator-selected variable. More commonly, cross-talk is reduced or avoided by choosing gaps between slices that are large enough so the excitation that "spills over" does not affect the nearest slice (Fig. 8-11).

If contiguous slices are needed, cross-talk can be avoided by acquiring two sets of images. First, half the image slices are acquired with 100% gaps between them (e.g., 5 mm thick with 5 mm gaps). Then the other half of the image slices are obtained during

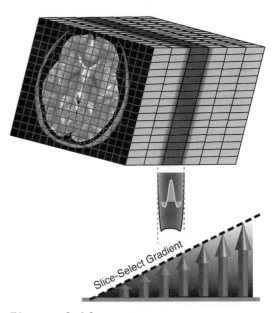

Figure 8-10
Cross-excitation. Because the range of frequencies of a radio pulse is not precise, its slice profile is less than perfect. Thus, adjacent tissue outside the intended image slice is partially excited.

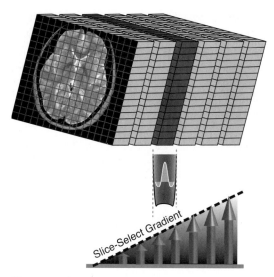

Figure 8-11
Cross-excitation is avoided by using gaps between image slices.

a separate acquisition, filling in the gaps to achieve a contiguous set of image slices (Fig. 8-12). This is sometimes referred to as *concatenated acquisition*.

Magnetization Transfer

Magnetization transfer (MT) results from excitation of protons in macromolecules, such as those in proteins and membrane phospholipids, which do not contribute directly to signal intensity in MR images. However, this excitation affects magnetization of water protons bound to these macromolecules.

Macromolecular protons have a much broader range of resonant frequencies than those in free water. Radio pulses of several thousand kilohertz larger or smaller than the resonant frequency of water protons

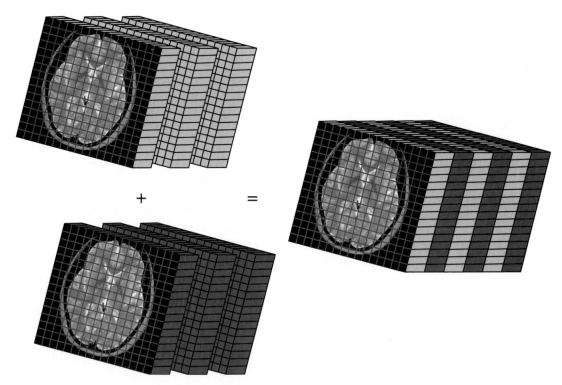

Figure 8-12
Contiguous slices free of cross-excitation can be obtained by interleaving two sets of slices, each with 100% gaps.

can therefore excite macromolecular protons and saturate their magnetization. This saturated magnetization is then transferred from the macromolecular protons to the surrounding water protons, thereby reducing the observable MR signal. The signal loss caused by this transfer of saturated magnetization is greatest in tissues containing abundant macromolecules.

The MT affects tissue contrast in multislice acquisitions, as radio pulses targeted to different image slices partially saturate the magnetization of all macromolecular protons within the volume of interest. Figure 8-13 illustrates the saturation of water, methylene (CH_2), and macromolecular protons by a radio pulse. The longitudinal magnetization of macromolecular protons can also be saturated deliberately by applying appropriate saturation pulses before each excitation pulse (see Chapter 14).

Solid tissues lose substantial signal intensity because of MT, whereas fluid and adipose

tissue do not. This loss of signal intensity is generally greater for tissues that have long T1 relaxation times because their longitudinal magnetization recovers more slowly after saturation. In many (but not all) situations, MT contrast resembles T2 contrast, as both tend to depict tissues with abundant macromolecules as having low signal intensity. The effects of cross-talk and MT contrast when using the fast spin echo technique are illustrated in Figure 8-14.

Time Considerations

One might think that the TR of a simple multislice pulse sequence would be as short as the TE multiplied by the number of slices; that is, as soon as an echo is sampled at the TE, the next slice could be excited. Thus, with a TE of 5 msec, a TR of 60 msec should be long enough to obtain 12 image slices. In practice, however, the number of slices obtained is often half this number or even fewer. Several additional factors contribute to reducing the time within a TR available for exciting slices and generating echoes.

An MR echo is not instantaneous; rather, it occurs over a period of a few milliseconds, during which time the frequency-encoding gradient is on. TE refers to the time of the echo peak; echo sampling begins before the TE and continues after the TE. Once the echo is sampled, there is still transverse magnetization, which, if excited by the next radio pulse, can lead to unwanted signals that degrade the image. Thus, after echo sampling is completed, a series of crushing, spoiling, or rewinding gradients is applied to eliminate this magnetization or otherwise prevent it from producing image degradation. Furthermore, excitation takes several milliseconds, and the gradients themselves may take several hundred microseconds to change amplitude, all of which adds to the minimum imaging time.

The overall efficiencies of single-slice and multislice two-dimensional Fourier transform (2D-FT) techniques are comparable; that is, for a given TE, the spatial resolution,

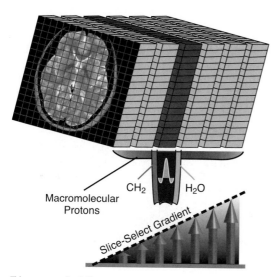

Figure 8-13

Range of frequencies within an image slice for H_2O (*light gray*), CH_2 (*dark gray*), and macromolecular (*shaded*) protons. H_2O and CH_2 protons have similar frequency ranges, corresponding to those of the excitation pulse. The frequency range is much greater for macromolecular protons, so they are excited by every excitation and refocusing pulse, including those targeted to other slices. This excited magnetization is then transferred to nearby H_2O protons.

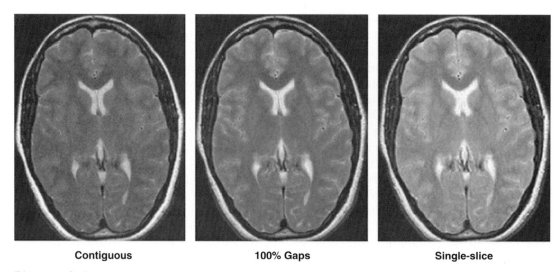

| Contiguous | 100% Gaps | Single-slice |

Figure 8-14
T2-weighted fast spin echo image of the brain obtained using contiguous multislice (*left*), interleaved acquisitions with 100% gaps (*middle*), and single-slice techniques (*right*). Cross-excitation is eliminated by using 100% gaps, resulting in increased signal intensity and improved contrast between gray and white matter. With the single-slice technique (*right*), cross-talk and magnetization transfer are both eliminated, further increasing the signal intensity of both gray and white matter.

number of signal averages, and number of image slices during single-slice and multislice acquisitions require about the same amount of time. For example, a single-slice technique might allow acquisition of one image slice per second, whereas a comparable multislice technique might require 20 seconds to acquire a stack of 20 image slices. Both techniques require 20 seconds to acquire the entire volume of interest.

With the single-slice technique described above, 10 images have been completely acquired after 10 seconds. With the multislice technique, however, 20 images have been partially acquired after 10 seconds and no acquisition has been completed. If severe motion occurs during a 20-image acquisition, one image is degraded with a single-slice technique, whereas all images are affected with the multislice technique. This is one reason why single-slice techniques tend to be less sensitive to motion artifact than multislice techniques. Motion sensitivity is explored further in Chapter 10.

Because time is required for magnetization to recover following each excitation due to T1 effects, more signal can generally be collected at longer TRs. Thus, multislice sequences usually have much higher SNR and are superior to single-slice sequences for many applications, especially in essentially stationary tissues such as the brain or extremities.

Three-Dimensional Fourier Techniques

Fourier transformation involves using data from the frequency, phase, and amplitude of waves to compute a detailed spatial map, or image. Thus far we have restricted our discussions to 2D-FT imaging, which involves using frequency-selective excitation of one or more discrete image slices and then encoding a two-dimensional image via phase encoding in one axis and frequency encoding in the other (Figs. 8-7 and 8-8).

Alternatively, it is possible to construct a three-dimensional picture using a single frequency-encoding gradient for localization along one in-plane axis and phase encoding for the other two axes. This process, whereby multiple signals are acquired using different values of phase-encoding gradients along two axes, is termed *three-dimensional Fourier transform* (3D-FT) imaging. The pulse sequence annotation for 3D-FT is illustrated in Figure 8-15, and the events are shown graphically in Figure 8-16.

A three-dimensional data set resulting from 3D-FT techniques is usually defined by

an in-plane field of view (FOV) (e.g., 20 cm^2) and matrix (e.g., 256×192) and by the number and thickness of image slices (often called *partitions*). This is similar to the description of 2D-FT images, except that 2D-FT slices may be separated by gaps whereas 3D-FT partitions are contiguous. The process by which image slices or partitions are defined is different for 2D-FT and 3D-FT techniques, however. With 2D-FT techniques, image slices are *selectively excited* using a slice-select gradient, whereas with 3D-FT techniques volume partitions are *encoded* using a phase-encoding gradient in exactly the manner that one axis of an image is phase-encoded. A three-dimensional representation of k-space for 3D-FT techniques is shown in Figure 8-17.

Although cross-talk due to cross-excitation is primarily a problem for 2D-FT acquisitions, there are other forms of cross-talk that occur between slices during a 3D-FT acquisition and, in fact, between pixels in any MR image. The Fourier encoding process creates a highly complex pattern of cross-talk that appears as prominent artifacts, such as "edge-ringing" in plane, and in a more subtle manner between slices in 3D-FT studies. These artifacts are most prominent when the number of phase-encoding steps in plane or the number of 3D slices is small.

With 2D-FT imaging, the excitation pulse is targeted to a single-image slice by the slice-select gradient, and each resulting echo contains signals from throughout that single slice. With 3D-FT imaging, however, each excitation pulse excites the entire volume, and *each resulting echo contains signals from throughout the entire volume.* Thus, each image, and each pixel within each image, is based on a much greater number of MR signals for 3D-FT techniques than for 2D-FT techniques. For this reason, 3D-FT techniques generate images with a much higher SNR than do 2D-FT single-slice images of comparable voxel size and other imaging parameters (Fig. 8-18). On some occasions, however, the longer TR of 2D-FT *multislice* techniques allows an SNR comparable to that of 3D-FT techniques.

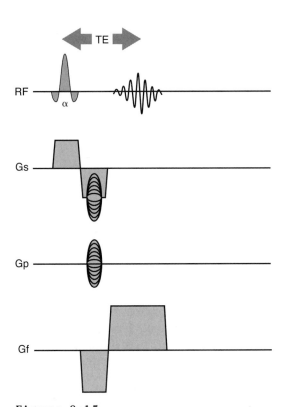

Figure 8-15

Pulse sequence for three-dimensional Fourier transform (3D-FT) volume acquisition. The volume is selected by the slice-select gradient (Gs), the rephasing lobe of which has variable strength. Thus, there is phase encoding in both the phase-encoding and slice-select axes.

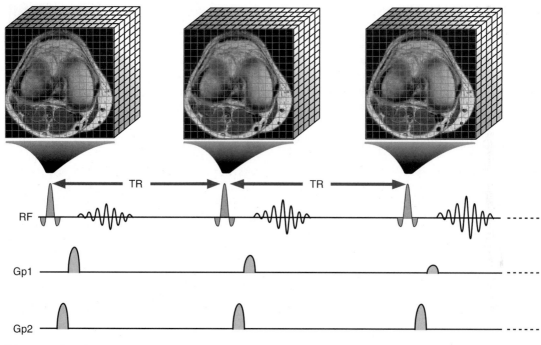

Figure 8-16
Three-dimensional Fourier transform (3D-FT) volume acquisition. The entire volume is excited by each excitation pulse. TR is the time between successive excitations and is therefore usually much shorter than the TR for 2D-FT multislice acquisitions. Phase encoding is performed in two axes.

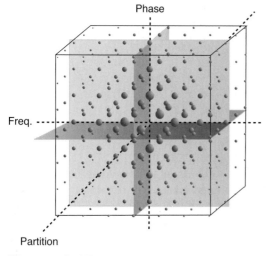

Figure 8-17
Three-dimensional map of k-space. Each point in k-space is represented by a sphere. Each echo provides a line of data along the frequency-encoding axis.

Although the entire imaged volume of a 3D-FT acquisition is excited by each excitation pulse, the pulse is usually transmitted during application of a gradient. The purpose of this gradient is to restrict the excitation to the volume of interest to prevent artifacts from unintended excitation of tissue outside the volume of interest. This gradient is referred to as a *slab-selective gradient*.

In general, the increased imaging time of 3D-FT relative to 2D-FT techniques is equal to the number of partitions. A general comparison between 2D-FT single-slice, 2D-FT multislice, and 3D-FT techniques is presented in Table 8-1. Most other parameters, such as TE and total acquisition time for a volume of interest, do not differ significantly.

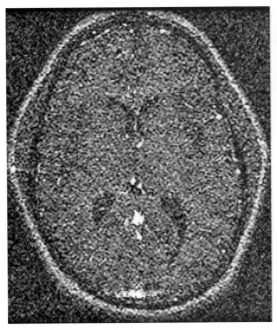
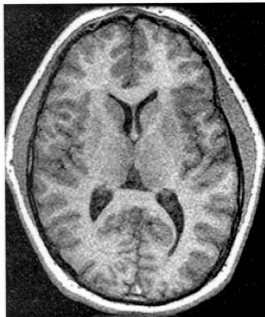

2D Spoiled GRE   **3D Spoiled GRE**

Figure 8-18
A comparison of two-dimensional (2D) (*left*) and three-dimensional (3D) (*right*) spoiled gradient echo 25/5/45°
images. For both techniques, 1.5 mm thick slices were imaged. The signal-to-noise ratio is much better with the
3D technique.

Zero-Fill Interpolation in the Slice-Encoding Axis

In Chapter 7 we discussed zero-fill interpolation, which involves adding zeros to the periphery of k-space to increase the number and decrease the size of the pixels calculated for MR images. For 3D-FT acquisitions,

zeros can be added to k-space in the periphery of the slice-encoding direction, which increases the number and decreases the thickness of the image slices created.

Most commonly, zero-fill interpolation is used to double the number of image slices reconstructed following a given 3D-FT acquisition. This has no effect on the

Table 8-1 ■ GENERAL FEATURES OF 2D-FT SINGLE-SLICE, 2D-FT MULTISLICE, AND 3D-FT TECHNIQUES

Parameter	2D-FT single-slice	2D-FT multislice	3D-FT
TR	Short	Intermediate/long	Short
SNR	Low	Intermediate/high	High
Cross-excitation	None	Possible	None
Magnetization transfer	Usually none	Some/substantial	None
Motion sensitivity	Low	Substantial	Substantial

2D-FT and 3D-FT, two- and three-dimensional Fourier transform; SNR, signal-to-noise ratio.

acquisition time, though the time for reconstructing the data often increases. Although no real additional data are acquired, the resulting image slices correspond to smaller increments of the patient's anatomy. Some describe the resulting data set as consisting of overlapping images of thickness defined by the acquisition of real data prior to zero filling. This is analogous to the creation of additional pixels via in-plane interpolation; although the image matrix is finer, there is blurring that prevents the additional pixels from depicting additional data. Generally, however, zero filling is a more accurate method for interpolation than simple pixel interpolation.

▼
Essential Points to Remember

1. For single-slice acquisitions, a slice is excited repeatedly, changing the phase-encoded value until echoes of all values have been obtained. During this period, no additional slices are excited.

2. Single-slice acquisitions are most appropriate when a short or minimal TR is acceptable or desirable.

3. Two-dimensional multislice acquisitions involve exciting several slices using a particular value of the phase-encoding gradient, usually without reexciting the first slice until after all other slices have been excited.

4. Two-dimensional multislice acquisitions are most appropriate when a longer TR is considered desirable or necessary to increase the SNR of tissues that have long T1 relaxation times.

5. Partial saturation of protons in an image slice during excitation of an adjacent image slice (cross-excitation) reduces the effective TR for the pulse sequence and the SNR of the resulting image. Cross-excitation may also add systematic artifacts.

6. Protons in macromolecules are partially saturated by radio pulses targeted to different image slices. This saturated magnetization is transferred to nearby water molecules, reducing the signal intensity of tissues with abundant macromolecules without affecting the signal intensity of free fluid or lipid. This phenomenon is called *magnetization transfer.*

7. Anatomical coverage and imaging efficiency can be similar for single-slice and multislice acquisitions so long as the rates at which signals are acquired are comparable.

8. Single-slice acquisitions are usually less sensitive to motion than multislice or 3D-FT acquisitions. A brief episode of motion that occurs during a multislice or 3D-FT acquisition may degrade every slice of that acquisition.

9. The 2D-FT techniques involve selecting slices by applying a magnetic field gradient during excitation radio pulses. 3D-FT techniques involve exciting the entire volume and then encoding partitions by applying a second series of phase-encoding magnetic field gradient pulses along the slice-select axis.

10. With 3D-FT techniques, every echo contains information about every voxel throughout the entire volume.

11. After a 3D-FT acquisition, zeros can be added to the periphery of k-space in the slice-encoding direction. This increases the number and decreases the apparent thickness of image slices reconstructed.

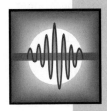

Chapter 9

Signal-to-Noise Ratio and Spatial Resolution

Magnetic resonance (MRI) pulse sequences can be chosen with great flexibility to optimize contrast between two or more tissues. Once this is done, most other choices relate to the competing concerns of the signal-to-noise ratio (SNR), spatial resolution, and acquisition time.

Signal-to-Noise Ratio and Spatial Resolution

We have considered the sources of magnetic resonance (MR) signals and the manner by which these signals provide information to be encoded into MR images. The images can be degraded by *noise*, which consists of random or systematic errors caused by (1) imperfections in the MR system, (2) the process by which images are acquired, or (3) factors arising from the patient, such as motion. In a properly operating MR system, the dominant sources of noise are thermal processes within the patient, and patient motion. In general, increasing the volume of data (signal) and decreasing the amount of noise optimizes image clarity. This relationship between data and noise is expressed as the SNR. It is always desirable to increase the overall SNR of an image, but it is commonly prevented because of important tradeoffs between the SNR, spatial resolution, and acquisition time.

Pixel and Voxel Size

Spatial resolution refers to the size of the volume elements (voxels) that make up the image. A *voxel* is a three-dimensional unit of an image consisting of a width in two axes; the third axis is the image slice thickness (Fig. 9-1).

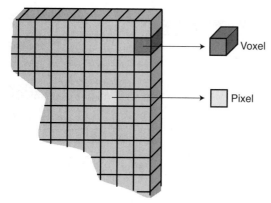

Figure 9-1
A voxel represents the volume of tissue that is depicted as a pixel in a two-dimensional (2D) image.

The in-plane spatial resolution is determined by the size of the picture elements (pixels) that make up the image. The size of each of these pixels is determined by dividing the area of the image by the number of pixels. For example, an image with a 200 × 200 mm field of view (FOV) has an area of 40,000 mm². If the image matrix is 256 × 256 pixels, it results in a total of 65,536 pixels, each with an area of 0.6 mm². If the slice thickness is 5 mm, the volume of each voxel is 3 mm³.

For an image with a given FOV and slice thickness, spatial resolution can be increased by dividing the image into a larger number of smaller pixels (Figs. 9-2 and 9-3). Alternatively, for an image with a given number of pixels, higher spatial resolution can be obtained by choosing a smaller FOV (Figs. 9-4 through 9-6). Using a denser matrix or smaller FOV involves acquiring an image of smaller voxel size.

The ability to resolve small structures is determined by the in-plane resolution and the slice thickness. Even with fine in-plane resolution, small structures can be obscured if their signal intensity is averaged with that of surrounding tissues, called *partial volume*

Figure 9-2
Effect of matrix size on spatial resolution. A finer matrix (*top row*), results in smaller, more numerous pixels for a given field of view, improving spatial resolution. The images at the *left* show an object consisting of the letter S enclosed in an oval; the images at the *right* depict the pixels that are darkened if they contain part of the object. The intensity of the darkening is less with the lower-resolution image (*bottom right*) because a smaller proportion of each voxel contains part of the object than those in the higher-resolution image (*top right*). In the lower-resolution image (*bottom right*), all but two pixels in the region of the object contain part of the object and are thus darkened, so the structure of the object cannot be resolved.

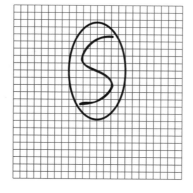
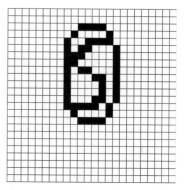
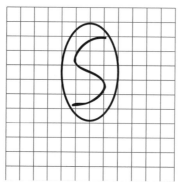
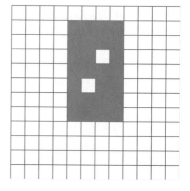

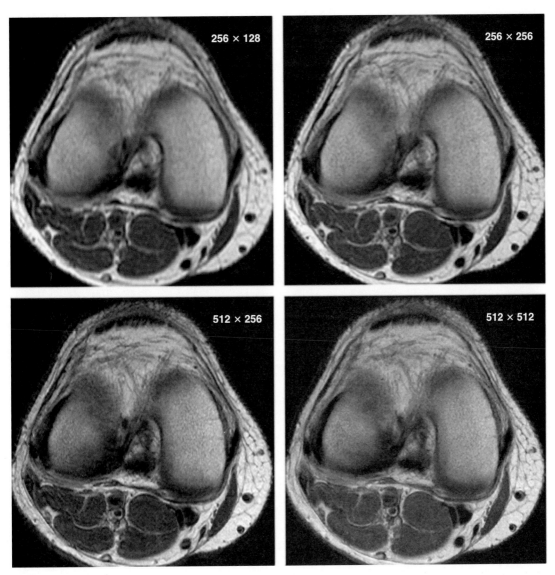

Figure 9-3
Axial T1-weighted images of the knee with increasing spatial resolution. As the matrix is increased from 256 × 128 to 512 × 512, finer anatomical structures can be resolved; however, the smaller pixel size also renders image noise more conspicuous.

averaging (Fig. 9-7). The direct effects on spatial resolution of three common user-selected pulse sequence parameters that determine voxel size, assuming that the other parameters are not changed, are described in Table 9-1.

Voxel size cannot be decreased with impunity, frequently forcing operators to settle for an image with less spatial resolution than might be desired. Decreases in voxel size are generally associated with decreases in the SNR and increases in the acquisition time (discussed later). Overall, therefore, improvements in spatial resolution come at the cost of a loss in the SNR.

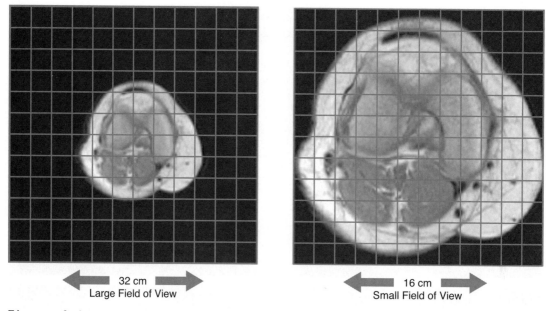

32 cm
Large Field of View

16 cm
Small Field of View

Figure 9-4

Effect of the field of view (FOV) on pixel size. The use of a smaller FOV (e.g., 16 cm^2) results in smaller pixels and finer spatial resolution without changing the number of pixels. Although the number of pixels in the entire image is not changed, more pixels are used to depict the object of interest in the 16 cm^2 FOV image. Each pixel represents a smaller volume of tissue.

SNR Versus Spatial Resolution

Voxels are volumes of tissue from which the pixels of an image are derived. The clarity of an image is best when the signal data for each voxel are much greater than the unwanted random or systematic fluctuations that combine to create image noise. As an image is divided into smaller voxels to increase spatial resolution, the volume of data used to create the signal in each voxel decreases. As the volume of data determining voxel signal values decreases, the relative importance of noise increases. Thus, an image composed of small voxels has the desirable attribute of high spatial resolution but with the potentially deleterious attribute of a low SNR.

The relationship between voxel size and the SNR may seem counterintuitive. The total volume of data in an image is not reduced when it is divided into smaller voxels, and noise does not necessarily increase. Why, then, does the SNR decrease when an image is divided into smaller voxels?

It may help to look at the following example. Consider a group of 100 persons, each 66 inches tall. If the accuracy of our measurement, limited by noise, is ± 1 inch, the range of measurements is 65 to 67 inches. If errors are random, it is likely that the average measured height of this crowd is close to 66 inches. If the same group is divided into smaller groups of 10 persons each, the effect of this imprecision in measurement is likely to be greater. For example, in one group the height of four persons might be underestimated and the height of one might be overestimated, yielding a mean of 65.7 inches. In another group, overestimation of four heights and underestimation of one would yield a mean of 66.3 inches, a difference between these two groups of more than 0.5 inch. As an extreme example, if each "group" contained only one person, groups could differ from each other by as much as 2 inches. The random variability between groups is therefore considerably greater if the groups are small than if they

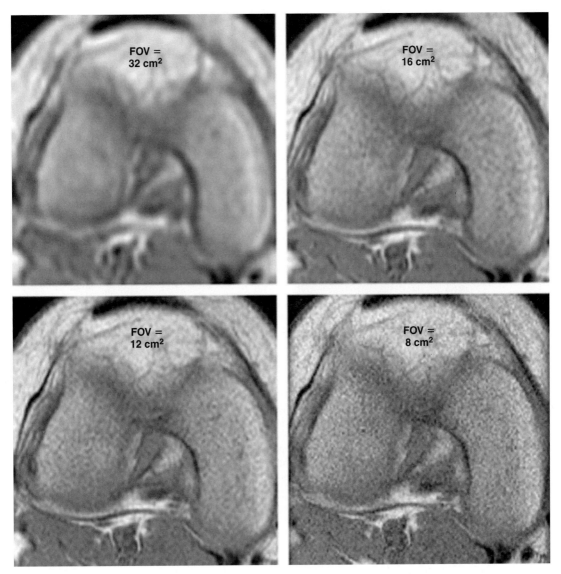

Figure 9-5
Effect of variation in the FOV on axial T1-weighted images of the knee. The images have been magnified so anatomical structures are of comparable size. As the FOV decreases from 32 cm² to 8 cm² while maintaining the matrix at 256 × 60, smaller structures can be resolved; however, image noise increases because of the smaller pixel size.

are large owing to the smaller volume of data from each small group.

Another example is illustrated in Figure 9-8. A 12 × 12 grid was constructed by randomly assigning values of 1 to 6. A value of 3 was added to the central 36 squares. The random variation is greater than the minimally darker shade of gray in the center of Figure 9-8, so it partially obscures it. When groups of nine contiguous pixels are averaged to form larger pixels, the random variations become less than the difference in shades of gray.

In conclusion, there is a direct relationship between voxel size and the SNR. When all other factors are held constant, decreasing the voxel size decreases the SNR. In other words, for each application it is usually necessary to balance the desire for both high spatial resolution and an adequate SNR.

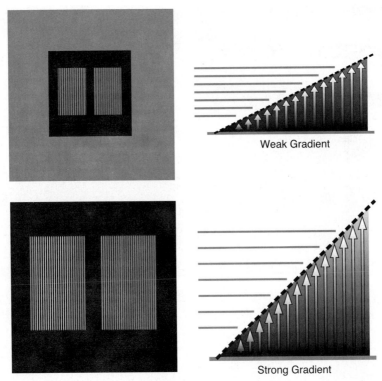

Figure 9-6
Effect of gradient strength on spatial resolution. In this example, the *black squares with vertical lines* represent the areas of interest and the larger *gray square* (*top*) represents surrounding space in the image that is of no interest. The use of a stronger frequency-encoding gradient (*bottom*) results in greater frequency differences between two points. This results in smaller pixel size and finer spatial resolution. If the same number of pixels along the frequency-encoding axis is depicted, the image has a smaller FOV because each pixel is smaller; hence, small structures are resolved. A square image is maintained by also increasing the strength of the phase-encoding gradient (see Phase Encoding, Chapter 6).

Table 9-1 ■ EFFECT OF ACQUISITION MATRIX, SLICE THICKNESS, AND FIELD OF VIEW ON VOXEL SIZE AND THEREFORE ON SPATIAL RESOLUTION	
Pulse Sequence Parameter Change	**Effect on Spatial Resolution**
Increased acquisition matrix	↑
Increased slice thickness	↓
Increased field-of-view	↓

Sampling the Signal

Number of Samples

The MR signal is a complex radio wave with a combination of frequencies, phases, and amplitudes. The phases of the wave come together in a momentary crescendo at the

Figure 9-7
Effect of slice thickness on axial magnetic resonance (MR) images of the knee. As slice thickness is increased from 3 to 8 mm, all other factors being constant, the larger voxels improve the signal-to-noise ratio (SNR). However, it becomes more difficult to perceive fine detail; and spatial resolution is degraded owing to a larger voxel size.

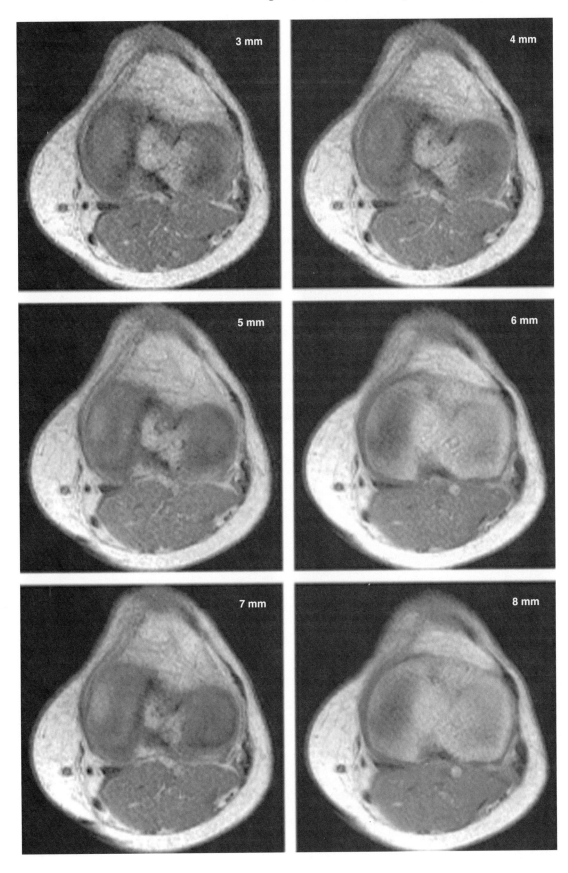

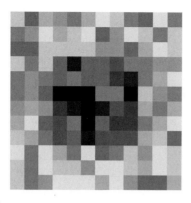
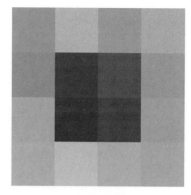

Figure 9-8
When nine adjacent pixels from the image (*left*) are averaged mathematically to produce larger pixels (*right*), random variations in noise are deemphasized, allowing the dark square at the center of the image to be depicted with greater clarity.

peak of each echo. Each echo is sampled for a finite period, usually a few milliseconds, during which time it is converted to digital data by a process called *analog-to-digital conversion* (ADC) (Fig. 9-9). Each sample consists of a portion of the analog signal that is digitized and represented by a point in k-space. Remember that a point in k-space does not correspond to a specific point in physical space. However, the *number* of points along a given axis of k-space corresponds to the number of pixels along that axis of the image.

This number can be increased to increase the spatial resolution of the MR image by spending more time sampling the echo (Fig. 9-10). Each echo can be sampled for a longer time during a similar gradient application (e.g., 8 msec rather than 4 msec per echo). This increases the *number of samples* per echo. Although it does not increase the *number of echoes* that must be sampled, the sampling of each echo takes longer. This increases the echo time (TE) if the echo is sampled at the same rate (Fig. 9-11). Alternatively, rather than sampling longer, it is possible to increase the number of samples obtained during a given sampling time by sampling faster (Fig. 9-12).

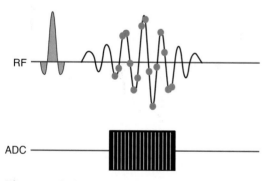

Figure 9-9
The echo is sampled for analog-to-digital conversion (ADC). In this example, 16 samples are indicated by *gray circles* in the radiofrequency (RF) signal and by *white vertical lines* in the ADC. This situation would lead to a frequency-encoding resolution of 16.

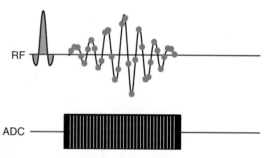

Figure 9-10
The echo is sampled for ADC at the same rate as in Figure 9-8 but for twice as long, obtaining data for a frequency-encoding resolution of 32. RF, radiofrequency.

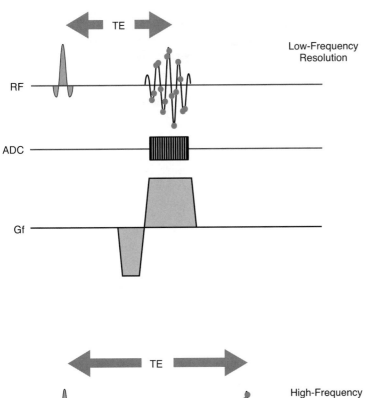

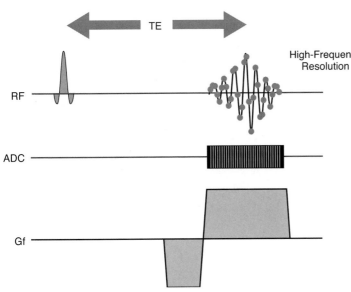

Figure 9-11
Doubling the number of samples per echo from 16 *(top)* to 32 *(bottom)* without changing the sampling rate doubles the frequency-encoding resolution and doubles the sampling time. The longer application of the frequency-encoding gradient (Gf) allows longer sampling of the echo, including more data from the tails. This increases the echo time (TE). ADC, analog-to-digital conversion; RF, radiofrequency.

Sampling Rate (Bandwidth)

The rate at which an echo is sampled is referred to as the *sampling bandwidth,* or sampling rate. As the sampling bandwidth (rate) decreases, the sampling time increases for a fixed number of points along the readout axis (Fig. 9-13) if the frequency-encoding resolution is not changed. In a simplified example, an MR image with a resolution of 256 in the frequency-encoding axis requires 256 samples of each echo. If the entire echo is sampled at a rate of 32 kHz (32,000 samples per second), 8 msec is

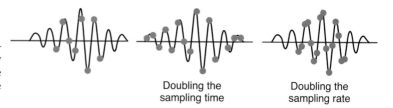

Figure 9-12
Data acquisition in the frequency-encoding axis can be increased by doubling the sampling time or the sampling rate. Each sample of the wave is indicated by a *gray dot*.

Doubling the
sampling time

Doubling the
sampling rate

needed to digitize the 256 samples. If the sampling bandwidth is reduced to 16 kHz, 16 msec is needed.

A reduced sampling bandwidth results in less sampling of high-frequency noise, which is excluded from the sampling range when the bandwidth is decreased (Fig. 9-14). The decreased noise sampled potentially improves the SNR proportional to the square root of the change in sampling time.

The SNR of tissues with a short T2 relaxation time may not be increased by the use of the low-bandwidth technique. If the T2 relaxation time is comparable to or shorter than the sampling time, it may not be possible to detect additional signal by sampling longer, as the signal may decay markedly during sampling (Fig. 9-15). For this reason, images of tissues with short T2 relaxation times (e.g., muscle) may show blurring and a decreased SNR when they are acquired using long sampling times (reduced sampling bandwidth).

Sampling Bandwidth, Gradient Strength, Field of View, Resolution

Sampling bandwidth, gradient strength, FOV, and spatial resolution are closely related. In this section we consider these interrelationships, discussing the effects of changing one factor while holding the others constant. The interrelationships can be understood best by remembering how the frequency-encoding gradient encodes position and determines the location of data in k-space.

To maintain a constant FOV and pixel size in an image, changes in the sampling

bandwidth must be complemented by proportional changes in frequency-encoding gradient strength (Fig. 9-14). This is because the location in k-space (spatial resolution) is proportional to the product of the gradient amplitude and time: the "area" of the gradient. For example, if the sampling bandwidth is reduced by half, the gradient strength must also be reduced by half and the gradient duration (sampling time) doubled; these changes compensate for each other, so the

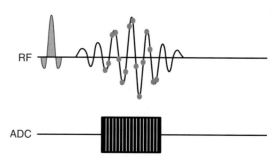

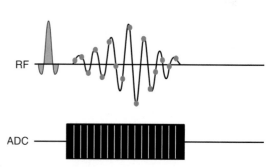

Figure 9-13
Relationship between the rate and duration of echo sampling. The same number of samples are obtained for ADC at *top* and *bottom*. The sampling rate at the top is twice as rapid, so sampling takes half as long. RF, radiofrequency.

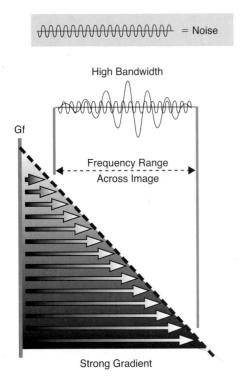

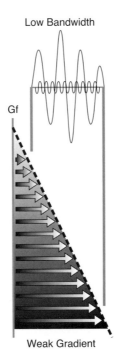

Figure 9-14

For a given FOV the frequency range across the frequency-encoding axis of an image is greater with a high sampling bandwidth than with a low one. Thus, the frequency-encoding gradient (Gf) is weaker for low bandwidth techniques. Less noise is sampled with the low bandwidth technique, so the SNR is higher.

area of the gradient, and therefore the coverage in k-space, is not changed.

Spatial resolution can be increased by keeping constant the number of *locations* along the frequency-encoding gradient while increasing the *strength* of that gradient. This reduces the FOV, thereby reducing the pixel size and increasing resolution. Let us consider why increasing the gradient strength reduces the FOV. Use of a stronger frequency-encoding gradient increases the differences in frequency between two particular points and decreases the physical distance between two particular resonant frequencies. With a stronger frequency-encoding gradient, small distances can be resolved better because they correspond to greater differences in frequency. Therefore, the spatial resolution improves as the gradient strength increases. If the number of samples remains constant, increasing the gradient strength results in a smaller image FOV.

The FOV can be reduced also by changing the sampling bandwidth, even if the gradient strength does not change though the gradient must be left on for a longer time. If the gradient strength remains unchanged while the sampling bandwidth is reduced, the FOV and pixel size are reduced by a proportional amount. Thus, reducing the bandwidth can reduce the pixel size (increasing the spatial resolution) without increasing the gradient strength. If the FOV and bandwidth are both reduced, the bandwidth per pixel (the frequency difference between pixels) does not change. For many applications, changes in the FOV correspond to proportional changes in bandwidth, so a high bandwidth is generally associated with a large FOV and vice versa.

Artifacts Associated with Reduced Bandwidth

For many applications, the major disadvantage of a reduced sampling bandwidth is the increased time needed for sampling each echo. It causes significant increases in echo

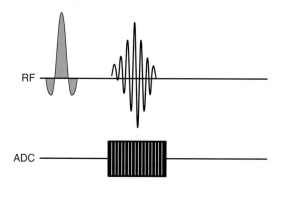

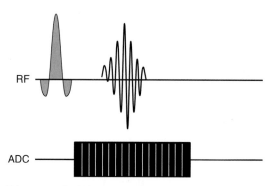

Figure 9-15

The sampling bandwidth (sampling rate) at the *bottom* is half that at the *top*, doubling the sampling time. Much of this sampling occurs during the tails of the echo, where the signal is negligible.

time (TE) (Fig. 9-10), which can introduce unwanted T2 or T2* contrast into an otherwise T1-weighted image (T2* contrast is discussed in Chapter 4). Additionally, greater image degradation from physiological motion or decay of signal can occur during the longer TE. An increased sampling time usually leads to increased acquisition time or a decreased number of image slices at a given TR (Fig. 9-17). Note also, as discussed in Chapter 7, that if the readout is made long compared to T2* the images are degraded by blurring.

Increased chemical shift misregistration artifact is another disadvantage of a reduced sampling bandwidth. The frequency (chemical shift) difference between water and methylene (CH_2) protons is constant at a given field strength, unchanged by variations in the sampling bandwidth. However, because weaker frequency-encoding gradients are used when the sampling bandwidth is reduced, the difference in frequency from one *pixel* to the next is reduced. A given chemical shift difference thus causes a shift of more pixels when the sampling bandwidth is reduced (Fig. 9-18).

As an example, the chemical shift between water and CH_2 protons at 1.5 T is approximately 225 Hz. If 256 frequency-encoding steps are used with a sampling bandwidth of 32 kHz, the chemical shift misregistration is approximately 2 pixels (32,000 Hz/256 pixels = 125 Hz/pixel; 2 pixels = 250 Hz). If the sampling bandwidth is reduced to 16 kHz, each pixel represents 62.5 Hz, so the chemical shift of 225 Hz represents about 4 pixels. If the sampling bandwidth is reduced by half, the chemical shift misregistration is doubled (Figs. 9-18 and 9-19).

Chemical shift artifact and, to a certain extent, motion artifact become more severe as the field strength is increased. However, the signal strength overall is greater at higher field strength. An SNR similar to that of high field strength can be achieved at low field strength by reducing the bandwidth. However, the increased SNR resulting from the reduced bandwidth is accompanied by exacerbated chemical shift misregistration, motion, and susceptibility artifacts. Thus, using a reduced sampling bandwidth has been referred to as a form of "magnetic field strength compensation," rendering the SNR and artifacts at low field strength more similar to those seen at high field strength. This tradeoff still usually favors the high field strength system. Specifically, the signal strength is directly proportional to field strength, whereas the SNR increases only as the square root of the bandwidth reduction. Additionally, the use of a lower bandwidth requires slower sampling, which increases the TE and acquisition times.

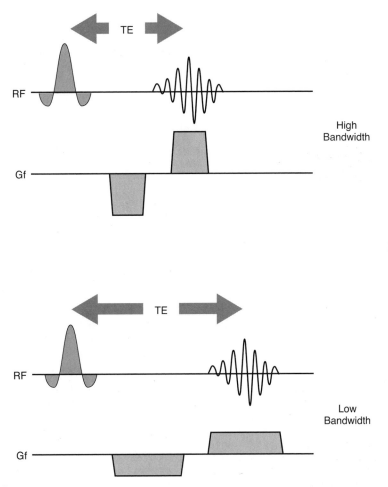

Figure 9-16
The use of a low bandwidth (*bottom*) requires a longer sampling time and therefore a longer TE.

Table 9-2 summarizes the general effects of individual parameter changes on the SNR, assuming all other parameters are held constant.

Simple Equation for the SNR

To summarize some of the major determinants of the SNR, we conclude with this simple equation:

$$\text{SNR} = K \times B_0 \times \text{voxel volume} \times \sqrt{\text{sampling time}} \quad (1)$$

Translation: The SNR is proportional to the volume of tissue in each voxel and to the square root of the time spent sampling the data. The factor B_0 represents the field strength. Doubling the field strength, on its own, approximately doubles the SNR. The proportionality term, K, includes the pulse sequence effects of TR, TE, flip angle, T1, T2, and so on.

The other terms, voxel volume and sampling time, are also computed easily.

$$\text{Voxel volume} = \frac{\text{Slice thickness} \times \text{FOV}}{\text{Nx} \times \text{Ny}}$$

$$(2)$$

$$\text{Sampling time} = \frac{N_{\text{phase}} \times \text{NSA}}{\text{bandwidth}}$$

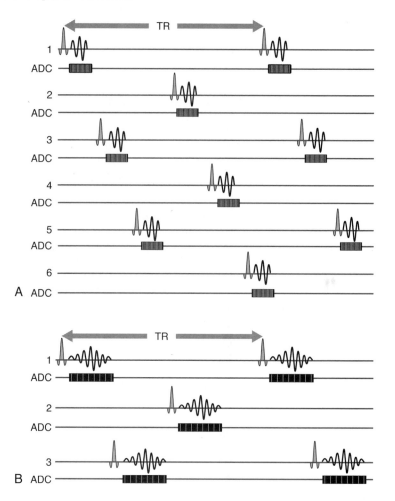

Figure 9-17
Compared to a high sampling bandwidth *(A)* a low sampling bandwidth *(B)* involves slow sampling and long TE, resulting in a longer time between excitations of different image sections. Therefore, with a low sampling bandwidth, fewer image sections can be obtained at a given TR.

Translation: The voxel volume depends on the slice thickness and field of view, and it becomes smaller as the numbers of pixels in x (Nx) and y (Ny) are increased. The sampling time is the product of the number of phase-encoding lines and the number of averages per line (NSA) divided by the bandwidth.

Cutting the bandwidth by a factor of two, for example, doubles the sampling time and therefore increases the SNR by about 1.4 (square root of 2). Likewise, doubling the NSA (e.g., averaging two data collections instead of using only one) doubles the sampling time and improves the SNR by a factor of the square root of 2.

A more complex example of the relationship between spatial resolution, SNR, and acquisition time involves increasing the spatial resolution by doubling the number of phase-encoding lines. This is accomplished by doubling the number of phase-encoding views obtained. According to equation 2, this involves reducing each voxel size by half as well as doubling the total number of echoes obtained, which in turn doubles the sampling time. According to equation 1, doubling the sampling time increases the SNR by the square root of 2. However, doubling the number of phase-encoding views also involves reducing the voxel volume (V) by half; according to equation 1, this *reduces*

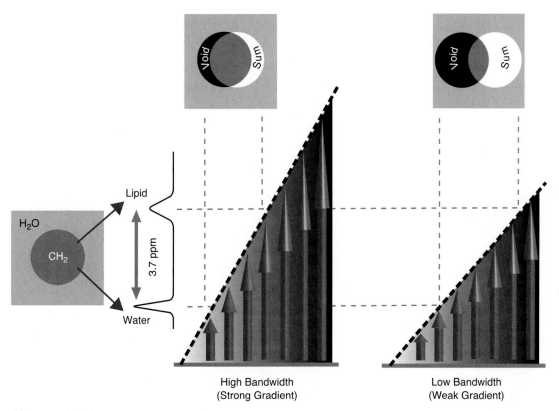

High Bandwidth
(Strong Gradient)

Low Bandwidth
(Weak Gradient)

Figure 9-18
The frequency difference between lipid and water corresponds to a shorter distance along a strong frequency-encoded gradient (Gf) (high bandwidth, *left*) than it does along a weak frequency-encoded gradient (low bandwidth, *right*). Therefore, the misregistration on an image obtained with low bandwidth (*right*) corresponds to a greater portion of the image than it does with high bandwidth (*left*).

Table 9-2 ■ SUMMARY OF THE EFFECTS FOR VARIOUS PULSE SEQUENCES

Pulse Sequence Parameter Change	Effect on SNR
Increased slice thickness	↑
Increased total field-of-view	↑
Reduced (rectangular) phase field-of-view	↓
Increased TR	↑
Increased TE	↓
Increased frequency resolution	↓
Increased phase resolution	↓
Partial Fourier technique	↓
Fractional echo sampling	↓
Increased signal averaging	↑
Increased magnetic field strength	↑
Increased sampling bandwidth	↓
Use of local receiver coil	↑

SNR, signal-to-noise ratio.

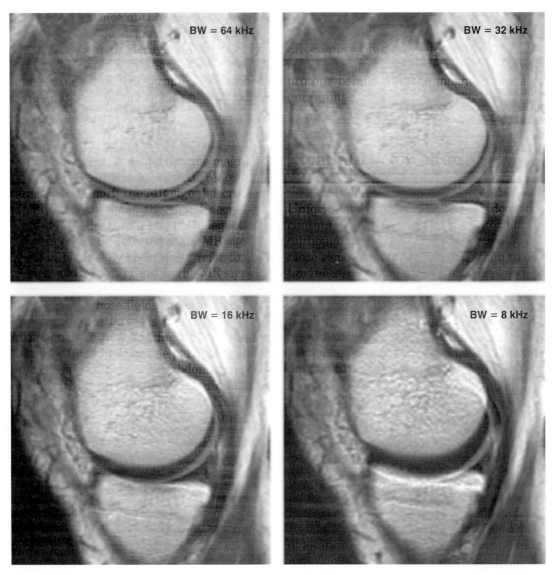

Figure 9-19
As the sampling bandwidth (BW) is decreased from 64 kHz to 8 kHz, the SNR improves. However, the images are increasingly degraded by severe chemical shift misregistration artifact along the frequency-encoding (superoinferior) axis, obscuring intraarticular anatomy.

the SNR by a factor of 2. These two effects combined reduce the SNR by $\sqrt{2}$ ($2 \times \sqrt{2} = \sqrt{2}$), or 1.4. Thus, improving resolution in the phase-encoding axis by doubling the number of phase-encoding views reduces SNR by a factor of 1.4, even though more data have been obtained. Additionally, according to equation 1, doubling the number of echoes doubled the acquisition time. This example demonstrates that spatial resolution in MRI can be quite "expensive" in terms of both SNR and acquisition time. (Acquisition time is explored further in Chapter 10.)

▼

Essential Points to Remember

1. The SNR, spatial resolution, and acquisition time are image attributes that compete with each other; efforts to improve one of these features usually worsen the other two.

2. Decreasing the voxel size by decreasing the FOV improves spatial resolution but decreases the SNR.

3. Increasing the number of voxels by increasing the matrix improves spatial resolution, decreases the SNR, and increases the acquisition time.

4. Obtaining multiple signal averages increases the SNR and acquisition time.

5. If the FOV is held constant, increasing the sampling bandwidth requires a stronger frequency-encoding gradient.

6. Increasing the sampling bandwidth decreases the SNR.

7. Advantages of an increased sampling bandwidth include faster data acquisition, reduced blurring of tissues with short T2 relaxation times, and reduced artifacts due to chemical shift misregistration, magnetic field heterogeneity, and motion.

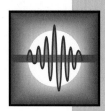

Chapter 10

Acquisition Time Reconsidered

If there is a single most important "currency" for tradeoffs between pulse sequence considerations, it is the acquisition time. Measures that increase spatial resolution or the signal-to-noise ratio (SNR) usually increase the acquisition time. Acquisition time limits the ability of magnetic resonance imaging (MRI) to depict, or resist, artifacts related to physiological events and administration of contrast media. Finally, a long acquisition time has significant adverse effects on patient tolerance and patient "throughput." The costs of a long acquisition time include suboptimal resolution, the SNR, control of artifacts, and the financial viability of an MRI center. Each radio pulse and each application of an imaging gradient, plus any necessary or unnecessary delays between them, take time. Whenever efforts to increase spatial resolution and the SNR prolong signal sampling or require sampling of more signals, the acquisition time increases.

Relationship to Spatial Resolution

Acquisition time is determined by the repetition time (TR) and the total number of signals sampled. Acquisition time is not affected by spatial resolution in the frequency-encoding axis when the TR remains constant; however, increasing the spatial resolution in the frequency-encoding axis often increases the duration of signal sampling, which increases the TE. An increased TE allows less time for exciting image slices. Thus, when all other acquisition parameters are unchanged, increasing the spatial resolution in the frequency axis decreases the number of slices that can be imaged during a given TR for two-dimensional (2D) multislice techniques. This is illustrated in a comparison of Figures 10-1 and 10-2. For a 2D single-slice technique or three-dimensional (3D)

117

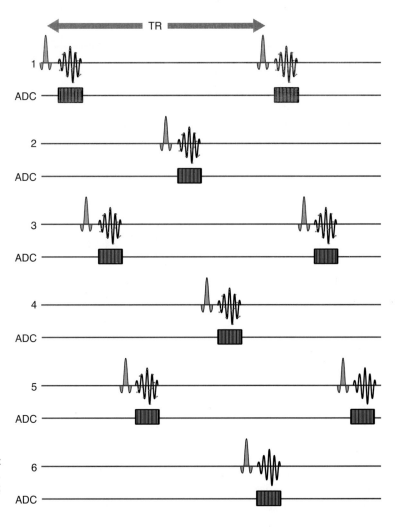

Figure 10-1
Multislice acquisition of six slices at 16 samples per echo. ADC, analog-to-digital conversion; TR, repetition time.

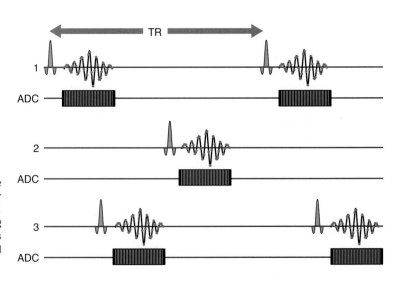

Figure 10-2
Multislice acquisition of three slices, obtaining 32 samples per echo. Compared with Figure 10-1 the duration of echo sampling has increased, which allows less time for obtaining additional slices during the TR.

techniques, the increased TE leads to slightly increased TR.

More 2D multislice images per TR can be obtained if the TE is reduced. Methods for reducing the TE include faster sampling of each echo and obtaining fewer samples per echo. Signals can be sampled faster using a larger sampling bandwidth, but this reduces the SNR. The number of samples obtained per signal can be decreased, but it decreases resolution in the frequency-encoding axis.

The effect of image slice thickness on the acquisition time of a 2D multislice pulse sequence is analogous to the effect of TE. Neither slice thickness nor TE directly affects the acquisition time when the TR is constant; however, both variables affect coverage in the slice-select axis. If slice thickness is reduced, more image slices are needed to cover the anatomy of interest, which requires either a longer TR or additional pulse sequence acquisitions.

The 3D technique is generally the most efficient for acquiring multiple images during a given period of time. Data acquisition can be continuous, with little, if any, dead time. Additionally, zero filling in the slice direction can be used to generate additional "overlapping" images. Although the TR values are usually small for 3D acquisitions, the fact that each echo contributes a signal to every image contributes to improving the SNR relative to comparable 2D techniques.

Relationship to k-Space

Each echo provides data for one horizontal line of k-space. Additional lines are obtained by repeating the acquisition using a different value for the phase-encoding gradient (Gp). The number of lines along the phase-encoding axis of k-space determines the number of pixels along the phase-encoding axis of the MR image. Each line of k-space and each MR signal requires additional time. Thus, reducing the spatial resolution

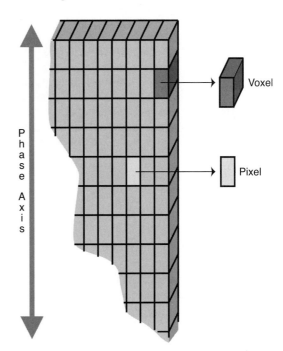

Figure 10-3
Representation of anisotropic pixel size, with reduced spatial resolution during the phase axis. If all other parameters are unchanged, the acquisition time would be half that of the image slice represented in Figure 10-1.

along the phase-encoding axis generally reduces the image acquisition time. The voxel matrix in such an image is illustrated in Figure 10-3, and the corresponding map of k-space is shown in Figure 10-4.

It is possible to reduce the acquisition time without changing the voxel dimensions by taking advantage of the special symmetry of k-space. For example, slightly more than half of the phase-encoding lines of k-space can be sampled, and the remaining phase-encoding values can be interpolated by filling them in with the complex conjugate of the sampled points, taking advantage of the symmetry of k-space. Phase artifacts are avoided by phase-correcting the entire data set based on sampling near the center of k-space. This method involves acquiring less than a single full acquisition for Fourier transformation, so it is referred to as a *partial Fourier technique* (Fig. 10-5).

Phase

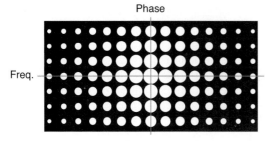

Freq.

Figure 10-4
A k-space representation of the image slice depicted in Figure 10-3.

Phase

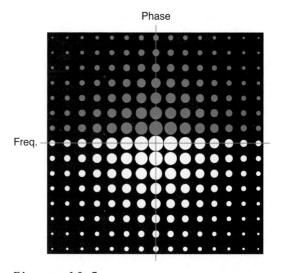

Freq.

Figure 10-5
A k-space representation of a partial Fourier image. Nearly half of the k-space is not sampled *(gray)* but is extrapolated on the basis of symmetry with the other half. The acquisition time is only slightly longer than that for Figure 10-4, although pixels are smaller and symmetrical.

Alternatively, slightly more than half of each signal may be sampled for analog-to-digital conversion (ADC). With this method, only part of k-space in the frequency-encoding axis is sampled directly, the remainder being interpolated. This method, referred to as *fractional echo sampling*, allows the use of a shorter TE (Figs. 10-6 and 10-7).

Some MRI techniques (e.g., echo planar, fast spin echo) involve creating images from more than one echo per excitation. Each echo is used to fill a line of k-space. The number of echoes acquired per excitation radio pulse is referred to as the *echo train*. For example, a pulse sequence that involves acquisition of four echoes and four lines of k-space after each excitation pulse is considered to have an echo train of 4. At a given TR and number of signals averaged, the total acquisition time is reduced by a factor of the echo train. For example, if the TR and averaging are held constant, the use of an echo train of 4 would reduce the acquisition time to one fourth that required for a single echo technique. Multiecho techniques are described in further detail in Chapter 13.

Relationship to Signal-to-Noise Ratio

The simplest method to increase the SNR is to obtain redundant additional data. The impact of random errors (noise) on a

measurement (signal) can be reduced by averaging two or more measurements. The signal intensity of a given pixel may be increased slightly by noise during one measurement and decreased slightly during another; averaging multiple signals reduces the impact of random noise on each pixel and on the image as a whole. For MRI this involves acquiring two or more signals, rather than only one, for each value of the phase-encoding gradient. This practice multiplies the image acquisition time by the number of averages. The number of signals sampled for each value of the phase-encoding gradient is generally referred to as the *number of signals averaged (NSA)* or the *number of excitations (NEX)*.

If two signals are obtained and added, the signal component of the SNR is doubled. Noise also increases but to a lesser extent; noise increases by the square root of the NSA because noise is random. Thus, doubling the NSA increases the SNR by $\sqrt{2}$, approximately 1.4. Therefore, the SNR can be improved by a factor of about 1.4 by doubling the image acquisition time.

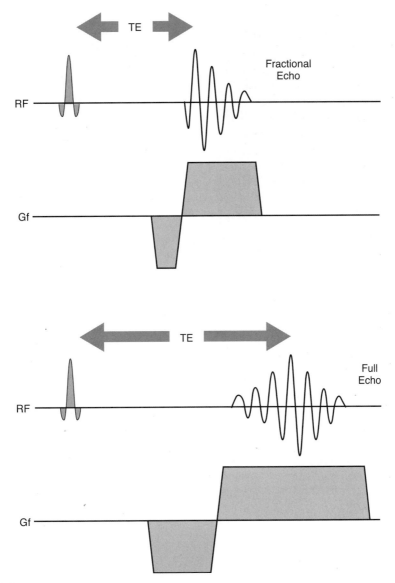

Figure 10-6
With fractional echo sampling (*top*), principally the latter portion of the echo is sampled. The peak of the echo can thus be sampled sooner than if the full echo were to be sampled (*bottom*), resulting in a shorter TE.

Simple Equation for Acquisition Time

Acquisition time = TR × Np × NSA/ETL (1)

where TR is the repetition time; Np is the number of phase-encoding views; NSA is the number of signals averaged; and ETL is the echo train length.

Translation. The acquisition time of a pulse sequence is determined by the time between excitations (TR) multiplied by the number of excitations. The number of excitations, in turn, is determined by the number of phase-encoding views (Np) and

Phase

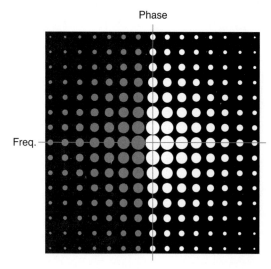

Freq.

Figure 10-7

A k-space representation of fractional echo sampling. Nearly half of the k-space (*gray*) is not filled directly, corresponding to the fraction of the echo that is not sampled. These k-space values are extrapolated based on symmetry with the other half. The resulting image slice has spatial resolution comparable to that of Figure 10-1, although the SNR is lower (fewer true data) and the minimum TE is lower (shorter echo sampling).

Table 10-1 ■ EFFECT OF VARIOUS PULSE SEQUENCE PARAMETERS ON ACQUISITION TIME

Pulse Sequence Parameter Change	Effect on Acquisition Time
Increased slice thickness	Decrease
Increased total field-of-view	No direct effect
Decreased (rectangular) phase field-of-view	Decrease
Increased TR	Increase
Increased TE	Increase
Increased frequency resolution	Increase
Increased phase resolution	Increase
Partial Fourier technique	Decrease
Fractional echo sampling	Decrease
Increased signal averaging	Increase

the number of signals averaged for each phase-encoding value (NSA), divided by the number of signals per excitation (ETL).

The effect on acquisition time of various pulse sequence parameters on imaging a given volume of interest, assuming other parameters are held constant, is summarized in Table 10-1. It must be remembered that the SNR, spatial resolution, and acquisition time are closely related, and that changing one parameter often affects the SNR as well as spatial resolution. For example, increased slice thickness reduces the imaging time only if the volume of coverage is kept the same. As another example, the total field of view (FOV) does not affect the imaging time if other parameters are held constant, but the spatial resolution and SNR do change.

▼
Essential Points to Remember

1. Increasing the number of frequency-encoded samples increases the spatial resolution in this axis but usually increases the TE. This in turn increases the minimum TR for 2D single-slice or 3D techniques, or it reduces the number of image slices obtained per TR for 2D multislice techniques.

2. Obtaining multiple signal averages increases the SNR and acquisition time.

3. Acquisition time can be reduced by incomplete filling of k-space (partial Fourier technique), extrapolating the missing values based on the special symmetry of k-space.

Chapter 11

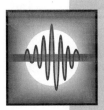

Receiver Coils

In the previous two chapters, we discussed how the signal-to-noise ratio (SNR) can be affected by changing the voxel size, image acquisition time, or sampling bandwidth (or a combination of these factors). Each of these changes involves making carefully considered tradeoffs between the SNR and other attributes of magnetic resonance (MR) image quality or acquisition time. None of these tradeoffs can be considered a "free lunch."

It is possible, however, to increase the SNR without increasing the voxel size or the acquisition time by using a local radio receiver coil configured better for a specific region of interest. In broadcast radio, we are usually interested in sensing signals at great and variable distances from the antenna. With magnetic resonance imaging (MRI), however, we are interested only in signals that arise within centimeters of the antenna. The local receiver coil is designed to detect radio waves and to transmit the

induced electrical current to the signal receiver, where the signal is processed and converted to digital data (Fig. 11-1). Most early local coils were flat receiver coils that were placed on the surface of the body part of interest. For this reason, local coils are often referred to as *surface coils*. Many local coils have been designed, however, to image deep structures optimally. This is accomplished by completely encircling the body part of interest or even inserting a local coil into a body cavity. Because of the wide range of specialized configurations that can be used, a more generic term, such as *local coils*, is more suitable.

There is a tendency to consider the use of local coils as a way of decreasing the image field of view (FOV) and thereby improving spatial resolution. Although local coils are often used as a component of a strategy for obtaining high-resolution images, the use of the local coil does not by itself directly affect voxel size. Voxel size is instead controlled

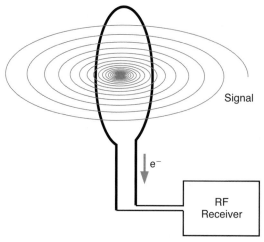

Figure 11-1

Simple loop radiofrequency (RF) coil for reception of magnetic resonance (MR) signals. The received radio signal induces electrical currents that are transmitted to the RF receiver.

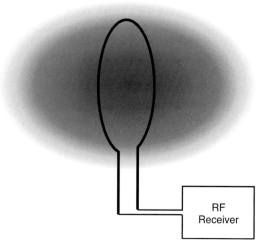

Figure 11-2

Sensitivity range of a simple loop coil. *Lighter shades of gray* distant from the coil indicate decreased sensitivity to MR signals.

by system sequence parameters, such as gradient amplitude. Local receiver coils, however, make smaller voxels practical, as they increase the SNR so a small voxel size can be sustained with reasonable signal levels.

One of the principal obstacles to improving the spatial resolution of MR images is its limited SNR. By definition, improving the spatial resolution involves reducing the voxel size, which in turn decreases the SNR. The major reason to use local coils is to improve the SNR for the region of interest. This increased SNR, in turn, allows the magnetic resonance operator to decrease the FOV, increase the image matrix without generating unacceptably noisy images, or both without generating unacceptable noisy images.

The importance of changes in the local receiver coil can be appreciated best by first reviewing some basic principles of MR signals and local receiver coils. The MR signal is strongest from tissue closest to the MR receiver coil (Fig. 11-2). Thus, a local coil is designed to be placed as close as possible to the region of interest. Larger local coils are sensitive to radio signals arising from a greater distance, so the diameter of a local coil must be increased to detect MR signals arising from deep tissues.

System noise and motion-induced noise in an image are present in all MR signals detected by the local coil and transmitted to the receiver. Thus, detection of MR signals from a larger region of interest results in more noise (Fig. 11-3).

An optimal SNR involves matching the size and shape of the local coil as closely as possible to the anatomy of interest. If the coil is too small, the signal is weak at the edges of the region of interest. If the coil is larger than the region of interest, noise is detected from tissue outside that volume. In other words, the SNR is less than optimal if the local receiver coil is fitted to a region larger or smaller than the region of interest.

The following two equations may be helpful for understanding the role of receiver coils and other parameters in influencing signal and noise.

$$\frac{\text{Signal}}{\text{Voxel}} = f(\text{T1, T2})(\text{coil-filling factor})(\text{voxel volume})(B_0) \quad (1)$$

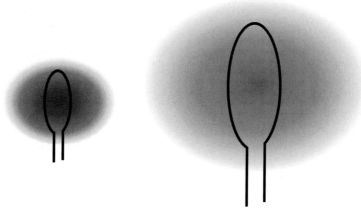

Figure 11-3
Sensitivity profiles of small- and large-loop RF coils. Sensitivity is greatest near the small coil, depicted as *dark shades of gray*. The larger coil has a lower signal-to-noise ratio (SNR), but its range extends over a larger volume.

Translation: The signal in each voxel depends on contrast factors such as T1 and T2, on the field strength (B_0), and on the size of the voxel (as the voxel volume increases, the signal increases). The *coil-filling factor* refers to the proximity of the signal sources to the radiofrequency (RF) receiver coil; f(T1, T2) is a function of T1 and T2.

$$\frac{\text{Noise}}{\text{Voxel}} = \frac{k(\text{coilfield of view})\sqrt{\text{bandwidth}}}{\sqrt{\text{total read out time}}} \quad (2)$$

Translation: The noise per voxel increases as the square root of the bandwidth and decreases with the square root of the readout (sampling) time. A larger coil detects noise over a larger region; k is a constant.

Transmit/Receive Coils

There are a few basic categories of local coils that can be used in appropriate situations. A single coil or coil array can be used for both transmitting the excitation and refocusing radio pulses and for receiving the MR signals. This involves switching the mode of the coil from transmission to reception, a procedure similar to the switching that occurs in sonic transducers for B-mode and pulsed Doppler ultrasonography. MR coils such as these are called *transmit/receive coils*.

Most currently used transmit/receive coils are circumferential (volume) coils used for body, head, or extremity imaging (Fig. 11-4). These coils are ideally suited for imaging entire objects or body parts they can encircle completely. One particular advantage of circumferential transmit/receive coils is the pleasing uniformity of signal intensity across the resulting MR images. Flat (surface) transmit/receive coils have been unsatisfactory for most clinical applications because the resulting signal intensity profile has a banded appearance that results from the variation in excitation flip angle.

Receive-Only Coils

Most successful flat or curved surface coils are receive-only coils. When such coils are

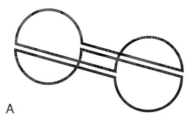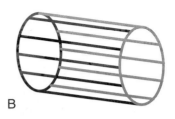

Figure 11-4
Two common geometries for transmit-receive volume coils: a saddle-shaped coil (*A*) and a birdcage coil (*B*).

A　　　　　　　　**B**

used, a separate coil is needed to transmit the excitation and refocusing radio pulses. In most current magnetic resonance imaging (MRI) units, the built-in "body coil" is used to transmit radio pulses, and the MR unit is set to receive signals from a local coil rather than from the built-in coil. Receive-only coils are ideal for superficial structures, but the signal intensity profile of images acquired when using these coils tends to be nonuniform unless images are acquired parallel to the plane of the coil. Uniformity perpendicular to the coil can be improved somewhat by using a curved, rather than flat, coil; but fall-off of signal intensity with greater distance from the coil is unavoidable. Software algorithms can also improve image intensity homogeneity, but some of them also reduce image contrast. Even if the intensity profile across an image is corrected, the SNR remains nonuniform, so that deep structures appear grainy.

Quadrature (Circularly Polarized) Coils

Quadrature coils are usually transmit/receive coils. This coil design transmits a radio pulse whose magnetization rotates in a full circle with the proton spins. (Standard "linearly polarized" coils along one axis do not. The radiofrequency (RF) pulse is varied only along one axis.) The advantages of a quadrature coil include a large reduction

in RF power deposition (because more of the RF energy is used for rotating the spins) and increased SNR (because the rotating transverse magnetization from the spins is measured around a full circle as it precesses). The increased SNR varies depending on the shape of the body part, but it can be as much as 40%.

Intracavity Coils

Optimizing the SNR for deep tissues has presented an enduring challenge to MR users and designers of MR equipment. One creative approach for imaging small structures deep within the body is to place a small receive-only surface coil in a body cavity on or near the surface of the structure of interest. Thus far, the most commonly used intracavitary coils have been intrarectal, for imaging the prostate gland, cervix, or rectal mucosa (Fig. 11-5). Intracavitary coils have also been investigated for use in the vagina, esophagus, and blood vessels.

Multicoil Arrays

The greatest challenge in coil design has been to maximize the SNR for a large region of interest. One approach is to optimize the size and design of a transmit/receive coil. This has

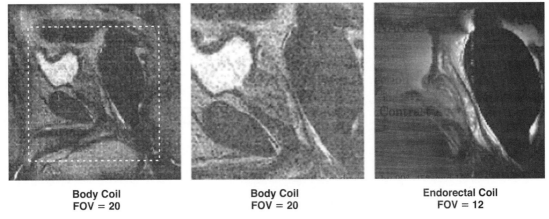

Body Coil
FOV = 20

Body Coil
FOV = 20

Endorectal Coil
FOV = 12

Figure 11-5

Sagittal fast spin echo T2-weighted images of the prostate, comparing the body coil and endorectal coil techniques. The body coil image was acquired with field of view (FOV) of 20 cm and magnified in the center image to correspond anatomically with the endorectal coil image, which was acquired with FOV of 12 cm. Tissue near the prostate has a higher SNR with the endorectal coil, even though the smaller FOV has resulted in smaller voxels. The SNR decreases with increasing distance from the endorectal coil.

been implemented most successfully for imaging the head and extremities. Because of the wide variety of body sizes and shapes, however, it has been far more difficult to image the pelvis, abdomen, and chest.

Another approach to increasing the SNR for large structures has been to combine two coils, typically placed parallel to each other and on either side of the body part of interest. This coil configuration is sometimes referred to as a *Helmholtz coil.* The MR signals detected by both components of this composite coil are processed together by one receiver. In effect, the two individual coil components are combined to produce a single large local coil that is sensitive to deep tissues at the expense of somewhat increased noise for depiction of superficial structures. In other words, a compromise is made relative to the use of a single surface coil that involves an improved SNR for deep structures and a decreased SNR for superficial structures. Compared to a standard transmit/receive body coil, SNR is typically improved for thin patients and is comparable for large patients; however, the signal intensity across the image is usually far less uniform than that obtained from conventional circumferential transmit/receive coils (Fig. 11-6). With multicoil arrays such as these, results are usually best when the separate coil elements are within one coil diameter's distance of one another.

Images acquired with multicoil arrays can be much improved if the signals detected by each of two or more coil components are processed separately by independent radio receivers. In this case, the processing can be arranged such that the noise contributions from each coil individually are not added. Separate sets of raw data are generated for each local FOV and are then combined in the final stages of image reconstruction. Each set of raw data reflects the SNR of one local coil. Thus, the added anatomical coverage provided by the coil array is not obtained at the expense of additional system noise. Multicoil arrays such as these are commonly referred to as *phased-array coils* (Figs. 11-7 and 11-8).

Currently, most phased-array coils are composed of four or more components, each transmitting detected signals to separate receivers. Phased-array coils with more

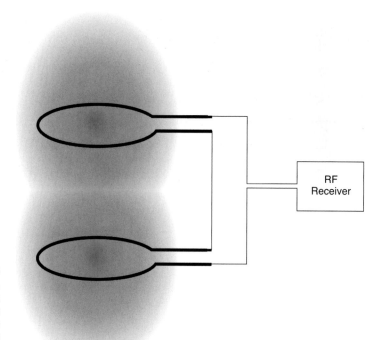

Figure 11-6
Helmholtz-type paired coil. Two paired loop coils detect signals, which are processed together by a single receiver. The effective size of the coil has been increased, so the volume of coil sensitivity has increased at the expense of the SNR near the coil.

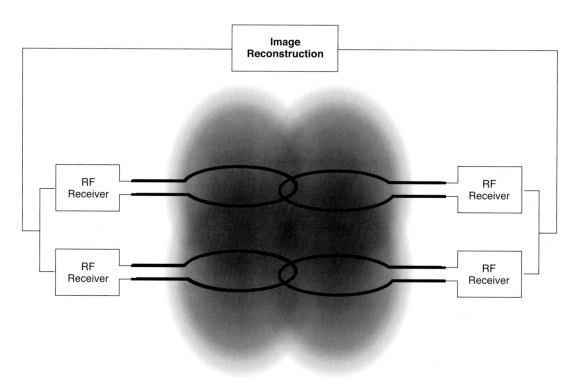

Figure 11-7
Four-element phased-array coil. Each coil detects signals, which are processed separately by four radiofrequency (RF) receivers. Images are reconstructed by combining data from each receiver. The SNR near each element is not diminished as it was with the Helmholtz-type coil depicted in Figure 11-6.

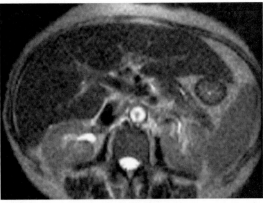

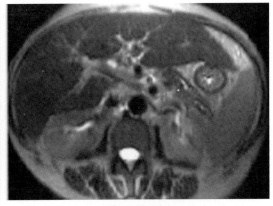

Body Coil   Phased Array

Figure 11-8
Comparison of single-shot fast spin echo images acquired using a standard-volume body coil (*left*) and a four-element multicoil phased-array coil (*right*).

elements are becoming more widely used, however, to allow more flexible use of parallel imaging techniques (see Chapter 17). Each component coil can be linear or quadrature, although the relative orientations of the coils must be optimized for successful implementation of the quadrature design. Like Helmholtz coils, phased-array multicoils may be more useful for thin body parts than for thick ones (Fig. 11-9). One significant disadvantage of a phased-array coil compared with a single circumferential transmit/receive coil is that signal intensity may be less uniform across the image. Generally, signal intensity is much greater at the surface of the coil than in deep tissues. An artifact originating from the motion of a structure near a coil can produce intense ghosts that degrade the entire image (Fig. 11-10). This problem, however, is not fundamental to the technology; and as processing algorithms improve, it should become a minor issue.

Nonuniformity of images acquired using phased-array coils can be reduced by image intensity correction software. One form of image correction involves reducing intensity differences between neighboring regions of pixels, although this may have the undesired result of reducing image contrast (Fig. 11-11). Another method involves measuring the intensity profile of the coil and using the resulting map to correct the image. With either correction technique the SNR within the imaging volume is not uniform with phased-array coils. Therefore, the conspicuity of lesions may not be uniform, so lesions deep in the body may be detected less frequently.

Another disadvantage of phased-array coils is the high cost associated with the need for two or more sets of radio receivers and signal-processing hardware rather than the single set needed for other coils. Additionally, the number of signals that must be detected per unit of time and incorporated for image reconstruction increases in proportion to the number of radio receivers used. For example, a four-coil phased-array setup involves processing four times as much data. Additional system memory may be necessary, and image reconstruction typically takes four times as much time. Once an MRI unit is equipped with the phased-array capability, however, the price of additional coils should not be much more than the price of new conventional coils.

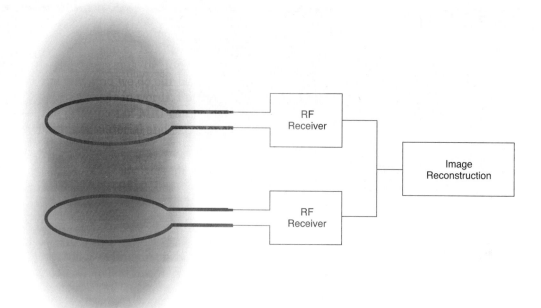

A

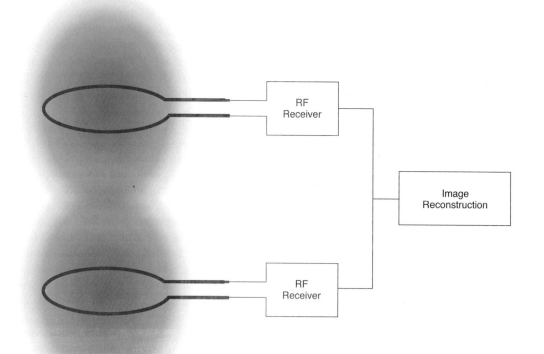

B

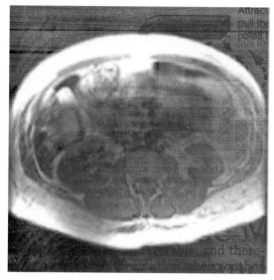
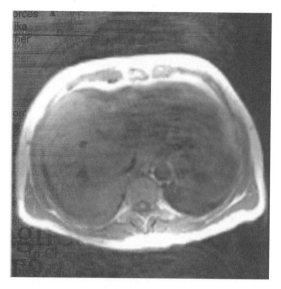

Figure 11-10

Image degradation due to anterior abdominal wall motion exacerbated by the use of a phased-array coil. T1-weighted spin echo 413/11 axial images acquired during respiration show high signal intensity of adipose tissue near the anterior and posterior components of the phased-array coil. The resulting artifact from anterior motion has produced high signal intensity curvilinear bands throughout the image.

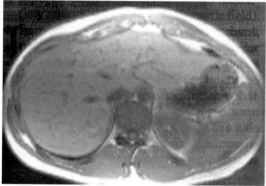
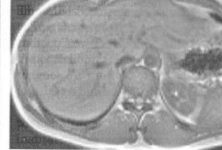

Uncorrected   **Corrected**

Figure 11-11

Image intensity correction. The T1-weighted gradient echo image (*left*) has less signal intensity in the deep tissues than it does anteriorly or posteriorly. *At right*, the image intensity correction has reduced the disparity, although tissue contrast has been degraded. Note the relative lack of contrast between the liver and the spleen in the corrected image (*right*) compared with the uncorrected image (*left*).

Figure 11-9

Effects of distance between coil elements for two-element phased-array coils. (*A*) If the distance between the two elements is small, as in thin patients or small body parts, the SNR is satisfactory throughout the volume of interest. (*B*) If the two elements are far apart, however, as in large patients or large body parts, the SNR at the center of the volume of interest may be suboptimal.

▼

Essential Points to Remember

1. Matching the size and configuration of the receiver coil with the body part of interest can increase the SNR.

2. Circumferential transmit/receive coils provide uniform signal intensity throughout most of the enclosed volume.

3. Flat or curved receive-only coils produce a high SNR for tissues close to the coil but a lower SNR for deep tissues.

4. As the radius of a receive-only coil decreases, the SNR close to the coil increases and the SNR deep to the coil decreases.

5. Optimal SNR over a large region of interest can be obtained using a multicoil array in which separate receivers process signals from each coil component (phased-array coils). This capability is expensive; and the data collection, processing, and reconstruction are complicated.

Chapter **12**

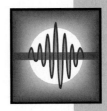

Magnetic Field Strength

In previous chapters we discussed how the signal-to-noise ratio (SNR) is affected by changes in spatial resolution, acquisition time, receiver bandwidth, and choice of receiver coils. In this chapter the influence of magnetic field strength on the SNR and other magnetic resonance (MR) characteristics are addressed.

Signal-to-Noise Ratio

As magnetic field strength increases, the imbalance in the number of protons in the parallel and antiparallel orientations increases, resulting in an increase in longitudinal magnetization. When an excitatory radiofrequency (RF) pulse is applied, it is this magnetization that is rotated into the transverse plane to become the MR signal. Therefore, the available MR signal increases

with field strength. Generally, although signal increases linearly with magnetic field strength (Figs. 12-1, 12-2, and 12-3), the SNR depends on a host of other factors, including relaxation effects and bandwidth.

It is essential, at all field strengths, to be aware of the many tradeoffs in the SNR so protocol adjustments can be made most appropriately. Voxel size, number of signal excitations, receiver bandwidth, and the receiver coil can be changed to produce noisy high-field images or crisp low-field images. Users of low magnetic field strength magnetic resonance imaging (MRI) instruments commonly increase the SNR by reducing the receiver sampling bandwidth. Conversely, users of high magnetic field strength MRI instruments may increase the receiver sampling bandwidth, which reduces many artifacts (especially chemical shift) and facilitates high-speed imaging. Therefore, the sampling bandwidth is typically lower on MRI instruments with a low magnetic field.

133

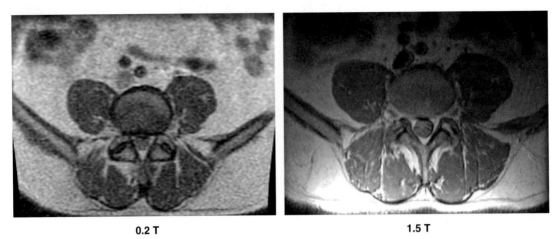

0.2 T   **1.5 T**

F i g u r e   1 2 - 1
Axial intermediate-weighted images of the lumbar spine, showing a lower signal-to-noise ratio (SNR) at 0.2 T (*left*) than at 1.5 T (*right*).

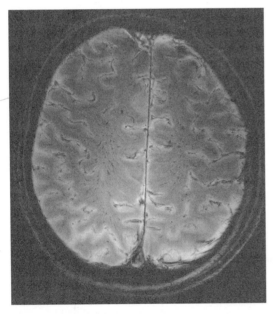

F i g u r e   1 2 - 2
A 1024 × 1024 image of the human brain acquired at 8 T. The image has high SNR despite the small pixels. (Courtesy of Allahyar Kangarlu, Ph.D., Department of Radiology, Ohio State University.)

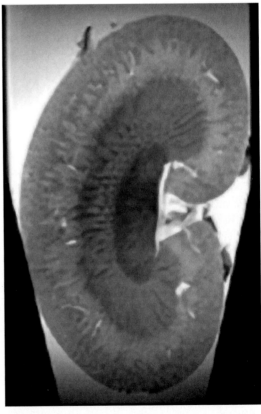

F i g u r e   1 2 - 3
Three-dimensional spoiled gradient echo image of a mouse kidney obtained at 12.0 T, with 100 × 100 × 100 μm voxels. (Courtesy of Sheng-Kwei Song, Biomedical MR Laboratory, Washington University School of Medicine.)

T1 Relaxation

The relationship of T1 to field strength is typically U-shaped (see Figure 3-7). The T1 is at its minimum when the motional energy of the spins is comparable to the energy difference between parallel and antiparallel orientations. At lower fields, the relaxation times of large molecules tend to be less than those of small ones because the motional energy is closer to the energy difference between the low- and high-spin magnetization states. At high field strengths, the difference between low- and high-energy states is larger, with the difference corresponding to the faster motion of small molecules. T1 therefore increases less for small molecules with high field strength. Temperature, which increases motional energy, has a significant effect on T1 as well, as the motion of all molecules is reduced at lower temperatures.

Unfortunately, there is no simple formula relating the T1 of any given molecule or tissue to field strength. Nevertheless, there is now considerable experience on which to rely to tabulate some of these relationships.

The effects of magnetic field strength on the T1 relaxation time are less pronounced for adipose tissue than for tissues rich in bound water. Therefore, as T1 relaxation times of most nonfatty soft tissues increase with field strength, the T1 differences between fatty and nonfatty tissues becomes more pronounced as well.

In summary, as the magnetic field strength increases, T1 relaxation times increase substantially for bound water, increase slightly for adipose tissue, and remain near constant for free water. Therefore, at high magnetic field strengths T1 contrast between free and bound water decreases, and the contrast between bound water and adipose tissue increases. Examples of T1 at 0.5 T and at 1.5 T and the ratio of the T1 values at the two field strengths are shown in Table 12-1. Table 12-2 describes the contrast between tissues at these two field strengths.

Chemical Shift

As discussed in Chapter 2, the MR frequency difference between spins caused by differences in their molecular environment is directly proportional to the main magnetic field. For example, the relative chemical shift between water and methylene (CH_2) protons, expressed as parts per million (ppm), is about 3.5, regardless of field strength. The frequency shift between water and CH_2, however, expressed as cycles per second (Hz), increases

Table 12-1 ■ REPRESENTATIVE T1 RELAXATION TIMES AT 0.5 T AND 1.5 T

Tissue	T1 at 0.5 T (msec)	T1 at 1.5 T (msec)	T1 ratio (1.5 T/0.5 T)
CSF (free water)	>4000	>4000	1.0
Skeletal muscle (bound/free water)	600	870	1.4
Gray matter (bound/free water)	656	920	1.4
Liver (bound/free water)	323	490	1.5
Adipose tissue	215	260	1.2

CSF, cerebrospinal fluid.
The T1 of cerebrospinal fluid (free water) is long and does not change appreciably with field strength in the clinical imaging range. Skeletal muscle, gray matter, and liver, rich in bound water, have significantly longer T1 values at 1.5 T. Adipose tissue also has longer T1 values at 1.5 T, but the magnitude of the change is less than that for bound water. In most cases, these trends are the same with the even higher field strengths that are coming into clinical practice.
Excerpted from the SMRI MResource Guide: 1994 edition: Wood ML, Bronskill MJ, Mulkern RV, Santyr GE: Physical MR desktop data. J Magn Reson Imaging 1993;3(Suppl):19–26.

Table 12-2 ■ T1 RATIOS AT 0.5 T AND 1.5 T BASED ON THE VALUES FROM TABLE 12-1

Tissues	T1 ratio at 0.5 T	T1 ratio at 1.5 T
CSF vs. gray matter	6.1	4.6
Skeletal muscle vs. adipose tissue	2.8	3.4
Skeletal muscle vs. liver	1.9	1.8

CSF, cerebrospinal fluid.
The relaxation rate effects favor reduced contrast between CSF and gray matter and increased contrast between skeletal muscle and adipose tissue as the field strength is increased. There is little change in the T1 ratios between skeletal muscle and liver with field strength in the standard clinical range.

with field strength. At 1.5 T protons precess at 63.86 MHz, so the MR frequency difference between water and CH_2 protons is 224 Hz.

$$63.86 \text{ MHz} \times 3.5/1{,}000{,}000 = 224 \text{ Hz}$$

At 0.3 T, the frequency difference between these protons is five times smaller than at 1.5 T, or only 48 Hz. Further both fat and water can be excited over a (narrow) range of frequencies that is only slightly dependent on field strength. Because the water and CH_2 resonances are so similar at low field strengths, it is particularly difficult to tune an excitation or saturation pulse to one peak accurately without affecting the other. For this reason, chemically selective techniques such as fat suppression or water excitation generally are not available at low field strengths. On the other hand, chemical shift misregistration artifact is proportionately lower at low field strengths.

As with techniques of chemically selective excitation, MR spectroscopy depends on the ability to distinguish among various chemical shifts. Therefore, MR spectroscopy is applied more successfully at high field strengths. As spectroscopy is typically limited by SNR, such acquisition also gain from the greater signal strength. In general,

MR spectroscopy is not implemented on MR systems with a field strength less than 1.0 T. On the other hand, the spectral line width (the range of frequencies over which the spectral signal is spread) depends inversely on the T2, which decreases slightly with field strength for many tissues. Furthermore, the susceptibility difference between tissues causes a frequency shift that is proportional to the field strength. Thus, the absolute field homogeneity is generally lower at high field strength, causing some difficulty in spectroscopic acquisitions and low bandwidth methods such as echo-planar imaging.

Choice of Field Strength

The increased MR signal available at high magnetic field provides options to increase spatial resolution, decrease the examination time, or both. Conversely, the low field strength MR user must be more concerned with maintaining an adequate SNR. Indeed, a high SNR is one of the greatest advantages of high magnetic field strength, and must be weighed against multiple disadvantages. The latter include generally higher purchase and maintenance costs, the requirement for increased radio pulse amplitudes, longer T1 relaxation times and reduced T1 contrast for some tissues, and increased sensitivity to artifacts due to chemical shift, magnetic field heterogeneity, and motion. The costs of high field strength MRI, however, can be offset by greater patient throughput and by more comprehensive examinations, whereas the potential for artifacts at high field strength can be decreased by the appropriate choice of imaging parameters and by artifact-reducing software.

Despite a steady stream of controversial reports, there simply is no optimal field strength for all applications. The best choice for a given user depends on a complex tradeoff of costs, applications, and nontechnical factors such as competitive pressures. As it becomes physically practical to engineer higher field strength instruments, there is a steady trend among research institutions to demand such devices. It would be a mistake to assume, however, that the mere availability of such scanners makes them the best choice for any given imaging center. Most importantly, users of MR—at any and all field strengths—must become familiar with the basic principles of MRI and with the methods for optimizing the diagnostic content of MR images on their equipment.

▼
Essential Points to Remember

1. The signal increases linearly with magnetic field strength, although other factors related to field strength cause the SNR benefit to be somewhat less.

2. Potential disadvantages of high magnetic field strength include higher costs, longer T1 relaxation times, and increased sensitivity to chemical shift, susceptibility, and motion artifacts.

3. Chemical shifts, such as that between water and CH_2 protons in triglycerides, are proportional to the field strength, so chemically selective techniques such as fat suppression are more successful at high field strengths.

4. MR spectroscopy is more successful at high field strengths because of the larger chemical shifts between peaks and the greater signal amplitude.

5. MR imaging parameters must be adjusted to adapt to changes in magnetic field strength. To compensate for low SNRs at low field strengths, adaptations include the use of larger pixel sizes, more averaging of signals, and lower bandwidths.

6. From a strict cost perspective, increasing the field strength may be a more expensive solution to a limited SNR than, for example, increases in the number of receiver coils or other improvements in system hardware. As field strengths beyond the current standard ranges are desired, the relative cost of high field units increases dramatically.

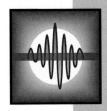

Chapter 13

Motion-Induced Artifacts

The sensitivity of magnetic resonance imaging (MRI) to motion allows the modality to be used for noninvasive depiction of blood flow and other physiological motion. This same sensitivity to motion, however, complicates the process of data acquisition and results in many artifacts in the magnetic resonance (MR) images produced.

The most successful method to avoid motion artifact is to prevent motion in the first place by having the patient suspend respiration and other voluntary motions during rapid image acquisition. Some images, however, cannot be acquired rapidly enough to allow suspended respiration; moreover, some patients cannot adequately control their movements, and cardiac-related motion cannot be suspended during image acquisition. Therefore, additional measures must be considered to limit the deleterious effects of motion on MR images.

An adequate understanding of the causes of motion artifacts allows a user to recognize these artifacts and to choose the best combination of methods to avoid them during various clinical applications. Each method of mitigating motion artifacts addresses a specific aspect of motion; no method is a "magic button" that eliminates motion artifact entirely.

There are two categories of acquisition errors that lead to motion artifacts. Errors can occur during the acquisition of each signal, resulting in phase shifts within each "view" (within-view errors). Errors also occur when the strength (amplitude) of the MR signal varies from view to view (view-to-view errors). These two categories of error are present to different degrees in different pulse sequences, and they are addressed by different artifact-reducing techniques. They are therefore addressed separately, along with corresponding techniques for artifact reduction.

139

Gradient-Induced (Within-View) Phase Changes

Each MR signal sampled is referred to as a *view*. Each view is sampled during a finite period of time, during which the rephasing lobe of the frequency-encoding gradient (Gf) is applied. The signal is formed by applying the rephasing lobe, which compensates for phase changes from the dephasing lobe of the gradient (see Gradient Dephasing and Rephasing, Chapter 6). Similarly, the slice-select gradient (Gs) has dephasing and rephasing lobes. The success of the rephasing components of frequency encoding and slice-select gradients depends on the absence of any phase changes other than those caused by the imaging gradients themselves. Motion is an important cause of such phase changes.

The dephasing and rephasing lobes of imaging gradients are each referred to as *unipolar gradients*. A pair of unipolar gradients such as these is designed to compensate for gradient-induced phase changes of *stationary tissue*. The dephasing caused by the initial gradient lobe is corrected because the rephasing lobe induces phase changes that are the exact opposite; hence, the net phase change for both lobes is zero. A unipolar rephasing lobe, however, cannot compensate for phase changes due to motion.

For example, consider the MRI signals that arise from blood flowing in a vessel. Here we assume that all blood within the vessel is flowing in the same direction at the same velocity (i.e., plug flow). During application of the dephasing lobes of the frequency-encoding or slice-select gradient the precessional frequency of protons in stationary tissue and blood changes depending on their location along the axis of these gradients. For stationary tissue, the changes in precessional frequency, and thus the phase changes, have identical magnitudes during the dephasing and rephasing gradient lobes. Therefore, the phase changes of stationary tissue are reversed during application of the rephasing gradient lobes, so at the peak of the echo time (TE) there are no phase differences. Flowing blood, however, moves between application of the dephasing and rephasing gradient lobes. Consequently, it experiences different gradient strengths during the dephasing and rephasing gradient lobes and the phase changes have different magnitudes (Fig. 13-1).

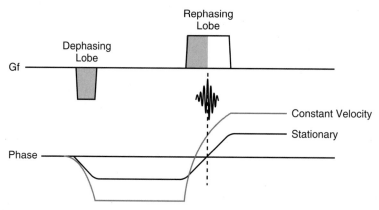

Figure 13-1

Phase changes for stationary and constant-velocity spins during application of the dephasing and rephasing lobes of the frequency-encoding gradient (Gf). For stationary spins, dephasing caused by the dephasing gradient lobe is corrected for by exactly opposite phase changes that develop when the rephasing lobe is applied with reversed polarity. For moving spins, however, the phase changes during these two gradient lobes are not identical, so phase differences persist at the expected TE.

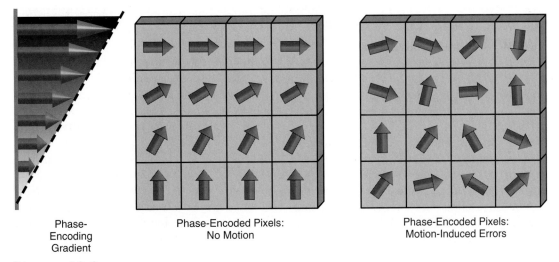

Phase-
Encoding
Gradient

Phase-Encoded Pixels:
No Motion

Phase-Encoded Pixels:
Motion-Induced Errors

Figure 13-2
The phase-encoding gradient is designed to impart uniform, predictable phase changes across its axis. They are used to encode position. Additional phase changes produced by motion lead to incorrect phase encoding.

If there were no phase-encoding gradient (Gp), the phases of all stationary MRI signals would be identical at the midpoint of the sampling time. The process of two-dimensional Fourier transform image reconstruction depends on applying a phase-encoding gradient so the phases of signals differ from one another depending on their location along this gradient. If the phase of an MR signal is altered by something other than the phase-encoding gradient, phase-encoding errors result. Motion during (and between) applications of imaging gradients results in uncompensated phase shifts, which result in phase-encoding errors (Fig. 13-2).

Appearance of Motion-Induced Artifact

Motion-induced phase-encoding errors manifest as artifacts along the phase-encoding axis regardless of the direction of the motion. The direction of the artifact is always along the phase-encoding axis because encoding along this axis is based on phase differences, and the phase differences

no longer accurately reflect position along this axis. This artifact is therefore sometimes referred to as a phase-encoding artifact. It manifests as altered (usually increased) signal intensity, often accompanied by reduced signal intensity of the moving structure itself. For example, consider an abdominal image that contains a high signal intensity gallbladder that moves during respiration. The effect is as if some of the intensity of this gallbladder is misrepresented at various locations along the phase-encoding axis.

If motion is entirely random, the location of the misrepresented signal intensity in the image varies randomly, and the artifacts are smeared along the phase-encoding axis. Frequently, however, motion is repetitive and periodic, such as the motion due to respiration or cardiac activity. Artifacts from periodic motion are more coherent and are located at regular intervals along the phase-encoding axis. The shape of these regularly spaced artifacts usually resembles that of the moving structure. Thus, artifacts that result from periodic motion during image acquisition are often referred to as *ghost artifacts* (Fig. 13-3).

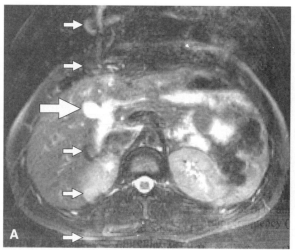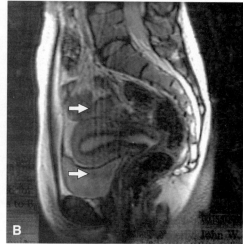

Figure 13-3
Examples of respiration-induced ghost artifacts on T2-weighted fast spin echo images. (*A*) Motion of the gallbladder (*large arrow*) during breathing has produced regularly spaced ghost images (*small arrows*). (*B*) Motion of the anterior abdominal wall has produced several curved lines (*arrows*).

The distance between ghost artifacts depends on the time between repetitive movements (TR) and the pattern of phase-encoding gradient changes. The distance between ghosts increases with the interval between movements and with the TR. For example, the distance between ghosts due to pulsatile flow increases as the TR or the time between heartbeats increases (i.e., as the heart rate decreases) (Fig. 13-4). When the TR is short enough that a motion is not repeated, a ghost artifact is not propagated throughout the entire phase-encoding axis. Rather, ghost artifacts on rapid images such as these may manifest as edge blurring.

Intravoxel Phase Dispersion

When tissue or blood protons in a voxel are all moving at the same velocity, they undergo identical phase shifts. This is true regardless of whether their velocity is constant. If the protons in a voxel have identical velocities, the net intensity of the MR signals is strong, but there are motion-induced phase shifts that cause artifacts along the phase-encoding axis of the image.

When protons in a voxel move at different velocities, however, there are several phase shifts in the voxel. Thus, the coherence of the magnetization and the resulting signal intensity are reduced. In this case, the signal intensities of the moving blood and the ghost artifacts are less intense than if all phase shifts were identical. The loss of phase coherence (and the consequent loss of signal intensity) that occurs when protons in a voxel move at different velocities or in different directions is referred to as *intravoxel phase dispersion*. Intravoxel phase dispersion is most common in blood vessels that have complex or turbulent flow or flow at the extreme periphery of a blood vessel adjacent to the vessel wall (Fig. 13-5). The rapid transition from high to absent flow at the periphery of a blood vessel often causes a signal void adjacent to the vascular wall.

Factors That Affect Within-View Phase Errors

Within-view phase errors are especially severe for high-velocity motion. Phase errors accumulate during the application of imaging

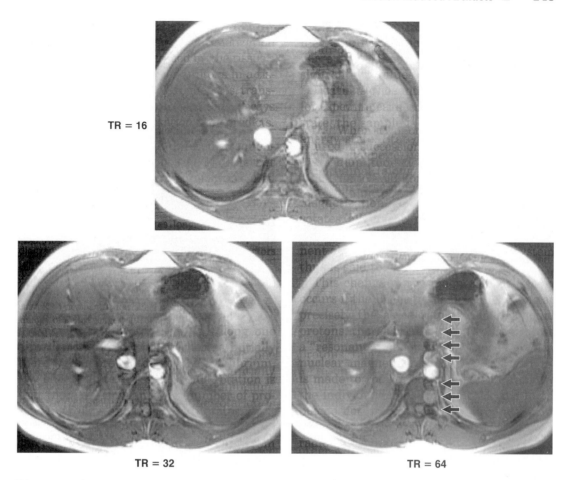

TR = 16

TR = 32

TR = 64

Figure 13-4
On single-section spoiled gradient echo images, the distance between the aorta and ghost artifacts (*arrows*) and the prominence of the artifacts increase with increasing repetition time (TR).

gradients, so the magnitude of the error increases if the imaging gradients are strong or are applied for long intervals (or both). The phase error grows during the interval between signal excitation and the sampling of its echo, so these errors increase with a longer TE.

As a single factor, strong imaging gradients would increase the severity of a motion artifact. In fact, however, the severity of a motion artifact generally decreases as the strength of the frequency-encoding gradient is increased because it is accompanied by an increase in the sampling bandwidth if the field of view is maintained. Increasing the sampling bandwidth decreases the sampling time. Therefore, increasing

the frequency-encoding gradient strength decreases the time available for motion to cause phase changes. If imaging efficiency is maximized, increasing the sampling bandwidth allows a reduced TE (or reduced time between echoes for pulse sequences when more than one echo is obtained per excitation radio pulse). The reduced TE (or interecho interval), in turn, further reduces the severity of the motion artifact. Thus, increasing the sampling bandwidth is a useful method for reducing the severity of the motion artifact. This beneficial effect of increased sampling bandwidth, however, must, be considered along with its adverse effect on the signal-to-noise ratio (SNR).

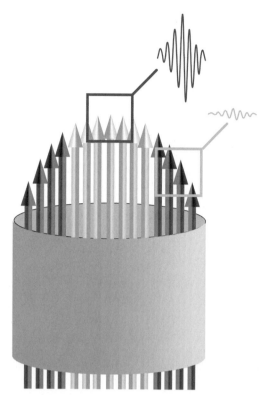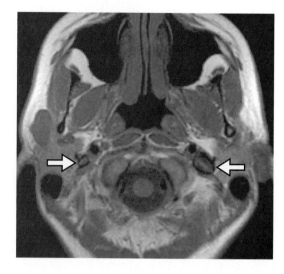

Figure 13-5

Intravoxel phase dispersion at the periphery of a blood vessel with laminar flow. *Left. Long arrows* represent faster flow. Flow velocity is high and nearly uniform at the center of the lumen, leading to little dephasing and therefore strong MR signals. Near the walls of the vessel the velocity decreases, and there is a wider range of velocities with each voxel. This produces a wider range of phase changes in each voxel, leading to lower MR signals. *Right. Arrows* indicate signal loss near the walls of the internal jugular veins, in this axial T1-weighted SE image of the neck.

Within-view phase errors are caused by phase momentum generated by imaging gradients, referred to as *gradient moments*. These gradient moments can be nulled by changing the pattern of the imaging gradients themselves, a strategy called *gradient moment nulling*.

Gradient Moment Nulling

The phase shift that results from motion during and between the application of imaging gradients can be thought of as the building up of momentum due to gradients, or a gradient moment. If the timing and duration of the gradients are altered appropriately, this gradient moment can be eliminated,

or nulled. Techniques whereby within-view phase errors are eliminated or reduced are properly called *gradient moment nulling techniques:* vendor-specific synonyms include motion artifact suppression technique (MAST), gradient moment rephasing (GMR), flow compensation (FC), and flow-adjustable gradients (FLAG). Clinical uses of gradient moment nulling include maintaining a high intravascular signal in the time of flight techniques and reducing the motion artifact in T2-weighted abdominal and spinal images.

Gradient moment nulling involves increasing the complexity of the dephasing and rephasing components of the imaging gradients. With gradient moment nulling, phase shifts of signals from both stationary and moving tissue that occur during the dephasing portion of the imaging gradient are reversed during the rephasing portion of the imaging gradient and are therefore nulled at the time of the echo. The resulting pattern of imaging gradient applications, referred to as the *gradient waveform,* includes more lobes than the simple unipolar dephasing and rephasing lobes of the "non-motion-compensated" gradient waveform we have considered thus far.

The simplest form of gradient moment nulling—nulling of the gradient's first moment—consists of replacing the unipolar gradient lobes with bipolar gradients for both the dephasing and rephasing portions of the gradient waveform. The gradient's first moment is the gradient momentum produced by constant velocity motion. Nulling of the gradient's first moment compensates for constant velocity motion that occurs between excitation and sampling of each signal (Figs. 13-6 and 13-7).

Higher orders of motion can be corrected by using increasingly complex gradient waveforms. The gradient's second moment refers to phase shifts that result from constantly changing velocity (acceleration), whereas the third moment refers to phase shifts from constantly changing acceleration (jerk). These higher orders of motion contribute less to the resulting phase shifts from complex motion. Correcting for them, however, requires increasingly complex and lengthy gradient waveforms. These complex waveforms require more time, increasing the TE, which in turn increases the artifact that results from uncompensated motion. In practice, the best results are usually achieved by nulling the gradient's first

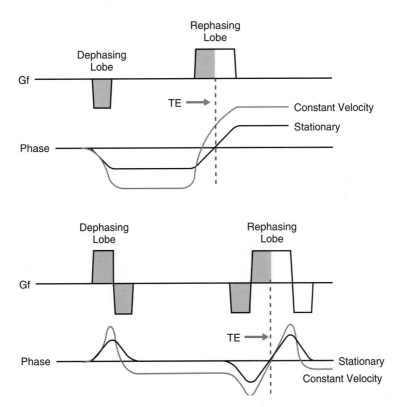

Figure 13-6
Phase changes for stationary and constant-velocity spins using simple bipolar gradients (*top*) and first moment nulling (*bottom*). At the echo time (TE) (*dotted line*), first moment nulling has eliminated phase changes for both stationary and moving spins.

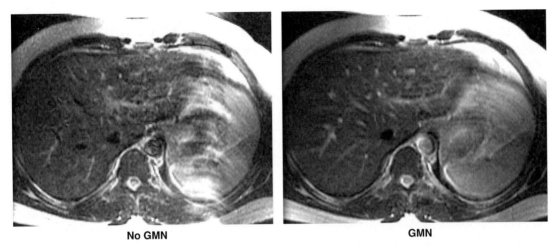

No GMN   GMN

Figure 13-7
Effects of gradient moment nulling (GMN) on a T2-weighted spin echo 2000/80 image. Artifact is less with GMN. Note that the aortic signal intensity is higher and there is less artifact due to its pulsatile flow.

moment and using the shortest possible TE or interecho interval. At best, the use of higher orders of gradient moment nulling yields marginal additional correction of motion artifact. In fact, if high sampling bandwidth and extremely short TE values (e.g., 2 msec or less) are used, the gradient moment may be so small that gradient moment nulling is not necessary.

Correction for constant velocity can reduce signal intensity loss from even highly pulsatile flow, such as that in the aorta or other arteries. This may seem surprising, as the flow velocity in these vessels is continually changing. Inspection of a typical arterial velocity waveform such as that obtained by Doppler ultrasonography or cardiac gated MR flow measurement techniques reveals

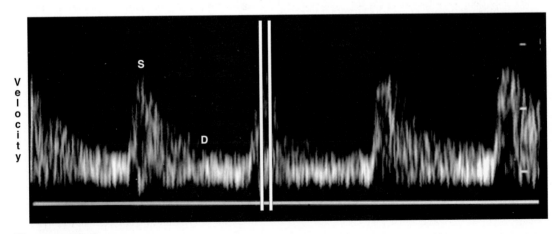

Velocity

Figure 13-8
Arterial Doppler ultrasonography tracing maps velocity along the vertical axis and time along the horizontal axis. Flow velocity varies from high during systole (S) to low during diastole (D). Velocity is not constant during any portion of the cardiac cycle; however, during intervals of a few milliseconds, as indicated by the *paired vertical lines*, there is little variation.

that arterial flow is, in fact, never constant (Fig. 13-8). Flow in the aorta accelerates rapidly to a sharp peak during systole, decelerates, and then is drastically reduced or disappears during most of diastole. Phase shifts from motion, however, occur *during the application of the dephasing and rephasing gradient lobes.* This brief period of time is even less than the TE, a small fraction of a second. Constant-velocity flow is, infact, a reasonably close approximation for the range of velocities that occur while sampling an echo. Thus, nulling the gradient's first moment compensates for most, but not all, of the phase shifts that occur between excitation and sampling of the resulting echo.

Even if all the phase shifts resulting from motion were entirely eliminated, as by infinitely complex and precise gradient moment nulling or infinitely short TE, artifacts from pulsatile flow and other forms of rapidly changing motion would not be eliminated unless other methods of artifact correction were used. This is because much of the artifact from inconstant motion results from view-to-view intensity changes rather than from within-view phase shifts. Gradient moment nulling is highly effective at reducing artifacts from within-view phase errors; however, some forms of motion, such as pulsatile flow, produce artifacts from view-to-view errors. Correction of view-to-view errors requires additional strategies.

View-to-View Intensity Errors

As established in Chapter 5, the intensity of signals is greatest when weak phase-encoding gradients are applied (for gross tissue contrast) and least when strong phase-encoding gradients are applied (for fine image detail). Fourier transform image reconstruction includes the assumption that the amplitude (signal intensity) of each echo is changed only by variations in the value of the phase-encoding gradient.

If motion occurs during data acquisition, the intensity of signals arising from a particular site may vary from view to view (signal to signal). The process of phase encoding by Fourier transform reconstruction does not account for these variations, so phase-encoding errors result. The effect of such errors is an artifact along the phase-encoding axis that is indistinguishable from those that result from within-view phase errors.

Let us consider, for example, view-to-view artifacts on an MR image of the abdomen that result from respiratory motion. During one view a particular voxel may contain hepatic tissue, resulting in moderately high signal intensity. During a later view, this same voxel may contain air, which has no signal intensity (Fig. 13-9). These variations

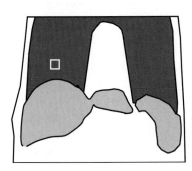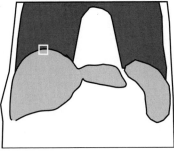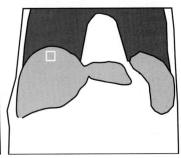

Figure 13-9
View-to-view changes due to the breathing motion of the interface between liver and lung. Signals from a given position in the image can be from lung, liver, or both, producing varying echo amplitude and thus incorrect phase encoding.

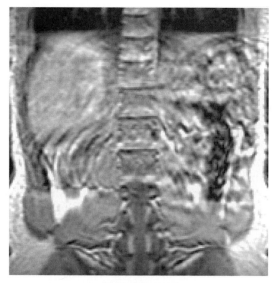 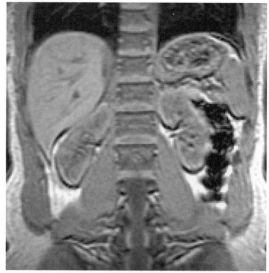

No Breath Hold   **Breath Hold**

Figure 13-10
Respiration-induced artifact on coronal T1-weighted spoiled gradient echo 100/1.8/80° images. Within-view errors are minimal because of the short echo time (TE). View-to-view changes during breathing produce ghost artifacts along the phase-encoding (left-to-right) axis that obscure image details. This can be corrected by breath holding (*right*).

in signal intensity result in phase-encoding mistakes, producing ghost artifacts that are distributed along the phase-encoding axis (Fig. 13-10).

As another example, let us consider high-velocity pulsatile flow. During systole, blood flows rapidly into the imaging volume, where a radio pulse excites it and an echo is sampled. Because this blood was outside the imaging volume during the previous excitation radio pulse, it entered the imaging volume completely unsaturated, with all of its longitudinal magnetization. During systole, therefore, blood has high signal intensity. During diastole, however, blood within the imaging volume is nearly stationary. It has been exposed to a series of excitation pulses, so longitudinal magnetization has recovered partially rather than completely. Therefore, the blood signal intensity is lower during diastole than it is during systole. The changing velocity of blood in the aorta leads to changing signal intensity, producing ghost artifacts from view-to-view intensity changes. These artifacts occur even if within-view phase errors are entirely eliminated.

Table 13-1 ■ EFFECTS ON WITHIN-VIEW AND VIEW-TO-VIEW MOTION-INDUCED ERRORS FOR VARIOUS FORMS OF MOTION

Type of Motion	Effect on Motion-Induced Errors	
	Within-View	View-to-View
Constant velocity motion	+++	−
Pulsatile flow	+++	+++
Complex motion	+++	+

The effects of different forms of motion are summarized in Table 13-1.

Strategies for Reducing Motion-Induced Artifacts

There are several strategies for reducing motion-induced artifacts. Some address artifacts due to both view-to-view intensity changes and within-view phase errors, whereas others are directed principally at one or the other of these basic causes. Strategies that reduce artifacts from both sources include averaging, cessation of motion (e.g., breath holding), reducing the signal intensity of the moving structures (e.g., suppressing the signal intensity of fat or of flowing blood), and reducing the time during which the center of k-space is filled (e.g., subsecond imaging). Gradient moment nulling is directed entirely toward reducing or eliminating artifact due to within-view motion. Strategies that reduce artifact principally due to view-to-view intensity changes include respiratory or cardiac monitoring (e.g., gating, triggering, or phase reordering).

Averaging

Averaging is a "brute force" method that decreases the conspicuousness of ghost artifacts without directly addressing the causes of within-view or view-to-view artifacts. Averaging works simply by increasing the signal intensity of the tissues of interest more than the signal intensity of ghost artifacts; this can be done because real tissue has a more consistent location along the phase-encoded axis than do the ghost artifacts (Fig. 13-11). Although body tissues may move

2 cm or more between views, it is far less than the changing position of ghosts, which may be located anywhere within the image along the phase-encoded axis.

In most situations, averaging is accomplished by acquiring two or more signals at each strength of the phase-encoding gradient before changing the strength of this gradient (Fig. 13-12). This results in each line of k-space being repeated two or more times before the next line is acquired.

This method of averaging is the simplest to implement because it does not increase the number of times the phase-encoding gradient strength is changed. The disadvantage of this averaging method is that the signal intensity of a pixel tends to be similar in two sequential views. For example, little motion occurs during a 6.5 msec TR, so averaging two successive views at this TR has only a minimal effect on reducing motion artifacts. In fact, because the time between lines of k-space is increased from 6.5 msec to 13.0 msec, some artifacts may even be intensified (Fig. 13-13).

In general, motion artifact is best corrected by averaging when all lines of k-space are acquired but before any is repeated (Fig. 13-12C). This method of averaging is not used commonly, however, because it involves more changes in the strength of the phase-encoding gradient and is therefore somewhat more demanding to implement.

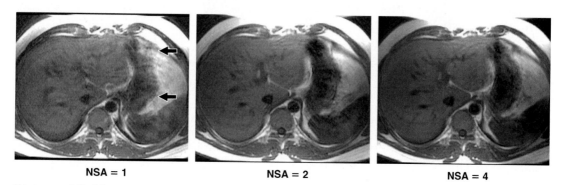

| NSA = 1 | NSA = 2 | NSA = 4 |

Figure 13-11
Effect of signal averaging on motion-induced artifact (SE 500/11). With no averaging (*top left*), the image is degraded by an artifact (*arrows*). With an increasing number of signals being averaged (NSA), the artifact is reduced and the signal-to-noise ratio (SNR) is increased.

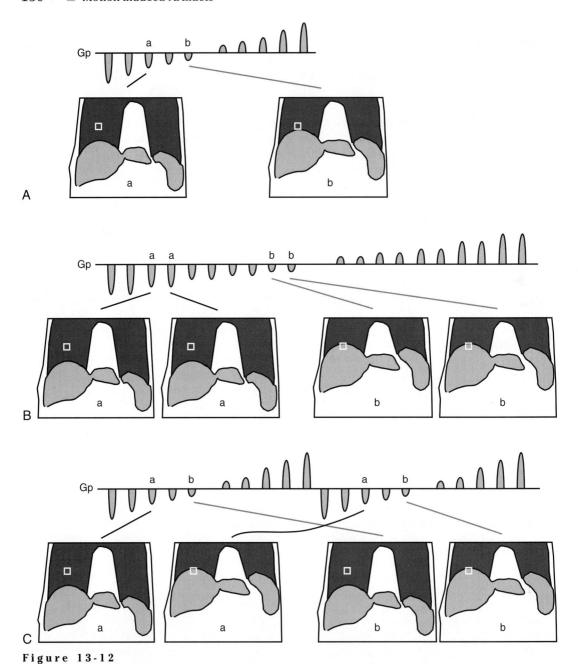

Figure 13-12

Effects of averaging view-to-view errors in rapidly acquired images. Two phase-encoding gradient (Gp) strengths are labeled (*a* and *b*). (*A*) Without averaging, there is little change between views *a* and *b*. (*B*) If each phase-encoding gradient strength is repeated twice before changing, there is little change, so little is accomplished by averaging; however, more time elapses between *a* and *b*, increasing view-to-view errors. (*C*) If each phase-encoding gradient strength is applied once before any is repeated, the views being averaged are different from one another. In this example, the average of both *a* views is identical to the average of both *b* views.

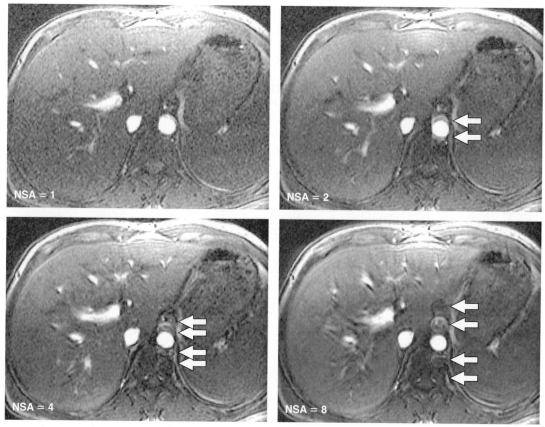

Figure 13-13

Effect of increasing the number of signals averaged (NSA) on artifacts from pulsatile aortic flow (*arrows*) on axial gradient echo images with a TR of 6.5 msec and a TE of 1.5 msec. With one signal average (*top left*), image acquisition is so rapid there is little motion artifact. As the NSA increases from one to eight, the SNR improves but the time increases between changes in the phase-encoding gradient strength. This increases the severity of the artifact and increases the distance between ghosts (*arrows*).

The major disadvantage of averaging is the longer time required. Thus, averaging is a viable option only for short pulse sequences, which include spin echo and gradient echo images with a short TR and T2-weighted images in which several echoes are obtained per excitation radio pulse (e.g., fast spin echo or turbo spin echo). Even with these techniques, other methods of artifact suppression are generally preferred when available owing to their greater efficiency. Additionally, the longer time required for pulse sequences with averaging may, in fact, lead to increased motion during acquisition and even to increased artifact.

Reduced Signal Intensity of Artifact-Producing Tissues

Ghost artifacts can be ameliorated by reducing the signal intensity of moving tissue. This method does not directly address the motion itself or the mechanism of motion artifact, but it reduces the magnitude of artifacts from both within-view and view-to-view errors. Saturating flowing blood before it enters the volume of interest via a spatially selective saturation pulse can reduce artifact. Such pulses reduce the signal intensity of both the blood within the vessel and ghost artifacts that arise from

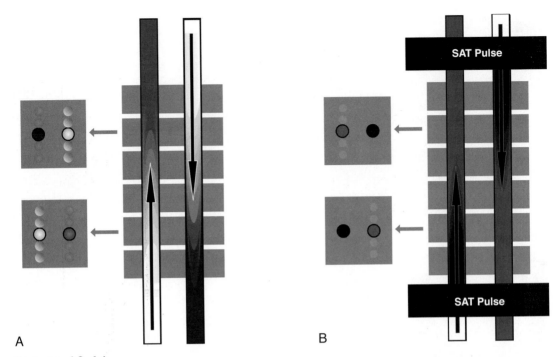

Figure 13-14
Spatial saturation pulses for reduction of flow-induced ghost artifacts in a two-dimensional (2D) multisection acquisition. (*A*) Stationary tissue is partially saturated by repeated excitations; however, blood that enters the imaged volume between excitations is fully magnetized and thus can produce greater signal intensity. The ghost artifact and increased signal intensity are greatest at entry sections (i.e., the first sections in the stack encountered by fresh, fully magnetized blood). (*B*) With saturation pulses (SAT pulses) above and below the imaged volume, in-flowing blood has less magnetization, rather than more, relative to stationary tissue. The vascular lumen in the entry sections therefore has the lowest signal intensity and exhibits the least artifact.

the blood (Figs. 13-14, 13-15, and 13-16). Spatially selective saturation pulses can also be used to reduce or eliminate signal intensity from moving structures other than blood. For instance, a saturation pulse can be applied to the anterior abdominal wall to reduce artifact from moving adipose tissue (Fig. 13-17, top).

Another form of saturation pulse commonly used to reduce motion artifact is *fat saturation,* a form of *chemically selective saturation.* Here, a radio pulse is designed to match the frequency of methylene (CH_2) protons in adipose tissue rather than the various tissues at a given position along an imaging gradient. Reducing the signal intensity of adipose tissue decreases the severity of the artifact generated by its

motion (Fig. 13-17, bottom). Spatially and chemically selective saturation pulses are discussed further in Chapter 15.

Cardiac and Respiratory Monitoring

Most methods of motion artifact reduction that are based on monitoring physiological motion are directed principally toward view-to-view intensity changes. The cardiac cycle can be monitored by electrocardiography (ECG) or impedance plethysmography (IPG). ECG monitoring allows more accurate determination of the phase of the cardiac cycle throughout image acquisition, as the

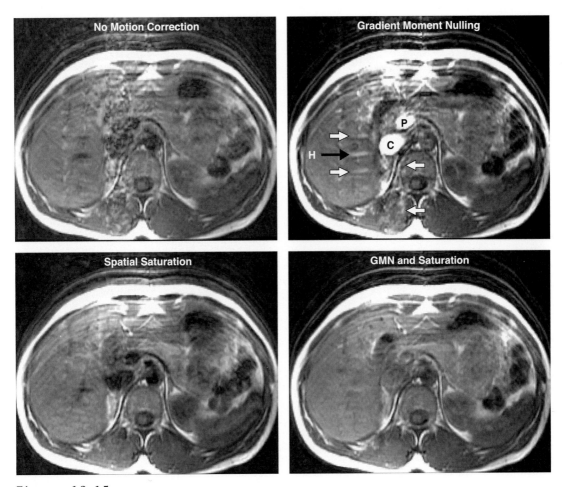

Figure 13-15

Effects of gradient moment nulling (GMN) and spatial saturation pulses on vascular ghost artifacts in the bottom sections of an axial SE 300/25 acquisition during quiet respiration. Without motion artifact correction (*top left*), there is severe image degradation along the phase axis (anteroposterior). With GMN (*top right*), signal loss from within-view errors has been corrected, increasing the signal intensity of the inferior vena cava (C), portal vein (P), and hepatic vein (H). These vessels have the highest signal intensity because this is the entry section for the inferosuperior flow direction of these vessels. There is still substantial artifact due to view-to-view changes from pulsatile flow in the inferior vena cava and hepatic veins (*white arrows*), although there is less artifact from the nonpulsatile portal vein. With spatial saturation (*bottom left*) the inferior vena cava and portal and hepatic veins are signal voids, and artifact from these vessels has been reduced. With the combination of GMN and spatial saturation (*bottom right*), the signal intensity of the vessels has increased slightly.

R-wave occurs immediately prior to ventricular systole. IPG is easier to implement and suffers less from artifacts due to extraneous cardiac or radiofrequency activity. However, there is a variable delay between ventricular systole and the capillary pulse sensed at the fingertip by the IPG lead. Therefore, IPG gating does not allow direct comparison between the phase of the cardiac cycle and the images themselves, and it does not permit strategies that restrict data acquisition to specific portions of the cardiac cycle, such as during diastole.

The respiratory cycle can be monitored by placing a bellows sensitive to respiratory motion around the upper abdomen.

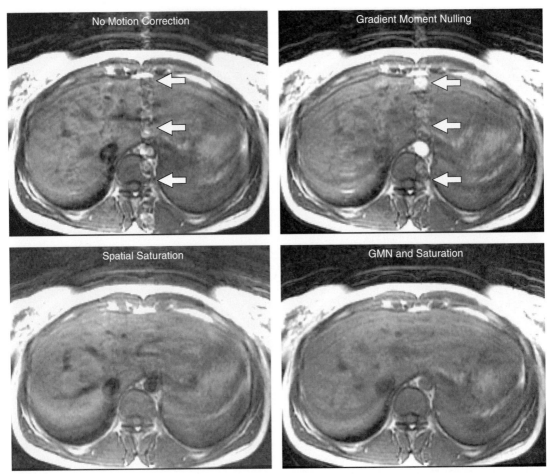

Figure 13-16

As in Figure 13-15, top sections. These are the entry sections for flow in the aorta, which produces a severe artifact (*arrows*). Gradient moment nulling (GMN) (*top right*) increases intraluminal signal intensity in the aorta but does not reduce ghost artifacts, which are caused primarily by view-to-view changes due to the pulsatile flow. Spatial saturation (*bottom left*) reduces the signal intensity of the aortic lumen and the artifacts. The combination of GMN and spatial saturation results in the least artifact, although vascular signal intensity is slightly higher.

Spirometry can also be used to determine a patient's pattern of respiration. More recently, a brief non-phase-encoded signal incorporated into the pulse sequence has been used to generate "navigator echoes" that depict the position of the diaphragm.

Some methods of motion compensation involve monitoring by the patient or MR operator. For example, patients can monitor their own breathing by signaling each breath to the MR operator, typically by squeezing a bulb. Alternatively, the operator can observe a tracing of the patient's respiratory pattern (respiratory waveform) and initiate image acquisition accordingly.

Gating and triggering techniques are used to ensure that the signal intensity in a given location is the same during each phase-encoding view of a particular image. These techniques reduce variations in view-to-view signal intensity. In some implementations, data are either discarded or not acquired

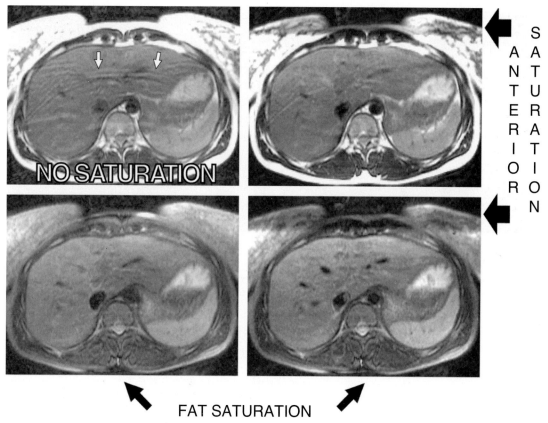

Figure 13-17
Effects of spatial saturation and fat saturation on respiration-induced ghost artifacts. This T2-weighted FSE 2000/120 image acquired during quiet respiration shows ghost artifacts (*top left*) due to motion of anterior adipose tissue. These artifacts are reduced by spatial saturation of the anterior abdominal wall (*top right*), by chemical (fat) saturation of adipose tissue (*bottom left*), or by combining the two methods (*bottom right*).

during periods of active motion (e.g., cardiac systole or respiratory inspiration) (Fig. 13-18). If this is done, actual motion during data acquisition is reduced, minimizing both within-view and view-to-view errors; however, the imaging time is prolonged when there are significant periods during which no data are acquired. A more efficient use of physiological triggering involves obtaining different slices of a multislice acquisition during different phases of the physiological cycle (Fig. 13-19). Alternatively, "cine" images can be obtained sequentially at a given location throughout the physiological cycle (Fig. 13-20).

With the techniques described above, data acquisition is discontinuous, with the pauses generally occurring during the QRS complex. This can cause longitudinal magnetization to vary from view to view, introducing artifacts. An alternative involves continuous acquisition of data, using the R wave to trigger a change in the phase-encoding gradient strength (Fig. 13-21). These techniques, if implemented successfully, eliminate most view-to-view variations. The severity of artifacts due to within-view errors on a given image depends on the amount of motion during that particular phase of the physiological cycle.

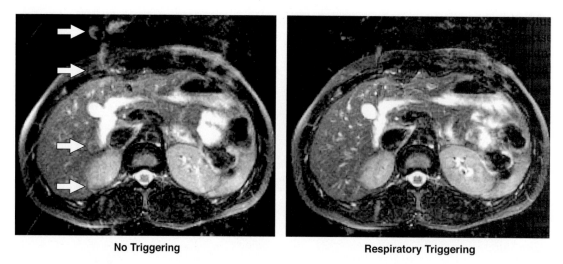

No Triggering   **Respiratory Triggering**

Figure 13-18
Respiration-induced T2-weighted FSE 3333/100 image shows an artifact due to motion of the gallbladder (*arrows*), which is eliminated by triggering data acquisition to periods of minimal motion (*right*) by monitoring via respiratory bellows.

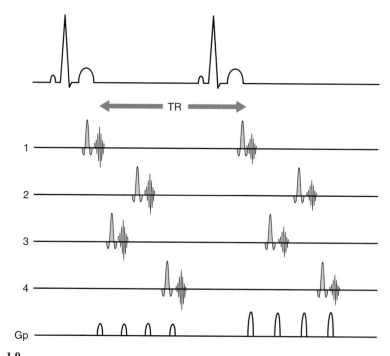

Figure 13-19
Multislice single-phase cardiac gating. Interleaved excitations of four slices are triggered by the R wave of an electrocardiographic signal. The value of the phase-encoding gradient (Gp) is changed after the next R wave. For a given image slice, all echoes occur during the same phase of the cardiac cycle. This minimizes artifacts from cardiac pulsations if the cardiac cycle is regular. Each slice is acquired at a different cardiac phase.

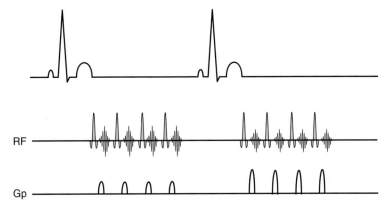

Figure 13-20
Single-section multiphase cardiac gating. Four excitations are obtained for each value of the phase-encoding gradient (Gp), resulting in four images of the same physical site at four phases of the cardiac cycle.

Specific techniques for cardiac imaging are discussed further in Chapter 30.

Suspending Respiration

The best way to avoid artifact due to respiratory motion is to avoid such motion during image acquisition. If the acquisition duration is short enough, the patient can voluntarily suspend respiration. With little effort, most patients can suspend respiration several times for 10 seconds or less. If the periods of suspended respirations are few, most patients can suspend respiration for 20 seconds. With active coaching, rehearsal before the actual imaging, and encouragement during image acquisition, most patients can suspend respiration for as long as 30 seconds. If oxygen is administered via nasal cannula before breath holding, patients can suspend respiration even longer.

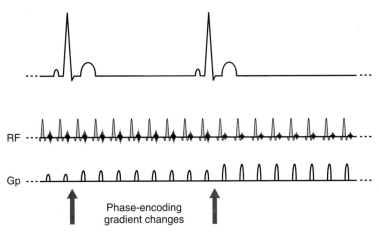

Figure 13-21
Continuous data acquisition with cardiac triggering. The TR is uniform throughout acquisition and is not related to the cardiac cycle. The value of the phase-encoding gradient (Gp) is changed at each R wave. The number of cardiac phases encoded is determined by the number of excitations that can occur during each cardiac cycle.

Suspension of respiration reduces artifacts from all abdominal contents, including bowel. In fact, ghost artifacts from the bowel are essentially eliminated by breath holding because peristalsis is usually slow and of small magnitude; however, antiperistaltic agents such as glucagon are useful for decreasing the blurring of bowel walls and for distending bowel lumens.

Subsecond Imaging

If satisfactory breath holding can be achieved, two-dimensional (2D) multislice or three-dimensional (3D) acquisitions are usually ideal, as these techniques allow images with a high SNR to be acquired efficiently (discussed in Chapter 8). Most images with an intermediate or long TR as well as 3D acquisitions, however, are highly sensitive to motion, so artifacts occur if breath holding is not successful. Additionally, these images often have prominent ghosts due to pulsatile flow. If a patient cannot successfully suspend respiration and other voluntary motion during image acquisition, the artifact can be reduced by using short-TR 2D acquisitions. If the TR is decreased, the flip angle should be smaller as well. The use of short-TR 2D techniques is an example of balancing low SNR and contrast versus reduced sensitivity to motion.

To reduce artifacts due to cardiac and vascular motion or gross body or limb movement, or for patients who cannot suspend respiration, image acquisition must be faster than that for breath holding. Even though substantial motion may occur during a 1-second acquisition, the motion artifact is severe only if the motion occurs during sampling of the center of k-space. Strategies for fast imaging are discussed more fully in Chapter 14.

Special Consideration of Pulsatile Flow

Although the velocity of pulsatile flow changes throughout the cardiac cycle, nulling the gradient's first moment and using the shortest possible TE generally eliminate most gradient-induced artifacts. The remaining artifacts are mostly due to view-to-view intensity changes. In other words, artifacts due to pulsatile flow on images with gradient moment nulling are caused mostly by the changing magnetization between systole and diastole.

During systole, high-velocity blood flow completely replaces blood between excitations, leading to high signal intensity. During diastole, however, slow or reversed flow leads to low signal intensity. This changing signal intensity produces phase errors and therefore ghost artifacts. With this basic cause of artifacts due to pulsatile flow in mind, we now review several parameters and their effects on these artifacts.

Saturation Pulses. Ghost artifacts can be reduced, but not eliminated, by the use of saturation pulses. Saturation pulses are most effective for rapidly flowing blood. Saturating the blood immediately before it enters the volume of interest during systole reduces its high signal intensity, which otherwise would have been unsaturated. However, during diastole, when there is little or no flow, blood entering the volume of interest is not saturated by a saturation pulse. Thus, the blood may exhibit more magnetization during diastole than during systole when saturation pulses are used. These view-to-view differences between systole and diastole produce artifacts, but they tend to be less severe than those that would have occurred had saturation pulses not been used.

A more effective method for eliminating signal intensity from flowing blood involves the use of double inversion recovery, sometimes referred to as "black blood imaging." This technique is described in greater detail in Chapter 15.

Contrast Enhancement. Gadolinium chelates and other T1-enhancing contrast agents reduce the T1 of blood, leading to faster recovery of magnetization after an excitation pulse. This increases the overall signal intensity of blood on T1-weighted images. In particular, the signal intensity of partially saturated blood during diastole is increased. The signal intensity of blood during systole does not change, however, as it is completely replaced between excitation pulses and thus is completely unsaturated. Because this blood is completely unsaturated, fast recovery after saturation (reduced T1) is not relevant. T1 reduction due to contrast enhancement increases the signal during diastole but does not affect the already-high signal intensity during systole; hence, the effect of contrast enhancement is to decrease the difference between the systolic and diastolic signal intensities. On images that have few within-view phase errors (e.g., rapid gradient echo images with a TE less than 3 msec), gadolinium administration may therefore *decrease* the severity of ghost artifacts by decreasing view-to-view errors (Fig. 13-22).

Within-view artifacts are more severe after contrast enhancement owing to the blood's higher signal intensity. Pulse sequences with a long TE or low sampling bandwidth, especially those that do not include gradient moment nulling, generally have more vascular artifacts after gadolinium administration.

Excitation Flip Angle. During systole, the use of a 90° flip angle produces maximal transverse magnetization and maximal signal intensity. At the time of the next excitation pulse, systolic blood in the image section is completely replaced and thus unsaturated. During diastole, however, blood is partially saturated and thus has less longitudinal magnetization if a 90° flip angle is used. The difference between systolic and diastolic magnetization is therefore maximized by the use of the 90° flip angle.

The longitudinal magnetization of diastolic blood flow at the time of each excitation pulse can be increased by using a smaller flip angle, as it decreases the amount of saturation by each excitation pulse. A smaller flip angle also reduces the amount of transverse magnetization formed from systolic blood flow. Thus, using a lower flip angle increases the signal intensity of blood flowing during diastole and decreases the signal intensity of blood flowing during systole, rendering them more similar to each other. This reduces the intensity of ghosts (Fig. 13-23).

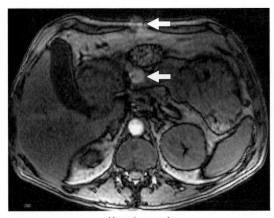
Unenhanced

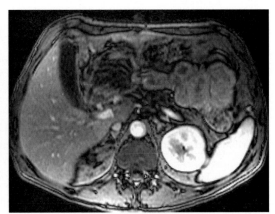
Post-Gadolinium

Figure 13-22
Effect of gadolinium enhancement on pulsation artifacts during breath-holding gradient echo T1-weighted images. Ghosts are prominent on the unenhanced image (*arrows*) but are less conspicuous "post-gadolinium" owing to decreased differences in systolic versus diastolic echo amplitudes.

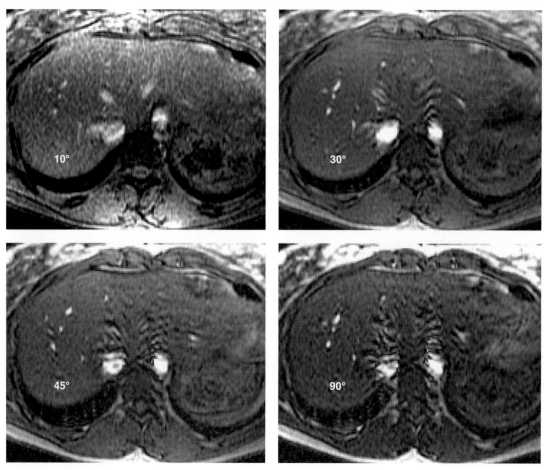

Figure 13-23
Effect of the excitation flip angle on artifact due to pulsatile flow using single-section gradient echo images with TR/TE values of 20/7. The artifact is increasingly severe as the flip angle increases owing to greater differences between systolic and diastolic echo amplitudes.

Table 13-2 ■ RELATIVE EFFECTIVENESS OF VARIOUS TECHNIQUES FOR MOTION ARTIFACT CORRECTION ON WITHIN-VIEW AND VIEW-TO-VIEW ERRORS AND ON MOTION-INDUCED BLURRING

	Effectiveness		
Artifact-Correction Technique	Within-View	View-to-View	Blurring
Gradient moment nulling	+++	−	−
Minimal TE	+++	−	−
Minimal TR	−	+++	+
Increased sampling bandwidth	+	−	−
Averaging	+++	+++	−
Spatial saturation	+++	+++	−
Physiological monitoring	−	+++	+++
Breath-holding	+++	+++	+++
Reduced flip angle	−	+++	−

Averaging. As described earlier, artifacts from pulsatile blood flow can increase in response to signal averaging, as the acquisition of data for the center of k-space is spread over a longer time. Artifacts from pulsatile flow can be reduced by completing the acquisition of the center of k-space as rapidly as possible (fast imaging), by spatial presaturation, or by cardiac gating, triggering, or reordering techniques. The effects of various artifact-correcting techniques on various components of motion-induced artifact are summarized in Table 13-2.

▼
Essential Points to Remember

1. Simple bipolar gradients do not correct for motion that occurs between the dephasing and rephasing gradient lobes—within-view phase errors.

2. Variable phase changes within a voxel lead to intravoxel phase dispersion, which manifests as decreased signal intensity.

3. Motion can cause the echo amplitude to vary from view to view. Phase-encoding errors due to this mechanism are called view-to-view intensity errors.

4. Unanticipated phase changes due to both within-view and view-to-view motion result in phase-encoding errors, which appear as artifacts along the phase-encoding axis.

5. Gradient moment nulling involves use of a more complicated gradient waveform that allows reduction of within-view phase errors. View-to-view errors are not affected.

6. View-to-view errors can be reduced by any measure that decreases the view-to-view variation of the signal amplitude from a given site within an image.

7. Methods for reducing view-to-view errors include arresting motion, applying spatial presaturation, gating or triggering data acquisition to the motion itself, or extremely rapid imaging.

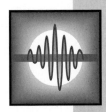

Chapter 14

Pulse Sequences: Gradient Echo and Spin Echo

Thus far we have introduced most of the components that combine to form the specific pulse sequences used in daily magnetic resonance (MR) practice. In this chapter we describe the basic classifications of pulse sequences created from these building blocks.

A basic gradient echo pulse sequence consists of an excitation pulse followed by measurement of a gradient echo. The echo is created by first dephasing the magnetization by applying the dephasing lobe of the frequency-encoding gradient (Gf) and then rephasing the magnetization by reapplying the gradient with reversed polarity. This results in a coherent signal.

Unspoiled Gradient Echo Techniques

Many gradient echo techniques achieve fast imaging times by using a short repetition time (TR). In fact, the TR is often comparable to or shorter than the T2 relaxation time of some of the tissues in the region of interest (Fig. 14-1). The presence or absence of residual coherent transverse magnetization at the time of the next excitation pulse affects the signal-to-noise ratio (SNR) and tissue contrast of the resulting image.

163

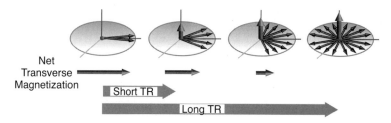

Figure 14-1
Relationship between persistent transverse magnetization and repetition time (TR). Transverse magnetization decays completely between excitations with a long TR. With a short TR, coherent magnetization may persist at the time of the next excitation.

First, let us consider a pulse sequence with a short TR, where residual transverse magnetization is present at the time of each successive excitation pulse. With each pulse, the transverse magnetization is rotated farther until it has been rotated a full 360°. The residual transverse magnetization adds to the longitudinal magnetization that has recovered from previous excitations (Fig. 14-2).

With such a pulse sequence, once a steady state has been established, there are two primary sources of longitudinal magnetization. As with other pulse sequences, longitudinal magnetization recovers after an excitation pulse at a rate determined by the tissue's T1. If transverse magnetization is still present at the time of each excitation pulse, this nondecayed transverse magnetization is rotated

back into the longitudinal plane, creating additional longitudinal magnetization.

The amount of residual transverse magnetization present at the time of each excitation pulse is determined by the TR and by the tissue's T2. The shorter the time between excitations (short TR), the less time there is for the transverse magnetization to decay. The slower the decay of transverse magnetization (long T2), the more residual transverse magnetization there is present at the time of each excitation pulse.

Pulse sequences in which transverse magnetization is present at the time of excitation pulses are considered *unspoiled*. Most commonly, these pulse sequences are gradient echo techniques, and the resulting images are called *unspoiled gradient echo images*.

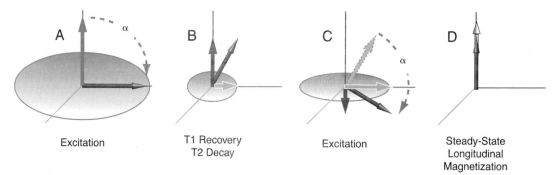

Figure 14-2
Rotation of persistent transverse magnetization into the longitudinal plane. (*A*) 90° Excitation. (*B*) T1 (recovery) and T2 (decay) relaxation. With a sufficiently short TR, the next excitation (*C*) rotates residual transverse magnetization (*light arrow*) into the longitudinal plane as it rotates recovered longitudinal magnetization (*dark arrow*) into the transverse plane. Steady-state longitudinal magnetization (*D*) (and thus the received MRI signal) therefore consists of contributions from both residual transverse (*light arrow*) and recovered longitudinal (*dark arrow*) magnetizations.

Commercial implementations of unspoiled gradient echo techniques include fast imaging with steady-state precession (FISP) and gradient recalled acquisition in the steady state (GRASS). With these pulse sequences, the use of a short TR decreases the amount of recovered longitudinal magnetization and increases the amount of residual transverse magnetization. These effects tend to balance each other for tissues with a long T2; hence for such tissues the signal intensity varies little with changes in TR (Fig. 14-3).

The echo time (TE) does not affect the amount of transverse magnetization present at each excitation pulse. The TE, the time between the creation of transverse magnetization and its measurement, determines the amount of transverse magnetization present *when the echo is measured*. However, after it is measured, transverse magnetization continues to decay, at a rate determined by the T2* (T2 plus the effects of magnetic field heterogeneity) of the tissue. The time available

for decay (before and after the TE) is determined by the time between excitation pulses, the TR. The time during which transverse magnetization decays *between excitation pulses* is not affected by whether the TE is immediately after the excitation pulse or immediately before the next excitation pulse. The amount of residual transverse magnetization present at the time of an excitation pulse is determined by the TR, not the TE (Fig. 14-4).

In images where residual transverse magnetization is rotated back into the longitudinal plane, variable dephasing by the phase-encoding gradient (Gp) can cause artifacts. The strength of the phase-encoding gradient is changed after each excitation pulse, allowing determination of the position of spins along this axis. As the strength of the phase-encoding gradient increases, it causes more dephasing, which decreases the overall strength of the resulting echo. If it is not compensated for, this variable

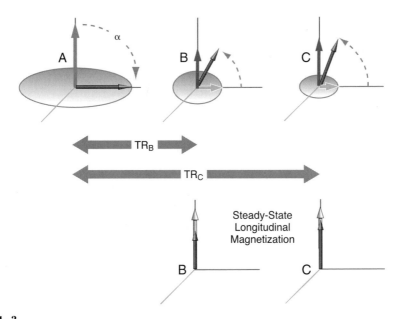

Figure 14-3

For unspoiled gradient echo techniques, the amount of equilibrium longitudinal magnetization may be similar at different TR values. (*A*) Transverse magnetization is created and longitudinal magnetization is saturated by a 90° pulse. (*B*) With a short TR there is abundant coherent transverse magnetization at the time of each excitation pulse, which is rotated back into the longitudinal plane. (*C*) With a longer TR more longitudinal magnetization is recovered but less residual transverse magnetization persists. In *B* and *C*, the *dark arrows* represent recovered longitudinal magnetization, while the *light arrows* represent refocused residual transverse magnetization.

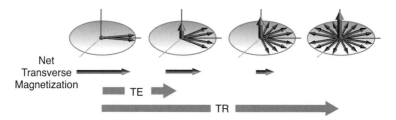

Figure 14-4
Decay of transverse magnetization after the echo time (TE). Coherent transverse magnetization is measured at the TE. During the remainder of the repetition time (TR) transverse magnetization continues to decay. The amount of transverse magnetization present during excitation is determined by the TR and the T2 of the tissue.

coherence of the transverse magnetization can produce artifacts.

The solution to this potential problem is similar to that for other imaging gradients. The phase-encoding gradient pulse can be considered a dephasing lobe. Then, just before each excitation pulse, a rephasing

lobe is applied to undo the phase encoding. This rephasing lobe of the phase-encoding gradient is often referred to as a *rewinding gradient* (Fig. 14-5).

On unspoiled gradient echo images, signal intensity is a function of the amount of longitudinal magnetization that has

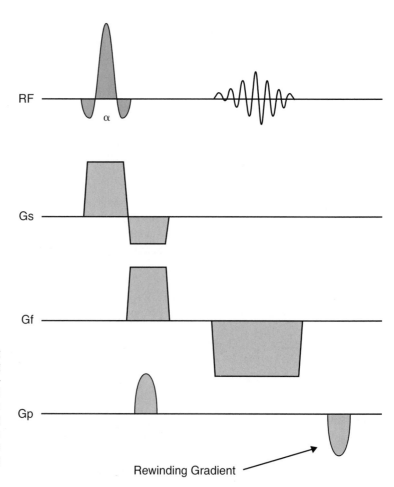

Figure 14-5
Rewinding gradient for reversing the effects of the phase-encoding gradient (Gp). Transverse magnetization is partially dephased by the phase-encoding gradient pulse. It is rephased by applying a rewinding gradient, which has identical magnitude but opposite polarity to the phase-encoding gradient.

Rewinding Gradient

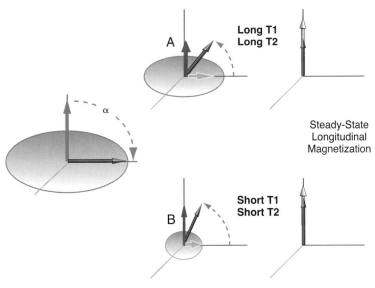

Figure 14-6

With unspoiled gradient echo techniques, tissues with a long T1 and a long T2 (*A*) may have signal intensity similar to that of tissues with a short T1 and a short T2 (*B*), as they have similar T2/T1 ratios. A long T1 results in little recovery of longitudinal magnetization between excitations, whereas a long T2 results in abundant, persistent transverse magnetization that is rotated back into the longitudinal plane. In contrast, a short T1 results in more recovery of longitudinal magnetization, whereas a short T2 results in less persistent transverse magnetization.

recovered between excitation pulses and the amount of transverse magnetization that persists. The amount of recovered longitudinal magnetization is greater for tissues with a short T1, and the amount of persistent magnetization is greater for tissues with a long T2. Thus, short T1 and long T2 each contributes to increased signal intensity on unspoiled gradient echo images. These images can thus be considered *T2/T1- weighted* (Fig. 14-6).

For most tissues, T1 and T2 tend to parallel each other; that is, tissues with a long T1 tend to have a long T2. Therefore, T1 and T2 contrasts tend to "compete" with each other, causing most tissues to have similar signal intensity on T2/T1-weighted unspoiled gradient echo images. For example, the liver has a short T1, which contributes to high signal intensity relative to most liver lesions; however, liver lesions and the spleen usually have a long T2, contributing to high signal intensity relative to the liver. The result of these two competing processes is relatively flat contrast and little differentiation between most tissues.

The tissues with the highest signal intensity on T2/T1-weighted gradient echo images are those in which T2 is as long, or almost as long, as T1. This is true of most fluids and lipids and causes fluid and adipose tissue to have especially high signal intensity on T2/T1-weighted images. As discussed in Chapter 4, T1 is the upper limit for T2; a tissue's T2 cannot be longer than its T1. T1 and T2 are equal if T2 relaxation is simply a return of transverse magnetization into the longitudinal plane, as for pure water. Additional decay of transverse magnetization occurs in solid tissues because of exchange of energy between spins, an exchange facilitated by association with nearby macromolecules. This causes T2 to be shorter than T1 for solid tissues, which in turn causes them to have low signal intensity on T2/T1-weighted gradient echo images (Fig. 14-7).

Further enhancement to unspoiled gradient echo images is achieved when the gradient waveforms are completely balanced, reducing the effects of motion. These balanced steady-state free precession techniques are discussed later in the chapter.

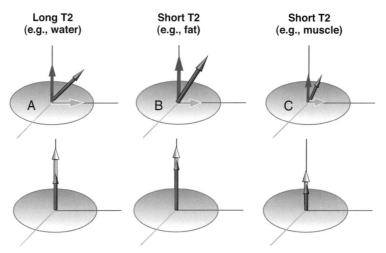

Figure 14-7

Effects of the T2/T1 ratio on equilibrium longitudinal magnetizations of unspoiled gradient echo images. Because both recovered longitudinal and persistent transverse magnetization contribute to equilibrium longitudinal magnetization, tissues with a long T1 and a long T2 (e.g., water, *A*) and a short T1 and a short T2 (e.g., fat, *B*) have similarly high T2/T1 ratios, and thus both have high signal intensity. Tissues with a long T1 and a short T2 (e.g., muscle and many other solid tissues, *C*) have lower T2/T1 ratios and thus lower signal intensity. In the bottom row, *dark arrows* indicate recovered longitudinal magnetization while *light arrows* indicate refocused residual transverse magnetization.

Spoiled Gradient Echo Techniques

Effective T1 contrast can be achieved on images where signal intensity is principally a function of the amount of longitudinal magnetization that has recovered between excitation pulses. T2 weighting that results from the rotation of persistent transverse magnetization into the longitudinal plane can obscure T1 contrast; this is undesirable if unambiguous T1 weighting is wanted. Thus, if T1 weighting is desired on short TR images, it is necessary to *spoil* the residual transverse magnetization before each excitation pulse. The residual transverse magnetization can be spoiled by applying a spoiling gradient that dephases the magnetization (Fig. 14-8). Because residual transverse magnetization is not returned to the longitudinal plane, spoiled gradient echo images generally have lower-equilibrium longitudinal magnetization, and thus lower SNR, than unspoiled gradient echo images (Fig. 14-9).

Most modern pulse sequences use an alternative method for spoiling the transverse magnetization: *radiofrequency spoiling*. This involves the use of excitation pulses designed to render the magnetization incoherent at the time of the next excitation pulse. By either method, spoiled gradient echo images can be obtained in which residual transverse magnetization does not affect image contrast. When the TR, TE, and flip angle are chosen appropriately, contrast can be heavily T1-weighted. Common examples of spoiled gradient echo techniques include fast low-angle shot (FLASH) and spoiled GRASS. A comparison of spoiled and unspoiled gradient echo images with TR values of 10 and 120 msec, respectively, is presented in Figure 14-10.

Some tissues look similar on T1-weighted and T2/T1-weighted images. Adipose tissue, for example, has high signal intensity on both images because 1/T1 (the relaxation rate) and T2/T1 are both high. Hemorrhagic and proteinaceous fluid may similarly have high signal intensity on both T1-weighted spoiled and T2/T1-weighted unspoiled

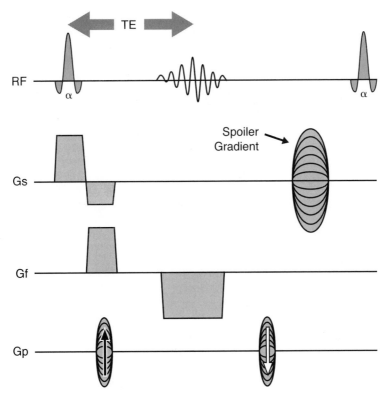

Figure 14-8
Spoiled gradient echo pulse sequence. Persistent transverse magnetization can be eliminated before each excitation by dephasing the transverse magnetization via a spoiling gradient.

gradient echo images. Simple fluid, however, has long T1 *and* T2 relaxation times, so 1/T1 is low whereas T2/T1 is high. Therefore, simple fluid has low signal intensity on T1-weighted spoiled gradient echo images and high signal intensity on T2/T1-weighted images.

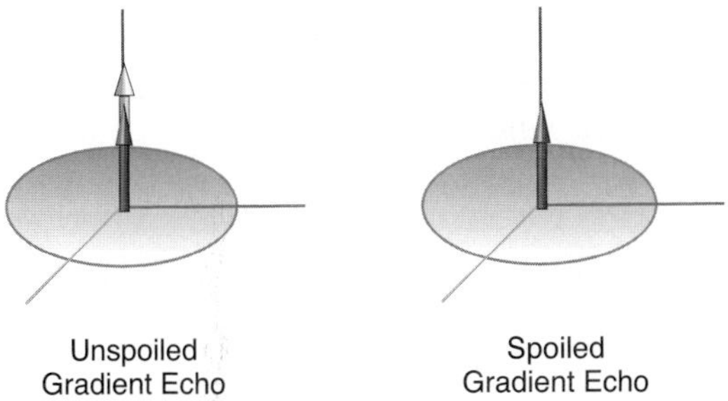

Repetition Time and Flip Angle: Effects on Tissue Contrast

The TR is a major determinant of the acquisition time for most pulse sequences. As the TR becomes shorter, the acquisition time decreases. A shorter TR affords less time for recovery of longitudinal magnetization. To achieve adequate T1 weighting on a spoiled gradient echo image using a 90° excitation pulse, the TR must be similar to or shorter than the tissue T1 relaxation times to be distinguished in the image.

Figure 14-9
Equilibrium longitudinal magnetization on unspoiled and spoiled gradient echo images. Spoiled gradient echo images have lower signal intensity because there is no residual transverse magnetization to contribute to equilibrium longitudinal magnetization.

Unspoiled Gradient Echo   Spoiled Gradient Echo

	10°	20°	45°	90°

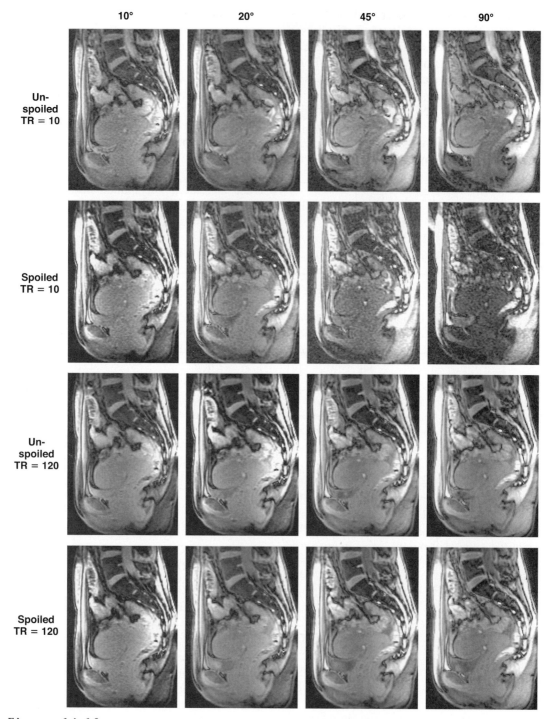

Un-spoiled TR = 10

Spoiled TR = 10

Un-spoiled TR = 120

Spoiled TR = 120

Figure 14-10

Sagittal gradient echo images of the pelvis with variable flip angles using unspoiled and spoiled techniques and repetition times (TRs) of 10 and 120 msec, respectively. With an unspoiled technique and a short TR, T2/T1 weighting increases with increasing flip angle, increasing the signal intensity of fluid. The signal-to-noise ratio (SNR) does not change substantially with different flip angles. With a spoiled technique, the SNR decreases substantially with increased flip angles at a TR of 10 msec. With the higher TR, the difference between unspoiled and spoiled images is less dramatic because there is greater decay of transverse magnetization during the TR; however, T1 contrast is better with the spoiled technique. (Note the lower signal intensity of urine and cerebrospinal fluid.)

If the TR is *much* shorter than the T1 relaxation times, the SNR may be decreased substantially unless the excitation flip angle is reduced along with the TR. For a given TR and T1 relaxation time, there is an excitation flip angle that can be used to obtain a maximal SNR (Ernst angle, as discussed in Chapter 3). As the TR decreases, the flip angle should generally be reduced if a comparable appearance is desired. Similarly, as the flip angle decreases, the TR generally decreases as well.

The TR values are short (less than 500 msec) for most currently used gradient echo techniques, so heavy T1 weighting can be readily achieved at most TR values used. The TR is therefore usually not the principal determinant of tissue contrast on gradient echo sequences (although the choice of TR can affect the image efficiency, SNR, and vulnerability to artifacts). For most gradient echo techniques, the excitation flip angle is a more important determinant of image contrast than is TR.

To optimize contrast between tissues with different T1 values, the excitation flip angle should be equal to or larger than the Ernst angle for the tissue with the shorter T1. In clinical practice, for a TR of 100 msec or more, an excitation flip angle of 60°–90° produces useful T1 weighting. As the TR is reduced below 100 msec, the flip angle should generally be less than 90°; and as it is reduced to 50 msec or less, for adequate T1-contrast and SNR the excitation flip angle should generally be held comparable to the TR (e.g., TR of 30 msec and flip angle of 30°). As the TR becomes even shorter, the flip angle is then higher than the TR (e.g., TR of 6 msec and flip angle of 15°). This "rule of thumb," of course, depends on the tissues being compared. For example, during magnetic resonance (MR) angiography (discussed in Chapter 23) higher flip angles are used so the magnetization of stationary tissue remains largely saturated.

For spoiled gradient echo images, reducing the excitation flip angle below the Ernst angle for all tissue T1 values of interest decreases the T1 weighting. For some applications this may be tolerable, or even desirable, if other contrast parameters (e.g., T2* or flow) are to be emphasized.

For unspoiled gradient echo images, changes in the TR and the flip angle have different effects on image contrast and the SNR. As the TR increases, less residual transverse magnetization remains at the time of each excitation pulse. In fact, with TR times longer than 200 msec, tissue contrast is similar on spoiled and unspoiled gradient echo images, except that on unspoiled images fluid has a higher signal intensity. As the TR decreases and more transverse magnetization persists at the time of each excitation pulse, the difference between spoiled and unspoiled gradient echo images increases.

For spoiled gradient echo images, the SNR decreases as the TR does. The loss of signal intensity follows directly from the logarithmic T1 relaxation curve; a shorter TR can be thought of as moving earlier and earlier along this curve toward the origin. For unspoiled gradient echo techniques, however, the effect on the SNR of reducing the TR is less profound because residual transverse magnetization increases with a shorter TR.

Echo Time: Effects on Tissue Contrast

As the TE increases, the signal intensity on the resulting image decreases because of decay of transverse magnetization. Transverse magnetization decays fastest for tissues with a short T2* relaxation time. Image contrast based on differences between tissues' rates of T2* decay is called *T2* contrast*. In spin echo pulse sequences, where magnetic field heterogeneity is corrected using a 180° refocusing pulse, TE is the parameter that directly affects T2 weighting. For gradient echo pulse sequences, TE is the parameter that directly affects T2* weighting, or sensitivity to susceptibility differences.

If the purpose of a pulse sequence is to accentuate the T1 differences between tissues, the TE should be kept as short as possible to minimize T2* contrast and artifacts from heterogeneous magnetic susceptibility. Another benefit of a short TE is to minimize signal loss from flowing blood on "bright blood" flow pulse sequences; however, the TE may be increased deliberately if T2* contrast is desired. T2*-weighted images may be useful for depicting calcifications, iron, and blood products as having low signal intensity.

Steady-State Free Precession

Each radio pulse in a gradient echo pulse sequence is usually intended to be an excitation pulse. Thus, we are usually concerned principally with the effects of this pulse on longitudinal magnetization; however, each radio pulse also affects the transverse magnetization that has not decayed during the TR.

Earlier in the chapter we discussed unspoiled gradient echo techniques, in which residual transverse magnetization is rotated back into the longitudinal plane, augmenting the signal intensity of tissues with sufficiently long T2 relaxation times. These techniques are also referred to as coherent steady-state free precession, or simply as steady-state free precession, techniques.

Each radio pulse, regardless of its flip angle, excites longitudinal magnetization and to some extent changes the rotational phase of transverse magnetization. This causes some refocusing of the transverse magnetization, although the extent of refocusing is less complete than with a 180° refocusing pulse in a typical spin echo pulse sequence. In other words, each in a series of radio pulses in a gradient echo pulse sequence creates transverse magnetization and refocuses transverse magnetization created by the preceding radio pulse. The refocusing of transverse magnetization by a radio pulse forms a spin echo, similar to the spin echoes formed in typical spin echo pulse sequences.

Let us review this information: Following a given radio pulse, a free induction decay (FID) is initiated. For most gradient echo techniques, the FID is sampled as a gradient echo, which is formed by first applying a dephasing gradient and then reapplying it as the frequency-encoding gradient with reversed polarity. Following the FID, the next radio pulse creates additional transverse magnetization but also refocuses the transverse magnetization created by the preceding radio pulse, creating a spin echo. The spin echo occurs at the time of the next radio pulse. The timing of the readout determines the extent of the contribution from each of these two echoes to the signal intensity in the resulting image. As the TR becomes sufficiently short, the tails of the FID and the spin echo merge, so a continuous signal exists with regular variations in amplitude. As the TR becomes progressively shorter, the amplitude variation becomes smaller.

Various steady-state free precession techniques can be used to generate different types of contrast, as discussed below.

T2-Weighting

If the TR is not sufficiently short, severe artifacts and image banding can occur owing to the amplitude variations of the gradient and spin echoes. Therefore, steady-state free precession techniques with TR >10 msec involve sampling the spin echo, but not the gradient echo, to achieve T2-weighting. As with conventional spin echo pulse sequences, the refocusing pulse occurs at the center of the TE, so the TE is double the time between the excitation and refocusing radio pulses. Because the time between the excitation and refocusing pulses is the TR, for T2-weighted steady-state free precession pulse sequences the TE is actually twice as long as the TR. For example, a typical T2-weighted steady-state free precession pulse sequence might have a TR of 30 msec and a TE of approximately 60 msec.

One problem when designing a steady-state free precession pulse sequence is that at the time of the spin echo the slice-select gradient and a radio pulse are both being applied. It is thus not possible to listen for an echo at the expected TE. One solution is periodically to miss an excitation pulse so an echo can be sampled at the TE. More commonly, the echo is sampled before refocusing is complete (Fig. 14-11). The

incomplete refocusing causes the image to be somewhat sensitive to T2* (susceptibility) contrast as well as to true T2 contrast. The sensitivity to susceptibility is based on the offset between the time of echo sampling and the time of complete refocusing of the spin echo, whereas the sensitivity to true T2 is based on the TE.

T2/T1 Weighting: Balanced Steady-State Free Precession

In some unspoiled gradient echo pulse sequences, as TR is minimized a true steady state of magnetization can be created where the FID and spin echo signals coincide and there is virtually constant magnetization present throughout the pulse sequence. Such a steady state depends on complete balancing of all gradients and centering the peak of the gradient echo exactly between each excitation pulse so the TE is exactly one half the TR (Fig. 14-12). The earliest implementation of this technique required application of several dummy pulses to

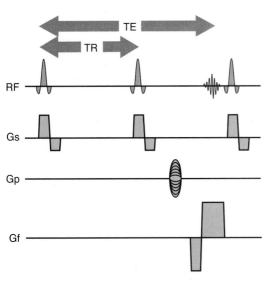

Figure 14-11
Steady-state free precession pulse sequence. Each radio pulse acts as an excitation pulse and a refocusing pulse for transverse magnetization created by the preceding pulse. A gradient echo is created by the readout gradient timed to occur in advance of the next radio pulse. This gradient echo is slightly offset relative to the spin echo, which coincides with the next radiofrequency (RF) pulse and application of the slice-select gradient (Gs).

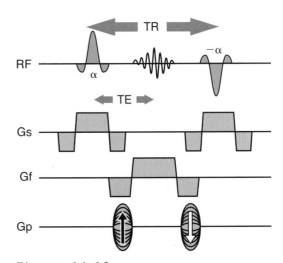

Figure 14-12
Balanced steady-state free precession pulse sequence. All gradient waveforms are balanced, the polarity of the excitation pulse is alternated, and the TE is exactly one half the TR.

attain the steady state. This interfered with its use as a fast imaging sequence. However, the steady state can be achieved more rapidly by applying a radiofrequency (RF) pulse at one half the flip angle, preceding the first excitation pulse by one half the TR. This RF pulse with half of the flip angle is repeated at the end of the pulse sequence to restore the longitudinal magnetization to its equilibrium position. A variety of techniques that take advantage of phase differences between water and lipid magnetizations can be used for lipid signal cancellation.

Balanced steady-state free procession optimizes the signal amplitude, so maximal signal strength is maintained. These images are highly sensitive to magnetic field heterogeneity; the best results are achieved with high field homogeneity and an extremely short TR. Typically, flip angles are rather large (e.g., 60° or more), and the TR may be as short as 3 msec or less. Such images have a high SNR and little sensitivity to motion, and they depict stationary as well as moving fluid as having high signal intensity.

The earliest images of this type were referred to as *True FISP*. Other terms are *FIESTA* (fast imaging employing steady-state acquisition) and *balanced fast field echo*. Unfortunately, the term "steady-state free precession" has been used to refer not only to these images but also to the T2-weighted techniques described above that sample only the spin echo, generating some confusion.

Spin Echo Techniques

The establishment of magnetic resonance imaging (MRI) during its first decade as an effective modality for clinical imaging was based principally on the success of spin echo pulse sequences for generating T1-weighted, T2-weighted, and intermediate pulse sequences. The spin echo pulse sequence is robust and highly tolerant of imperfections in the main magnetic field, imaging gradients, and radio pulses.

A spin echo pulse sequence is virtually identical to a simple spoiled gradient echo pulse sequence, as described above, with the addition of a refocusing pulse at the center of the TE. Optimal refocusing is achieved with the use of a 180° pulse, but smaller pulses are occasionally used to reduce demands on the pulse amplifier or to reduce the RF exposure to the patient. Because the refocusing pulse reverses the phase differences between spins at either end of the frequency-encoding axis, the rephasing lobe of the frequency-encoding gradient is applied with the same polarity as that of the dephasing gradient rather than with reversed polarity, as with gradient echo techniques.

Spin echo techniques are generally more tolerant of system imperfections than are corresponding gradient echo pulse sequences. Refocusing radio pulses not only eliminate phase differences caused by the frequency-encoding gradient itself but also correct for imperfections in the main magnetic field and for microscopic magnetic field gradients caused by heterogeneous magnetic susceptibility in the patient. The principal disadvantage of spin echo pulse sequences is the time required for application of the refocusing radio pulses and their accompanying slice-select gradients (Fig. 14-13).

Unspoiled and spoiled examples of 90° and 10° flip angles are used to illustrate high and low angles, respectively, for these gradient echo pulse sequences. The amount of T2 or T2* contrast with any of these pulse sequences is generally determined by the TE. Adequate T1 contrast with spoiled GRE or SE techniques depends on the use of a TR that is similar to or less than the T1 relaxation times of the tissues of interest. The suitability of the pulse sequences discussed in this chapter for providing T1, T2, T2*, and T2/T1 contrast is summarized in Table 14-1.

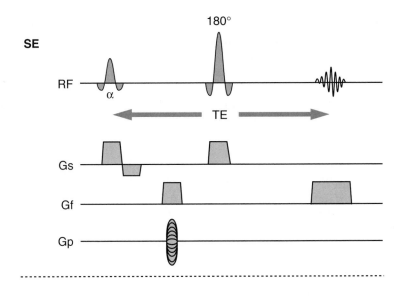

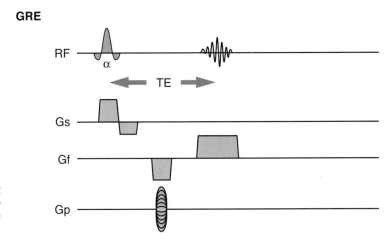

Figure 14-13
Comparison between spin echo (SE) (*top*) and gradient echo (GRE) (*bottom*) pulse sequences. The GRE pulse sequence does not include a 180° refocusing pulse or its accompanying slice-select gradient, so the TE can be shorter than for SE sequences.

Table 14-1 ■ POTENTIAL OF VARIOUS PULSE SEQUENCES FOR ACHIEVING T1, T2, T2*, OR T1/T2 CONTRAST

	Potential, by Contrast Mechanisms		
Pulse Sequence	**T1**	**T2 or T2***	**T2/T1**
Unspoiled GRE, 90°	–	T2*	+++
Unspoiled GRE, 10°	–	T2*	–
Spoiled GRE, 90°	++	T2*	–
Spoiled GRE, 10°	–	T2*	–
Steady-state free precession	–	T2 and T2*	–
Balanced steady-state free precession	–	T2 and T2*	+++
Spin echo	+++	T2	–

▼

Essential Points to Remember

1. Gradient echo images involve applying an excitation radio pulse and then forming an echo by reapplying the frequency-encoding gradient with direction reversed.

2. With some gradient echo techniques, tissues with a T2 similar to or longer than the TR have persistent transverse magnetization at the end of the TR. This unspoiled transverse magnetization is rotated back to the longitudinal plane by subsequent excitation pulses, and it thus contributes to image signal intensity. These pulse sequences are referred to as unspoiled gradient echo techniques.

3. For unspoiled gradient echo images, short T1 and long T2 relaxation times both contribute to increased signal intensity. These images are therefore T2/T1-weighted.

4. In unspoiled gradient echo images, fluid and fat tend to have high signal intensity, and most other tissues have intermediate signal intensity.

5. Spoiled gradient echo images are T1-weighted because residual transverse magnetization is spoiled at the end of each TR, before the next excitation pulse.

6. With longer TR or shorter tissue T2, residual transverse magnetization becomes less important, as does the difference between spoiled and unspoiled techniques.

7. Applying a rewinding gradient, which is a repetition of the phase-encoding gradient with reversed polarity, can reduce artifacts caused by residual transverse magnetization due to the varying strengths of the phase-encoding gradient.

8. For short-TR techniques, the SNR can be low if a 90° excitation pulse is used, as there is little time for T1 recovery. With a short TR, the SNR improves if the flip angle is smaller. As the TR increases, comparable contrast can be achieved by increasing the excitation flip angle.

9. On gradient echo images, decay of transverse magnetization is due to both T2 relaxation and local magnetic field heterogeneity. The combined contrast mechanism is T2* contrast. As the TE increases in the gradient echo images, contrast due to T2* differences increases.

10. In T2-weighted steady-state free precession techniques, each radio pulse serves as both an excitation pulse and a refocusing pulse for the previous excitation. The TE is about twice as long as the TR.

11. In unspoiled balanced gradient echo images with a shortened TR, a constant level of magnetization is reached that does not vary significantly throughout image acquisitions. These images generally have a high SNR, particularly of stationary as well as moving fluid, and little sensitivity to motion.

12. Spin echo techniques are similar to gradient echo techniques, except that a 180° refocusing pulse is applied at the midpoint of the TE (to correct for a heterogeneous magnetic field and chemical shift effects). Additionally, the rephasing lobe of the frequency-encoding gradient has the same polarity as the dephasing lobe, rather than the opposite.

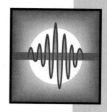

Preparatory Pulses, Including Fat Suppression

The repetition time (TR), echo time (TE), and excitation flip angle can be manipulated to alter T1, T2, or T2* contrast on gradient echo and spin echo images, as described in earlier chapters. Additional radio pulses applied before a pulse sequence can affect contrast in a variety of ways. These additional pulses are called *preparatory pulses* (Fig. 15-1). Common preparatory pulses include inversion, spatial saturation, chemically selective saturation, and magnetization transfer pulses.

Inversion Recovery

A 180° inversion pulse before one or more excitation pulses imparts strong T1 contrast. Such T1 contrast is in addition to the tissue contrast that results from the remainder of the pulse sequence itself. Ideally, no

transverse magnetization results from the inversion pulse. Rather, the 180° pulse only *inverts* the longitudinal magnetization, converting it from positive to negative (Fig. 15-2).

Once inverted, the negative magnetization begins to recover, initially toward zero and then toward its equilibrium positive value. The rate at which the longitudinal magnetization recovers is determined by its T1; that is, the rate of recovery following a 180° inversion pulse is 1/T1 (Fig. 15-3).

During the course of this recovery, a radio pulse excites the recovering longitudinal magnetization, creating transverse magnetization. The amount of transverse magnetization created depends on the magnitude of the longitudinal magnetization that had recovered after the inversion pulse. The time between the inversion and excitation pulses is defined as the *inversion time* (TI). Figure 15-4 diagrams the components of a basic spin echo inversion recovery pulse sequence.

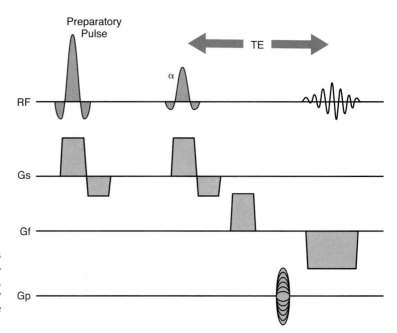

Figure 15-1
A preparatory pulse precedes the excitation pulse (α). A slice-select gradient (Gs) is applied, so the effects of the preparatory pulse are restricted to the desired image section.

The amplitude of the magnetic resonance (MR) signal created by the excitation radio pulse is determined by the absolute value of the longitudinal magnetization immediately before the excitation pulse. That is, negative and positive longitudinal magnetization, once excited, give rise to transverse magnetization with positive polarity (Fig. 15-5).

The amplitude of the positive longitudinal magnetization prior to each inversion pulse is determined by the amount of T1 recovery since the previous excitation pulse. This is maximal when the TR is long, so inversion recovery pulse sequences usually utilize a long TR. The principal determinant of tissue contrast on most inversion recovery pulse sequences is the TI. Figure 15-6 shows the contrast behavior for two representative tissues.

When the TI is long enough (i.e., at least 1 second or longer), the longitudinal magnetization of nearly all protons has time to

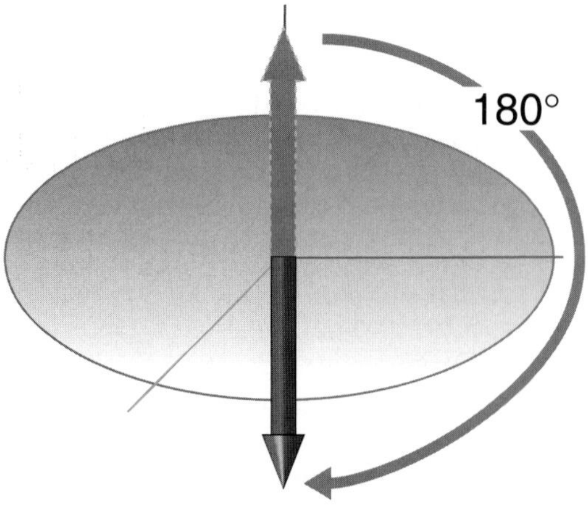

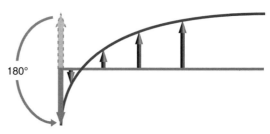

Figure 15-2
A 180° inversion pulse rotates equilibrium longitudinal magnetization from the positive to the negative longitudinal plane.

Figure 15-3
Following inversion by a 180° inversion pulse, longitudinal magnetization recovers logarithmically toward zero and then toward its original positive equilibrium level.

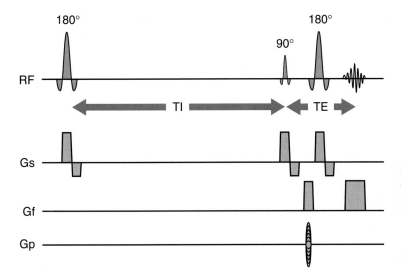

Figure 15-4
Spin echo inversion recovery pulse sequence. Each 90° excitation pulse is preceded by a 180° inversion pulse. The time between the inversion and excitation pulses is the inversion time (TI).

recover beyond zero. The contrast on inversion recovery images with a sufficiently long TI resembles that of T1-weighted spin echo or spoiled gradient echo images in that tissues with short T1 relaxation times have higher signal intensity than tissues with long T1 relaxation times, as these tissues have recovered more of their longitudinal magnetization.

The contrast between any two tissues with different T1 relaxation times can be optimized on inversion recovery images by choosing a TI such that the inversion pulse

occurs when the longitudinal magnetization of one of the tissues has recovered to zero but not beyond. On such an image, this target tissue has no signal intensity. The signal intensity of this tissue is said to have been *nulled*, and the TI needed to null the signal intensity from a given tissue is called the *null point* for that tissue. For example, an inversion recovery pulse sequence with a TI of approximately 600 msec allows time for the signal intensity from the spleen and many tumors to recover to zero at 1.5 T, nulling their signal intensity on these

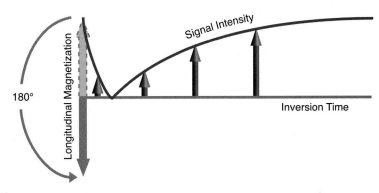

Figure 15-5
Transverse magnetization is created by excitation of either negative or positive longitudinal magnetization. Similar signal intensity can therefore result from excitation of either of these magnetizations. The signal intensity on an image reflects the *absolute value* of longitudinal magnetization at the time of the excitation pulse.

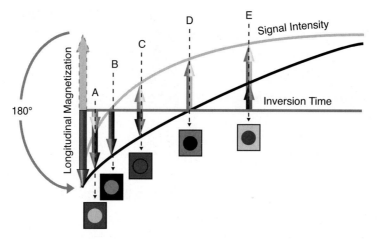

Figure 15-6

Inversion recovery tissue contrast at different TI values. The *light gray line* and *arrows* indicate a short T1 (e.g., solid tissue), whereas the *dark line* and *arrows* indicate a tissue with a long T1 (e.g., simple fluid). At the *bottom*, solid tissue is represented by the *boxes* and fluid by the *circles* within them. (*A*) With a short TI, solid tissue (*dark box*) has recovered farther toward zero and therefore has lower signal intensity than does fluid (*light circle*). (*B*) With a slightly longer TI, the solid tissue (*black box*) has relaxed to zero and therefore is a signal void. (*C*) With further prolongation of TI, the magnitude of the negative longitudinal magnetization of fluid is equal to that of the positive magnetization of solid tissue, so they are isointense except for a cancellation void at their interfaces. (*D*) With a longer TI, fluid (*black circle*) has relaxed to zero, depicted in the image as a signal void (*E*). With a longer TI, both tissues have positive longitudinal magnetization, which is greater for solid tissue.

images and producing effective contrast for detecting focal liver lesions. Similar contrast can be obtained at 0.5 T using an inversion recovery pulse sequence with a 400 msec TI. Figure 15-7 illustrates tissue contrast at various TI values.

On many inversion recovery pulse sequences, signal intensity can be ambiguous. That is, longitudinal magnetization of tissues with a short T1 may have recovered beyond zero to achieve positive longitudinal magnetization, whereas tissues with longer T1 may have merely recovered to a similar magnitude of negative longitudinal magnetization. The amount of transverse magnetization created by the excitation pulse is determined by the *magnitude* of the longitudinal magnetization without regard to its *polarity,* that is, without regard to whether the longitudinal magnetization is positive or negative. Thus, at a given TI a tissue with a short T1 may have an amount of positive longitudinal magnetization equal to the amount of negative magnetization of a tissue

with a longer T1. These two tissues have identical signal intensity, although their T1 values may be considerably different.

Fortunately, two tissues with different T1 values but identical signal intensities on an inversion recovery image may be distinguished from each other if they share a border because this border is depicted as a signal void. A signal void between two tissues on opposite sides of the null point on an inversion recovery image is referred to as a *bounce-point artifact* (Fig. 15-8). The bounce-point artifact may be quite useful for depicting otherwise isointense lesions within a tissue, such as liver lesions with a long T1.

Inversion recovery images with a short TI have become popular for many applications. This particular form of inversion recovery pulse sequence even has its own acronym, STIR [short tau (TI) inversion recovery]. The TI in STIR pulse sequences is usually chosen so the longitudinal magnetization of adipose tissue is nulled. Adipose tissue therefore has little if any

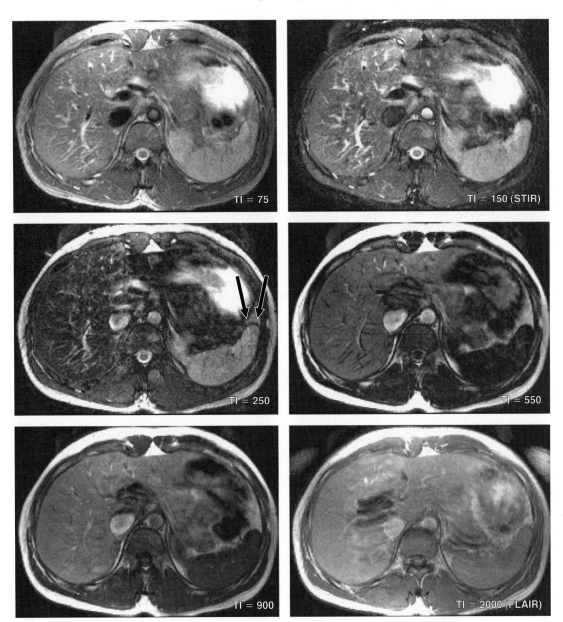

Figure 15-7

Effect of changing the TI on axial fast spin echo inversion recovery images of the abdomen (TR/TE 3750/30 msec). With a TI of 75 msec, longitudinal magnetization of all tissues is negative; tissues such as the spleen, gastric fluid, and cerebrospinal fluid (CSF) have a long T1 and therefore higher negative longitudinal magnetization than tissues with a shorter T1, which have relaxed closer to zero. With a TI of 150 msec, adipose tissue has relaxed to zero, whereas tissues with a longer T1 still have negative longitudinal magnetization. With a TI of 250 msec, adipose tissue has positive longitudinal magnetization, having relaxed past the null point, whereas spleen and fluid have negative longitudinal magnetization. Note the bounce-point artifact at the interface between the positive and negative longitudinal magnetization of, respectively, adipose tissue and the spleen (*arrows*). At this TI (250 msec), liver longitudinal magnetization is nulled. With a TI of 550 msec, splenic magnetization is nulled. With a TI of 900 msec, most magnetization is positive, and the contrast resembles that of a spin echo T1-weighted image. With a TI of 2000 msec, the longitudinal magnetization of CSF is near zero, whereas all other magnetization is positive.

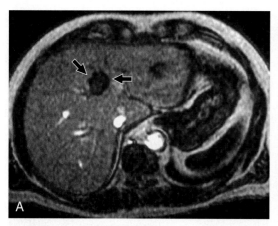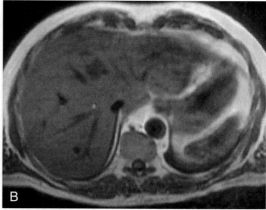

Figure 15-8

Bounce-point artifact on inversion recovery images. (*A*) Magnetization prepared gradient echo image with a TI of 550 msec. The spleen signal has been nulled. Liver magnetization has recovered past zero, and the magnetization of a cavernous hemangioma (*arrows*) is negative. The liver and hemangioma are nearly isointense, although their magnetizations are opposite, causing a signal cancellation artifact at their interface. (*B*) T1-weighted spin echo image showing absence of a signal void surrounding the hemangioma.

signal intensity on these images even in the absence of any chemical shift-selective technique (e.g., fat saturation). At 1.5 T, adipose tissue is nulled if the TI approximates 150 msec, whereas at 0.5 T the appropriate TI is approximately 100 msec.

STIR images are also particularly attractive because T1 and T2 contrast tend to be additive, rather than destructive, for most tissues; that is, tissues with a long T1 usually have a long T2 as well. With most pulse sequences, a long T1 leads to low signal intensity and a long T2 to high signal intensity. On STIR images, however, a long T1 causes less recovery toward zero than does a short T1, causing tissues with a long T1 to have higher signal intensity than those with a short T1. As in other images, a long T2 contributes to high signal intensity. Thus, a long T1 and long T2, which tend to occur together in tissues, both contribute to high signal intensity on STIR images.

On the opposite end of the spectrum of specialized inversion recovery pulse sequences are those in which TI is quite long (approximately 2 seconds). A TI such as this is chosen so that simple fluid, such as cerebrospinal fluid (CSF), is nulled.

These pulse sequences have been referred to as fluid-attenuated inversion recovery (FLAIR). Typically, FLAIR images have a long TE and are thus T2-weighted, although CSF and other simple fluids have no signal intensity because they have been nulled (Fig. 15-9).

Inversion recovery techniques are among the most powerful and flexible available for generating T1 contrast, with or without additive T2 contrast; however, except for STIR and FLAIR, inversion recovery images are not commonly used in clinical practice because they have less signal intensity and longer acquisition times than do comparable images without inversion pulses. Their signal intensity is lower because the additional T1 contrast on inversion recovery images is based on variable rates of decay during the TI; all tissues lose signal intensity during this time but at different rates. The acquisition time is usually longer for a given number of slices because during the TI additional image slices could have been acquired. Inversion recovery thus involves spending more time to achieve a lower signal-to-noise ratio (SNR).

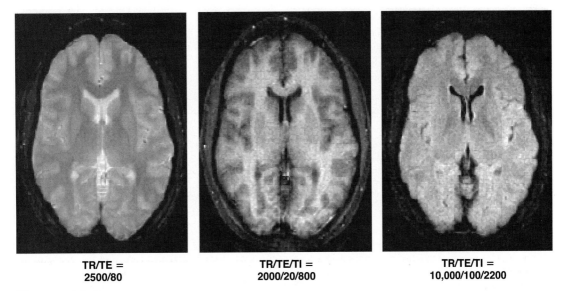

TR/TE = 2500/80	TR/TE/TI = 2000/20/800	TR/TE/TI = 10,000/100/2200

Figure 15-9
Multishot echo planar imaging comparing T2 weighting (*left*) with two echo planar methods for producing low signal intensity CSF. With a short TE and an 800 msec TI, there is substantial T1 contrast between gray and white matter, and the positive longitudinal magnetization of these tissues is greater than the value of the negative longitudinal magnetization of CSF. With a longer TR, TE, and TI (*right*), contrast between gray and white matter is T2-weighted, and the signal intensity of CSF has been nulled. This image is an example of fluid-attenuated inversion recovery (FLAIR).

Spatially Selective Saturation

One popular form of preparatory pulse is a *spatially selective saturation pulse,* which saturates the magnetization from a certain region of tissue from which signal intensity is not desired. This is done by selectively exciting the region and then applying a dephasing gradient to spoil the transverse magnetization (Fig. 15-10). The magnetization in the unwanted region is now saturated. A subsequent excitation pulse, targeted to the slice of interest, produces signal intensity only from the desired tissue. Commonly, there is one saturation pulse before each excitation pulse (Fig. 15-11), although some fast imaging techniques include several excitation pulses per saturation pulse.

The most common application of spatially selective saturation pulses is to saturate magnetization from flowing blood or moving tissue (see Chapter 13). These saturation pulses are usually targeted outside the volume of interest. The magnetization of blood is thus reduced substantially before it enters the image slice, so it has less signal intensity than it would otherwise. The excitation radio pulses delivered to tissue in the image slice thus generate more signal intensity from the stationary tissue than from the saturated blood that flows into the slice. The blood vessels in the slice of interest thus have lower signal intensity and produce less artifact than on comparable images without spatial saturation pulses. Saturation pulses may also be targeted in an image slice to reduce unwanted signal intensity arising from blood vessels in the image slice itself or from moving adipose tissue.

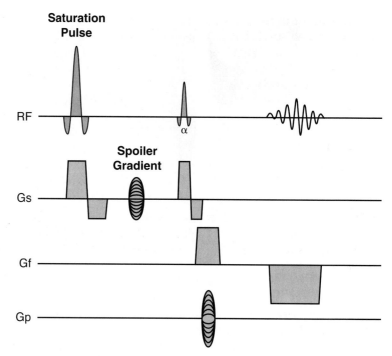

Figure 15-10
Spatially selective saturation. A spatial saturation radio pulse is targeted to a particular volume of tissue by simultaneously applying a slice-select gradient. The transverse magnetization created by this radio pulse is then dephased by a spoiler gradient.

Double Inversion Nulling of Blood Signal

The success of spatial presaturation pulses for reducing the signal intensity of blood depends on the velocity and orientation of the blood flow. It is often not possible for a given saturation pulse to be targeted so it saturates all desired blood signal, especially in complex structures such as the heart. A more successful technique involves a set of two inversion pulses.

First, a 180° inversion pulse is applied without an associated imaging gradient, inverting magnetization throughout the imaged volume. Such an inversion pulse is referred to as a *nonselective inversion*. Next, a second inversion pulse is applied during application of the slice-select gradient. This second pulse imparts an additional 180° rotation (360° total) to the spins in the slice, returning magnetization to its equilibrium state. Spins outside the slice, however, remain inverted. A TI is then chosen to allow the blood magnetization to recover to zero (about 650 msec at 1.5 T).

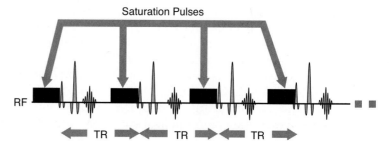

Figure 15-11
Spin echo pulse sequence with one saturation pulse prior to each excitation pulse.

During this time the nulled blood washes into the imaged slice, so that following excitation of the slice the blood is darkened more successfully than possible using simple spatial saturation.

Chemically Selective Saturation or Inversion

Saturation pulses may be targeted to certain chemical shifts rather than to spatial regions. Currently, most chemical shift saturation pulses are nonselective; that is, they are applied in the absence of imaging gradients. For example, a radio pulse with a narrow range of frequencies corresponding to the resonant frequency of methylene (CH_2) protons in adipose tissue excites these protons but has little effect on water protons (Fig. 15-12). Next, a spoiler gradient dephases the transverse magnetization created by the CH_2-selective excitation pulse (Fig. 15-13). After such a *fat saturation pulse* and the subsequent spoiler gradient, an excitation pulse creates transverse magnetization principally from water, so the signal intensity in the resulting image is mostly from water. With most current techniques, imaging gradients are turned off during application of chemically selective pulses. Therefore, chemical saturation is reapplied each time a

slice is excited, affecting all slices each time (Fig. 15-14).

The excitation flip angle of a fat saturation pulse should optimally be larger than 90° because of the short T1 of CH_2 protons in adipose tissue. Following a fat saturation pulse, longitudinal magnetization recovers so rapidly that by the time the excitation pulse occurs there is substantial recovery of lipid longitudinal magnetization. The lipid longitudinal magnetization that recovers during the time between the saturation and excitation pulses can produce substantial lipid signal intensity on the resulting image. A saturation pulse greater than 90°, however, rotates longitudinal magnetization more than 90°, so recovery to zero may occur by the time the excitation pulse is applied. In this way, lipid magnetization can be minimized. The exact optimal fat saturation flip angle varies depending on the interval between the saturation and excitation pulses, but typically it is between 100° and 130° (Fig. 15-15).

The effectiveness of fat suppression can be improved if fat and water magnetizations are out of phase when the echo is sampled. If fat and water are in phase, any incompletely saturated lipid signal adds to the water signal on the resulting image. If these magnetizations are out of phase, however, unsaturated lipid signal interferes destructively with the water signal, reducing the overall signal intensity of adipose tissue on the final image (Fig. 15-16).

A variation on the notion of selectively exciting lipid magnetization beyond zero is called spectral inversion recovery (SPIR) or spectral inversion at lipids (SPECIAL). With this technique, lipid magnetization is selectively inverted without affecting water magnetization. Then during the TI, lipid magnetization relaxes toward zero, at which time the excitation pulse occurs. Because lipid magnetization at this time is zero, only water is excited. The water magnetization was not inverted, so contrast between tissues that do not contain lipid is not affected. Other than causing suppression of lipid signals, the lipid-selective inversion does not affect the contrast of the resulting image.

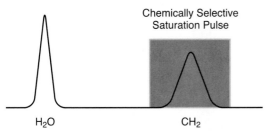

Figure 15-12
Chemically selective saturation. A chemically selective radio pulse with a frequency matching that of the undesired protons is applied to the entire volume of tissue, without a slice-select gradient. In this example, CH_2 protons are saturated (fat suppression).

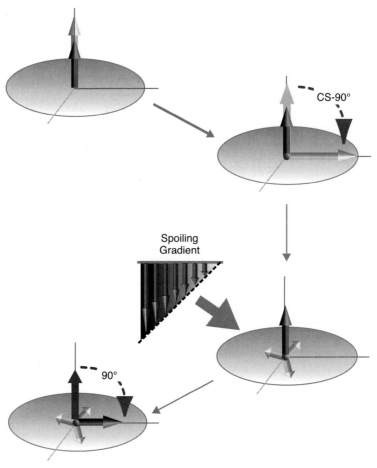

Figure 15-13

Fat saturation. A chemically selective pulse excites CH_2 magnetization (*light arrows*). The resulting transverse magnetization is then dephased by a spoiler gradient. Next, an excitation pulse excites the remaining water longitudinal magnetization (*dark arrows*), generating signal primarily from water protons.

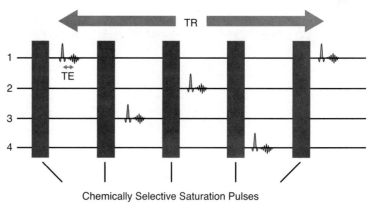

Figure 15-14

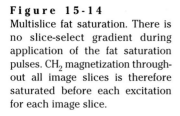

Multislice fat saturation. There is no slice-select gradient during application of the fat saturation pulses. CH_2 magnetization throughout all image slices is therefore saturated before each excitation for each image slice.

Chemically Selective Saturation Pulses

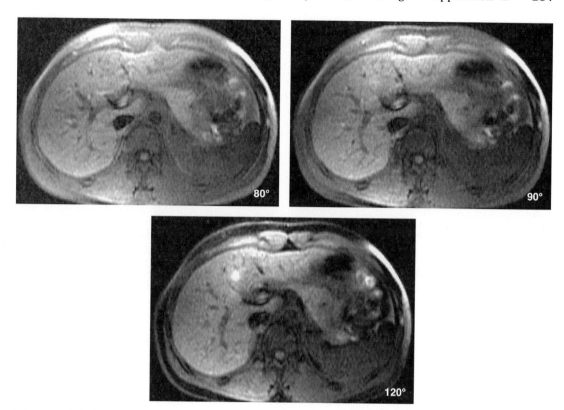

Figure 15-15

T1-weighted spin echo images showing improved fat suppression as the flip angle of the fat saturation pulse increases to 120°. A nonuniform magnetic field has caused suboptimal fat suppression, especially in the left anterior superficial region.

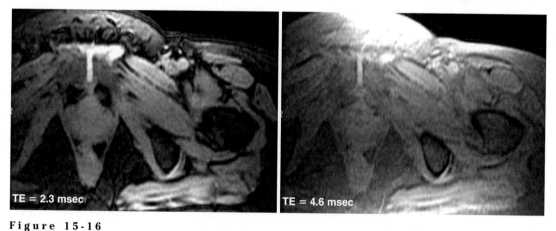

Figure 15-16

Improved fat suppression on opposed-phase, compared with in-phase, gradient echo images at 1.5 T. In a dual gradient echo sequence, fat suppression is superior on the first echo image [opposed-phase at 2.3 msec (*left*)] because of cancellation between water and unsuppressed lipid magnetizations. On the second echo image [in-phase at 4.6 msec (*right*)], unsuppressed lipid magnetization adds to the signal, reducing the effectiveness of fat suppression.

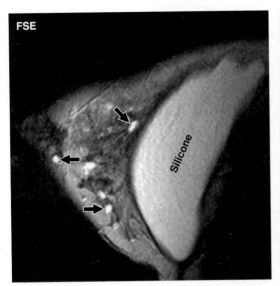 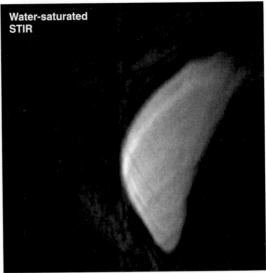

Figure 15-17
Silicone-only image obtained by combining short TI inversion recovery (STIR) and chemically selective water saturation. The T2-weighted fast spin echo (FSE) image (*left*) depicts adipose tissue, cysts (*arrows*), and silicone in a breast prosthesis as having high signal intensity. With a combination of water saturation and STIR techniques, the signal intensities due to water and fat are both suppressed, leaving only the silicone signal in the image.

Chemically selective saturation can be combined with other magnetization preparation techniques. For example, inversion recovery and chemically selective preparatory pulses can be combined to produce silicone-only images in patients with prosthetic breast implants. The STIR technique can be used to null the signal from adipose tissue, and chemically selective saturation can be used to suppress the signal from water. The only remaining signal is from silicone, which has a chemical shift different from that of CH_2 or water (Fig. 15-17).

Water Images Generated without Preparation Pulses

There are chemical shift selective methods for creating images that depict only water. They resemble fat-saturated images but do not involve any preparatory pulses.

Dixon Techniques

"Dixon techniques" utilize in-phase and opposed-phase images, as described in Chapter 5. Briefly, in-phase images are those where H_2O (water) and CH_2 (fat) magnetizations are in phase with each other, so their signals are additive. In opposed-phase images, the phases of water and CH_2 magnetizations are opposite, so they interfere destructively. In-phase and opposed-phase images can be obtained from separate acquisitions or as part of a double-echo technique. For example, at 1.5 T, following a single excitation pulse two gradient echoes can be formed and measured, with TE values of about 2.25 msec (opposed-phase) and 4.50 msec (in-phase).

For many applications, a simple comparison between these two images is a powerful method for characterizing tissue. The two images also can be used to generate calculated images that depict only water or fat. If the in-phase image is "water + fat" and the opposed-phase image is "water – fat," adding them together produces an image that is "water + water" (i.e., entirely a water signal). This image resembles a fat-suppressed image. If in-phase and opposed-phase images are subtracted, the resulting calculated image is one of fat alone, as if it were water-suppressed. Techniques that generate calculated images from two source images are referred to as *two-point Dixon techniques*.

Compared with fat suppression, calculated water images are less dependent on a highly homogeneous magnetic field and do not require a radiofrequency (RF) pulse targeted narrowly to CH_2 magnetization. Therefore, calculated water images can be generated by a magnetic resonance imaging (MRI) system with a field strength that is too low for effective fat saturation (Fig. 15-18).

There are two important disadvantages to Dixon techniques. One is that they require acquisition of two images and therefore are not as fast as single-acquisition fat-suppressed techniques. Another problem is that the two images may differ in respects other than the water-fat phases. In particular, the TE values of the two images are usually different, so tissues with a short T2 or T2* may display incorrectly. Even if an in-phase spin echo image is coupled with an opposed-phase gradient echo or offset spin echo image with identical TE values, T2* differences are depicted more prominently in the latter.

A more robust method for calculating water or fat images that corrects for T2* differences is the *three-point Dixon* technique. This technique utilizes three images where the phase difference between the first and third is 360°. For example, at 1.5 T, gradient echo images with TE values of 2.25 msec (opposed phase), 4.50 msec (in phase), and 6.75 msec (opposed phase) can be used. However, these images require more time, and the calculations are more complicated, than those for the two-point Dixon images.

Dixon techniques usually utilize gradient echo images, varying the TE to achieve in-phase and opposed-phase effects. It is also possible to use modified spin echo techniques. One method involves two acquisitions, one of which is a standard spin echo image, where the refocusing pulse occurs at one half the TE, resulting in a completely refocused spin echo. During the other acquisition, the refocusing pulse is offset from the middle of the TE, so the echo peak is sampled at an interval from the spin echo that corresponds to a 180° difference in the fat-water phase. At 1.5 T this means that it is about 2.25 msec before or after the time of complete refocusing.

It is also possible to use a double echo technique, where the first echo is a refocused spin echo, and the second, nonrefocused echo occurs at an interval that corresponds to the fat-water opposed phase. This method has been implemented on some 0.3 T systems; the initial spin echo may have a TE of 16 msec, and the second echo occurs 11 msec later, so the water and CH_2 magnetization phases are opposed. One significant problem with this method is that a tissue may have lower signal intensity on the second (opposed-phase) image because it contains water and fat, or because it has a short T2*. In other words, heterogeneous chemical shift and heterogeneous susceptibility can each cause signal intensity loss with this method unless it is implemented as a three-point Dixon technique.

Spatial-Spectral Selective Excitation

The major disadvantage of selective saturation is that an additional excitation pulse and spoiling gradient are needed. This requirement adds significantly to the acquisition time. First, lipid magnetization is excited throughout the imaged volume (i.e., without a slice-select gradient); the transverse magnetization created is then spoiled, and the remaining unsaturated (primarily water) signal is excited during application of the slice-select gradient. Because of the additional time required for

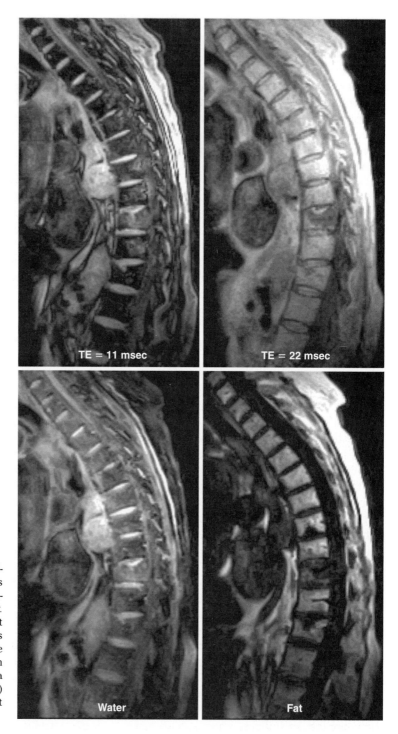

Figure 15-18
Example of two-point Dixon calculation of water and fat images from opposed-phase and in-phase images at 0.3 T. *Top left.* The first echo of a dual gradient echo image, with TE = 11 msec, is opposed-phase. *Top right.* The second echo, with 22 msec, is in phase. Addition of the raw data yields a water image (*bottom left*) and subtraction yields a fat image (*bottom right*).

the saturation process prior to each excitation pulse, fewer image slices can be excited during a given TR.

Slice-selective excitation of only water, called *spatial-spectral excitation* (or *spectral-spatial* excitation), is preferable in some respects, but it generally has not been possible with a single excitation pulse. The frequency range of a single RF pulse is chosen so it corresponds to the frequency range specified by the slice-select gradient, making sure the water and lipid in the selected slice are excited. This has not allowed use of a single RF pulse for selectively exciting water or fat.

Spatial-spectral excitation, usually used for selective excitation of water, has been implemented using composite pulses. It consists of several pulses that, in sum, provide the desired amount of rotation to water magnetization while adding to zero for CH_2 magnetization.

The spacing between these RF pulses is set as the time for water and CH_2 magnetization to reach 180° phase difference. At 1.5 T, this is about 2.25 msec. The initial excitation pulse rotates transverse magnetization from both water and CH_2 protons; the second pulse adds to the rotation of water but provides reversed rotation to CH_2 because of its phase change relative to water. When all pulses are completed, water has been excited, but the excitation of lipid magnetization has been nulled so no lipid transverse magnetization is created.

In one implementation of spatial-spectral excitation, a 90° excitation is achieved using three pulses (of 22.5°, 45.0°, and 22.5°). This is referred to as a 1-2-1 composite pulse because the middle pulse induces rotation double that of the first and third. Alternatively, four pulses of 11.25°, 33.75°, 33.75°, and 11.25° can be used, a 1-3-3-1 combination. At 1.5 T, because the pulses must be spaced by 2.25 msec, a 1-3-3-1 combination requires at least 7 msec.

As the number of component pulses increases, the precision of water excitation and CH_2 nulling increase, at the expense of increased time. The increased time not only reduces the efficiency of data acquisition (information per unit time) but also increases the TE and therefore the sensitivity to susceptibility artifacts. The 1-2-1 and 1-3-3-1 combinations have been most commonly used for clinical applications (Fig. 15-19). Although a shorter TE can be obtained using a 1-1 pulse, fat suppression is often inadequate (Fig. 15-20).

In clinical practice, spatial-spectral excitation is most useful for providing effective fat suppression as an alternative to fat saturation in two-dimensional (2D) multislice acquisitions, as it eliminates the need for multiple fat saturation pulses. In applications where the TE must be minimized (e.g., heavily T1-weighted dynamic contrast-enhanced examinations), the necessary increase in TE is prohibitive, and segmented spectral inversion is generally preferred.

Magnetization Transfer

In Chapter 7 we discussed how magnetization from macromolecular protons is saturated by radio pulses that do not correspond to the resonant frequency of water and lipid protons in an image slice. The saturated magnetization is then transferred to water protons near these macromolecules, producing decreased signal intensity from tissues that contain bound water. This process, referred to as *magnetization transfer* (MT), does not affect protons in free water or lipid molecules.

If signal intensity from tissues rich in bound water is not desired, it can be reduced by applying saturation pulses targeted to macromolecular protons. These MT saturation pulses may consist of strong pulses targeted to frequencies above or below that of the water and lipid protons in the desired image slice (Fig. 15-21).

Alternatively, a series of pulses may be targeted to the slice of interest that imparts a total of 0° or 360° of rotation to free water and lipid. Because T2 of macromolecular protons is only a fraction of a millisecond, the transverse magnetization created by exciting these protons decays so rapidly it is not returned to equilibrium by the series of pulses. Therefore, water and lipid proton magnetization is not affected, but magnetization from macromolecular protons is saturated (Fig. 15-22). By either method, MT pulses decrease the signal intensity of tissues that contain bound water (Fig. 15-23).

MT pulses are sometimes used in clinical settings where suppression of soft tissue is desirable. One example is suppression of brain or other tissue to accentuate pathological tissue that enhances after

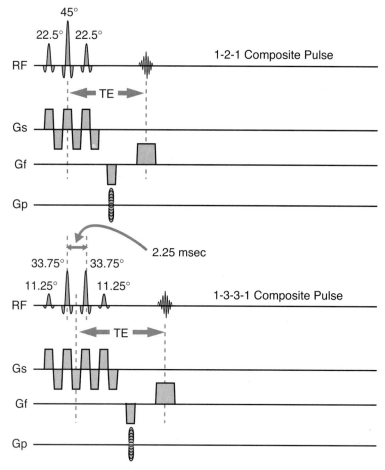

Figure 15-19

Pulse sequence diagrams for spatial-spectral excitation using 1-2-1 (*top*) and 1-3-3-1 (*bottom*) composite 90° pulses. At 1.5 T, the pulse components are 2.25 msec apart. The TE is defined as the interval between the midpoint of the composite pulse and the echo peak.

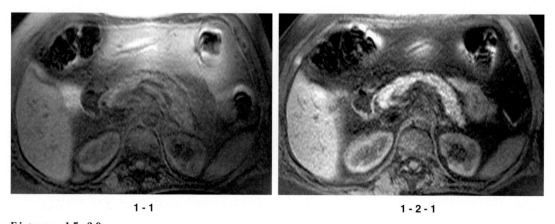

Figure 15-20

Abdominal images obtained at 1.5 T using spatial-spectral excitation, with a 1-1 composite pulse (*left*) and a 1-2-1 composite pulse (*right*). Although the TE is about 1.1 msec longer with the 1-2-1 pulse, the image quality is far superior.

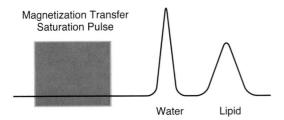

Figure 15-21
Magnetization transfer saturation pulse is applied at a frequency different from that of water or lipid, exciting the short T2 protons of macromolecules such as proteins.

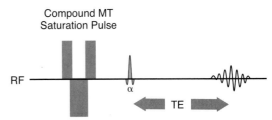

Figure 15-22
A series of pulses imparts a total of 0° rotation to water and lipid protons. The rotation of macromolecular protons is less precise, so their magnetization is partially saturated.

administration of gadolinium contrast agent; gadolinium shortens the T1 of the abnormal tissue so it recovers faster following magnetization transfer. Brain and other soft tissues may also be suppressed by MT pulses to accentuate time-of-flight effects; because most of the blood

is free fluid, it is relatively unaffected by MT pulses. Another application of MT pulses is to suppress the cartilage signal to improve its contrast relative to synovial fluid. The major disadvantage of MT pulses is that they tend to prolong the acquisition time.

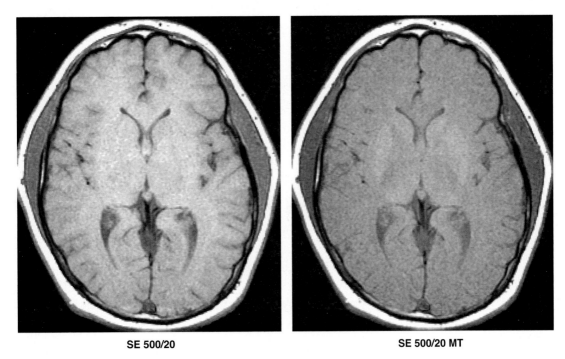

SE 500/20   SE 500/20 MT

Figure 15-23
Effect of magnetization transfer (MT) preparatory pulse on the SE 500/20 image of the brain. With the MT saturation pulse, brain parenchymal signal intensity is reduced, especially that from white matter.

Magnetization-Prepared Rapid Gradient Echo Techniques

The preparatory pulses described thus far have been applied once before each excitation pulse. Applying these preparatory pulses and associated gradients takes time. If each excitation pulse is preceded by a preparatory pulse, the number of image slices that can be acquired during a given TR decreases. The decrease in number of slices per TR or increase in acquisition time may be particularly severe for inversion recovery techniques, as data often are not acquired during the TI.

Single-Preparatory Pulse Sequences

The efficiency of magnetization-prepared pulse sequences can be improved greatly if each preparatory pulse can prepare the magnetization for more than one excitation pulse. In fact, it is possible to obtain a fast 2D acquisition that is preceded by a single preparatory pulse (Fig. 15-24). This is generally feasible only if the TR is short, as for gradient echo techniques with a TR of less than 10 msec.

Because of the short TR, small flip angles (usually 30° or less) are necessary.

Alternatively, high flip angles can be used with balanced steady-state free precession techniques (as discussed in Chapter 14), and these images can be preceded by preparatory pulses. Without preparatory pulses, these short TR gradient echo images may have little tissue contrast. In fact, the preparation pulse may be the primary determinant of tissue contrast on these images. Inversion recovery preparatory pulses can be used to acquire heavily T1-weighted images in less than 2 seconds. Examples of rapid inversion recovery–prepared gradient echo images are shown in Figure 15-25. Preceding rapid gradient echo images with spatial, chemical shift, or MT presaturation pulses can also change their appearance.

T2-weighted gradient echo images can be acquired by applying a preparatory *series* of pulses. This series typically begins with a 90° excitation pulse, which creates transverse magnetization. This is followed by a 180° refocusing pulse, which refocuses the transverse magnetization. Finally, a second 90° pulse returns the residual transverse magnetization to the longitudinal plane. The amount of transverse magnetization that is returned to the longitudinal plane depends on the T2 of the tissue. The time between the two 90° pulses is equivalent to the TE of a standard spin echo pulse sequence (Fig. 15-26).

Because contrast on the ensuing rapid gradient echo pulse sequence is affected by T2 differences among the tissues, these images are T2-weighted. T2-weighted

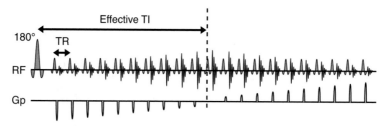

Figure 15-24

Inversion recovery-prepared rapid gradient echo pulse sequence. There is a single preparatory 180° inversion pulse before the remainder of the pulse sequence. Without this preparatory pulse there would be little tissue contrast. The inversion pulse generates T1 contrast based on the time between the inversion pulse and the weak phase-encoding gradients. This is the *effective* inversion time (TI), as the echoes that result from these weak phase-encoding gradients are used to fill the center of k-space.

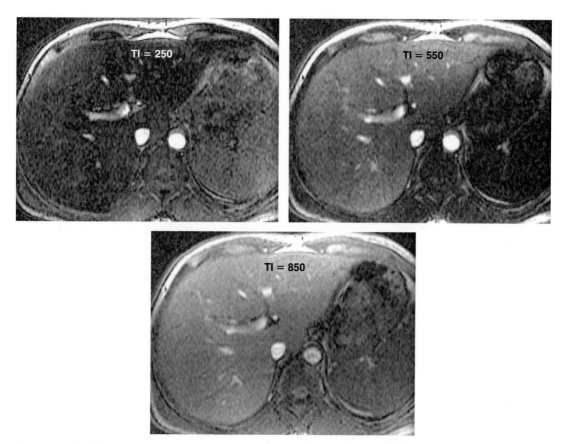

Figure 15-25
Inversion recovery–prepared rapid gradient echo images with the TI varying between 250 and 850 msec. The TR/TE/flip angle are 6.5/1.5/30°. For each image there is only one inversion pulse.

magnetization-prepared gradient echo images have not become popular because rapid T2-weighted images obtained by other techniques (see Chapter 13) generally have better image quality.

Phase-Encoding View Order

The increased efficiency afforded by using only a single preparatory pulse for magnetization-prepared gradient echo images

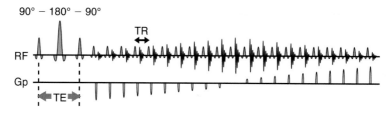

Figure 15-26
T2-weighted magnetization-prepared gradient echo pulse sequence. The initial 90° pulse creates transverse magnetization, which decays according to its T2. A 180° refocusing pulse corrects for magnetic field and chemical shift heterogeneity. A second 90° pulse rotates the persistent transverse magnetization back into the longitudinal plane. The magnetization available for the rapid gradient echo pulse sequence is therefore that of the tissues with a long T2, so the image is T2-weighted. TE is the time of the spin echo from the initial 90° excitation.

is not without cost. Throughout acquisition of the rapid gradient echo, which usually takes about 1 second, longitudinal magnetization recovers toward its baseline equilibrium value. Therefore, signals acquired at the beginning and end of the sequence have significantly different contrast. For example, consider an inversion recovery magnetization–prepared gradient echo sequence with a TI of 250 msec. The TI for the first echo is 250 msec, and that for the last echo is more than 1000 msec. This causes significant edge artifacts and image blurring and increases the importance of the order in which the phase-encoding gradient (Gp) strengths are changed.

As discussed in Chapter 6, image contrast is determined by the echoes with the weakest phase-encoding gradients. The timing relative to the preparatory pulse is therefore most important for the echoes with the weakest phase-encoding gradients. One way to ensure that the expected contrast is achieved is to obtain the echoes with weak phase-encoding gradients (i.e., the central lines of k-space) first. This order of filling k-space is referred to as *centric view order*; It is distinguished from the standard order used for conventional gradient echo and spin echo pulse sequences (*sequential order*), whereby phase-encoding gradient strength proceeds from the strongest negative one through zero and ends with the strongest positive one. Figure 15-24 shows the rapid inversion recovery–prepared gradient echo pulse sequence with sequential phase order; Figure 15-27 shows a comparable pulse sequence with centric view order.

The view order for acquiring three-dimensional Fourier transform (3D-FT) images is a bit more confusing than it is for 2D-FT images. In standard centric view order, *within a given plane of k-space*, lines may be filled in centric order (i.e., from the center to the periphery); then the next plane may be filled. Thus, many peripheral lines of k-space are filled before some lines near the center. A more robust centric order is termed *elliptical centric order*. This method of traversing 3D k-space begins at the central line and then circles through lines near the center in many planes before reaching more peripheral lines in any part of k-space.

Segmented Magnetization-Prepared Sequences

Tissue contrast can be controlled most effectively, and edge artifacts minimized, when more than one preparatory pulse is used. In a segmented variation of the magnetization-prepared gradient echo technique, several preparatory pulses are applied, each before a segment of the excitation pulses. With this modification, only a segment of the total number of views is acquired after each of several preparatory pulses. The variability of longitudinal magnetization among echoes is therefore decreased substantially. With such segmenting of the acquisition, the time that elapses during acquisition of each image is increased several-fold. Overall imaging efficiency is maintained by exciting additional slices during the intervals between a given slice's data acquisition and its next inversion pulse; however, the much longer acquisition time leads to greatly increased sensitivity to motion.

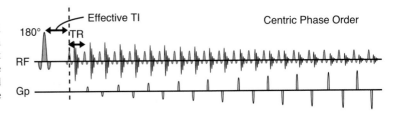

Figure 15-27
Inversion recovery–prepared gradient echo sequence with centric view order. The first echoes, with the weakest phase encoding, are the strongest and therefore determine the tissue contrast.

The segmented magnetization-prepared technique can be used for 2D multislice or 3D acquisitions. Segmented selective inversion of lipids is commonly used to provide efficient, homogeneous suppression of lipid signals for fast 3D gradient echo imaging. To reduce the TI, the inversion is reduced. For example, at 1.5 T, a TI of 150 msec is required for recovery to zero after a 180° inversion pulse, but the TI can be reduced to about 20 msec using a lower inversion pulse flip angle.

▼
Essential Points to Remember

1. Preparatory pulses are applied before an excitation pulse to alter tissue contrast or reduce the signal intensity of undesired tissues.

2. Examples of preparatory pulses are inversion, spatial saturation, chemical shift saturation, and MT saturation pulses.

3. A preparatory pulse can occur before every excitation pulse, before some pulses, or only once, before a rapid gradient echo pulse sequence (i.e., magnetization-prepared gradient echo techniques).

4. An inversion pulse rotates longitudinal magnetization 180°, converting it into negative longitudinal magnetization. Spins recover according to their T1, initially toward zero and then toward equilibrium positive magnetization. The time between the inversion and excitation pulses is the TI.

5. Following an inversion pulse and subsequent excitation pulse, the transverse magnetization created is positive, regardless of whether the longitudinal magnetization was positive or negative. Thus, the farther the positive or negative longitudinal magnetization is from zero, the greater is the resulting transverse magnetization.

6. Inversion recovery techniques can be used to null specific tissues based on their T1 values by choosing a TI so the inverted longitudinal magnetization has recovered to zero at the time of the excitation pulse.

7. Inversion recovery images where the TI is short enough to null the signal intensity of adipose tissue are called STIR images. On these images the signal intensity is greatest for tissues with a long T1, as the longitudinal magnetization of these tissues is farthest from zero.

8. On STIR images, a long T1 and long T2 both contribute to high signal intensity, rendering T1 and T2 contrast additive for most tissues.

9. Inversion recovery images with an intermediate TI can be heavily T1-weighted, depicting tissues with a long T1 as having low signal intensity.

10. On inversion recovery images with a TI of about 2000 msec, free water magnetization has relaxed to zero and is therefore nulled. These FLAIR images depict free fluid as having low signal intensity, even if they are T2-weighted owing to a long TE.

11. Spatially selective saturation pulses can be used to saturate flowing blood before it enters an image slice. It can also be used to saturate moving tissue to reduce its generation of artifacts.

12. Chemically selective saturation pulses have a narrow frequency range targeted to a specific population of protons (e.g., CH_2 protons in fat). The selectively excited spins are then spoiled, so there is little magnetization from these undesired protons at the time of the excitation pulse.

13. MT saturation pulses are targeted at frequencies other than those of water or CH_2. Macromolecular protons have extremely short T2 values and precess over an extremely wide bandwidth, so they are saturated by these off-resonance pulses. This saturation is transferred to nearby water molecules.

14. With magnetization-prepared gradient echo techniques, the contrast is determined by the *effective TI,* which is the time between the preparatory pulse and the acquisition of the center of k-space (using the lowest phase-encoding values).

15. Sequential phase-encoding order refers to beginning with strong negative phase-encoding values and progressing through zero toward high positive values.

16. *Centric phase-encoding order* refers to beginning with the weak phase-encoding values (center of k-space). With centric phase encoding, the effective TI corresponds to the delay between the preparatory pulse and the onset of the rapid gradient echo pulse sequence.

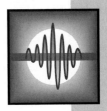

Chapter 16

Multiecho Techniques

Thus far, we have considered primarily pulse sequences in which each excitation pulse creates one signal, or echo. With such sequences, for example, 256 excitation pulses are needed to produce 256 echoes. A variety of multiecho techniques acquire more than one echo with each excitation pulse

Images with Multiple Image Contrast

Traditionally, magnetic resonance imaging (MRI) examinations have included three sets of images that emphasize the T1, T2, and proton density contrast behavior of the tissues of interest. The T1-weighted images are acquired using a short repetition time (TR). Both the T2-weighted and intermediate (proton density)-weighted scans have traditionally been acquired at a long TR, typically requiring several minutes to collect. An image with a long TR and a long echo time (TE) is relatively T2-weighted, whereas an image with a long TR and a short TE is intermediate-weighted. Repeating an entire acquisition once with a long TE and once more with a short TE doubles the total acquisition time. The long TR allows collection of many slices; but even so, there is substantial dead time between the excitation and collection of data from each slice. In particular, there is substantial dead time between an excitation pulse and sampling an echo with a long TE.

Fortunately, by applying one or more additional 180° pulses, it is possible to acquire multiple TEs following the same excitation. This, then, allows both intermediate- and T2-weighted scans to be collected in the same sequence, with no additional acquisition time required.

Consider collecting an intermediate-weighted data set with a spin echo pulse sequence having a TR of 2500 msec and a TE of 10 msec. At 5 msec after the 90° excitation pulse, a 180° radiofrequency (RF) pulse is applied, resulting in a spin echo at 10 msec. With a readout period of about 10 msec, data collection has been completed for a single k-space line from a single slice in about 15 msec (TE+0.5×readout period). This leaves a period of 2500–15 msec (nearly 2.5 seconds) before this slice needs to be excited again. Thus, 70 or more slices could easily be excited in an interleaved manner during this period; but even then much of the acquisition time would remain unused.

At the time of the spin echo (10 msec in this example), however, the spins are back in phase. If an RF pulse is applied 35 msec later (45 msec after the excitation pulse), for example, a second spin echo is formed, this time at a TE of 80 msec following the original excitation pulse, giving it stronger T2 weighting. A second line of raw data for each slice is collected during a period of

about 85 msec, leaving enough time still to interleave the collection of 30 or more slices. The end result of this process is that for each slice two lines of raw data are collected, with two contrast behaviors, contributing one line each to two images: one intermediate-weighted and one T2-weighted (Fig. 16-1).

The phase-encoding gradient is pulsed briefly prior to the first echo, resulting in phase dispersion along the phase-encoding axis that is the same for both the short and long TEs. Each line is typically acquired in the presence of a frequency-encoding gradient pulse. Because the second refocusing pulse effectively reverses the encoding of the first, whereas the data still encode the same line of k-space, the individual points are collected in reverse order so the image orientation is reversed along this line.

Techniques in which the first echo has a TE that is less than half the TE of the second echo are referred to as *asymmetrical double echo pulse sequences* (Fig. 16-1). These pulse sequences yield a second echo

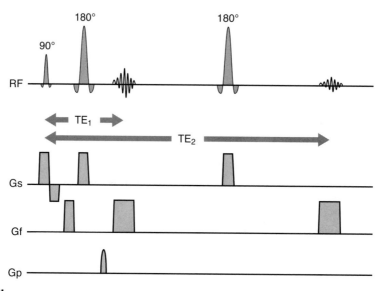

Figure 16-1
Double echo spin echo pulse sequence. Following excitation, two echoes, each refocused by a 180° pulse, are created by applying a rephasing frequency-encoding gradient (Gf) lobe for each. The second echo is of lower magnitude than the first owing to T2 relaxation. There is a single phase-encoding pulse, so the phase encoding is identical for both. Data from these two echoes are applied to different images with different TEs, one short and one long, yielding an intermediate-weighted image and a T2-weighted image.

with T2 weighting and a first echo with only minimal T2 weighting (intermediate weighting). For example, 180° refocusing pulses may be applied at 5 and 65 msec after the excitation pulse, producing echoes with TEs of 10 and 120 msec, respectively (65 msec after the excitation pulse corresponds to half the time between the TEs of 10 and 120 msec). Double echo pulse sequences, in which the second echo has a TE twice that of the first TE, are referred to as *symmetrical double echo pulse sequences* (Fig. 16-2). With symmetrical double echo sequences, the first echo image has more T2 weighting than does a first echo image acquired using the asymmetrical double echo technique.

The second echo of a symmetrical double echo technique tends to have less motion artifact than the second echo of an asymmetrical double echo technique. This is because gradient moment errors in the readout direction accumulated during the first half of the TE are compensated for by reapplying the gradients for the second echo, which results in nulling of the gradients' first moment (see Chapter 10). Figure 16-3 illustrates

images of the pelvis acquired with asymmetrical and symmetrical techniques.

Multiecho Conjugate Techniques

Multiecho techniques can be used to decrease the acquisition time in single images and generate images with different tissue contrast, as described above. With such techniques, different phase-encoding values are applied for each of the multiple echoes, so each echo fills a different line of k-space in the same image.

For such methods, some new terminology must be introduced. Each set of echoes that follows an excitation pulse is referred to as an *echo train*. The period during which these echoes are acquired is the *echo train duration,* and the number of echoes in the echo train is the *echo train length* (ETL). In this chapter, we discuss two common classes of multiecho techniques: the echo planar technique and the fast spin echo technique.

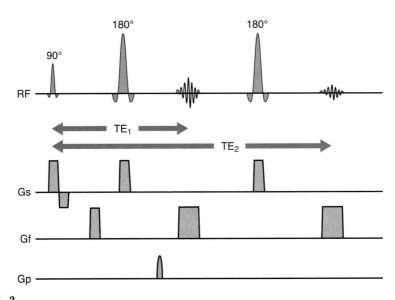

Figure 16-2
Symmetrical double echo pulse sequences. The first TE is half the second TE. The second 180° refocusing pulse occurs halfway between the two echoes, each of which has identical phase encoding.

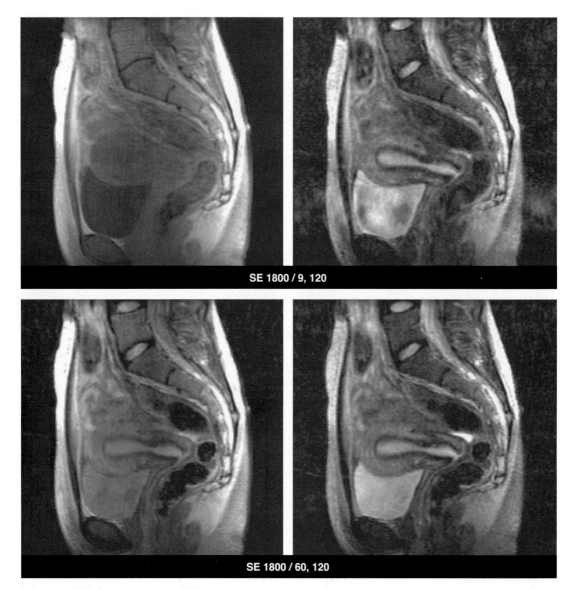

SE 1800 / 9, 120

SE 1800 / 60, 120

Figure 16-3
Double echo spin echo (SE) sagittal images of the pelvis using asymmetrical and symmetrical techniques. With the asymmetrical technique (*top*), the short TE of 9 msec for the first echo minimizes T2 weighting (note the low signal intensity of urine). With the symmetrical technique (*bottom*), both images are T2-weighted. Note that motion-induced artifacts are worse with the asymmetrical technique because of the intrinsic nulling of motion artifacts in symmetric echo acquisition.

Echo planar involves acquiring multiple gradient echoes following each excitation pulse, and fast spin echo involves acquiring multiple spin echoes following each pulse. Additional methods have been introduced that combine gradient and RF echoes. Rather than referring to the echo train length of an echo planar technique, it is more customary to refer to the number of "shots," where each shot refers to a separate *excitation* pulse. The number of signals in each shot, analogous to the echo train length, can be calculated by dividing the total number of phase-encoding values by the number of shots. In this book, we emphasize the features that the echo planar and fast spin echo techniques share, so we occasionally refer to the echo planar signals as echoes and describe the shots as echo trains.

Transverse magnetization decays throughout the echo train. That is, the transverse magnetization of any given tissue is different at the beginning of the echo train than at the end; each echo is acquired using a different TE.

As discussed previously, tissue contrast, as well as most signal intensity in an image, is dominated by the echoes acquired using the weakest phase encoding (the central lines

of k-space). These lines of k-space can be assigned to any position in the echo train by using the weakest phase-encoding value at this echo time. Thus, for a given echo train consisting of multiple TEs, the image contrast can be dominated by any of the included TEs. The TE of the echo acquired that uses a phase encoding of zero (representing the center line of k-space) is defined as the *effective TE* (TE_{ef}) (Fig. 16-4). The other echoes contribute less to image contrast and more to edge detail as the strength of the phase encoding increases. The TE_{ef} can be assigned to any echo in the echo train, including one at its beginning, middle,

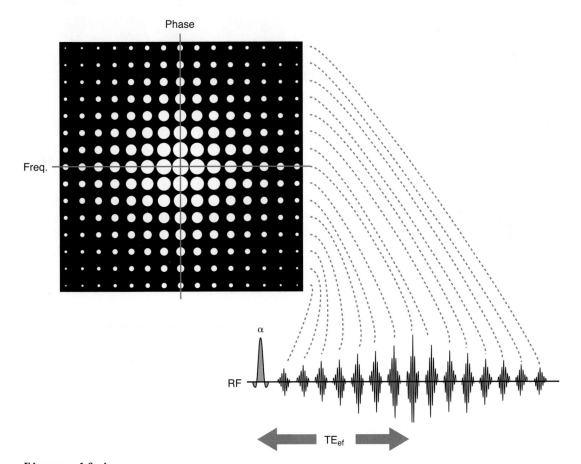

Figure 16-4
Filling of k-space for a single-shot multiecho technique. Each echo has different phase encoding. The strong phase-encoding values produce weak echoes, which fill the peripheral lines of k-space for fine detail, whereas the weak phase-encoding values produce strong echoes that fill the central lines of k-space and define the effective TE (TE_{ef}).

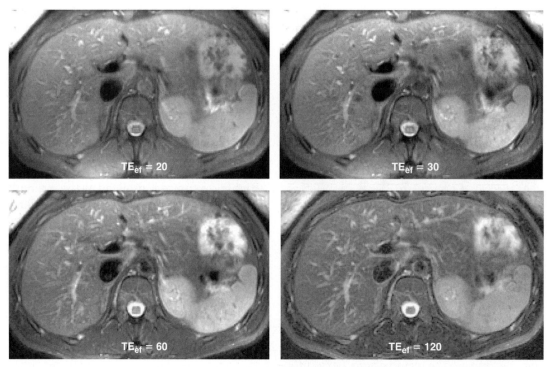

Figure 16-5
Axial fast spin echo images of the abdomen using a TR of 3000 msec and an echo train length of 16. For these images the timing of each of the 16 echoes in the echo train is identical, but the order of the phase encoding is changed so the TE_{ef} varies from 20 to 120 msec, increasing the T2 weighting.

or end. Thus, for a multiecho technique with a given echo train, there is a remarkable degree of flexibility in image contrast (Fig. 16-5). This flexibility is limited somewhat, however, by artifacts that arise from abrupt changes in signal intensity between adjacent lines of k-space.

Gross tissue contrast, at least for large objects, is not altered markedly by the presence of echoes with several TEs. The most significant artifacts of multiecho techniques are those that involve edge detail, including blurring of edges and ghost artifacts. For similar acquisition parameters and matrix, multiecho images are blurrier than their single-echo counterparts.

Blurring of multiecho images is caused by decay of transverse magnetization during the echo train. Thus, blurring is most severe for tissues with short T2s because the transverse magnetization of these tissues varies most during the echo train. Generally, images are blurriest and ghost artifacts most severe when the effective TE is near the beginning of the echo train, that is, when the TE_{ef} is short and the echo train is long.

Echo Planar Imaging

Echo planar imaging (EPI) techniques involve acquiring multiple gradient echoes per excitation. The most familiar version of such a multiecho technique is a single-shot technique in which all the gradient echoes used to form an image are obtained after a single excitation pulse. This can be accomplished by oscillating the Gf rapidly, producing numerous gradient echoes (Fig. 16-6).

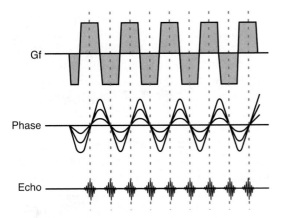

Figure 16-6
Multiple echoes can be created using the echo planar technique by oscillating the Gf. The transverse magnetization is refocused at the center of each lobe of this gradient, producing the echo.

Several methods have been used to change the amount of phase encoding of signals during the acquisition. Currently, the most common method is to "blip" the phase-encoding gradient repeatedly prior to each signal measurement. Unlike with conventional spin echo or gradient echo techniques, the strength of the phase-encoding gradient pulse is not changed. Instead, the phase-encoding of each blip is additive, so successive echoes appear in different lines of k-space (Fig. 16-7).

Single-shot echo planar images are among the most rapidly acquired magnetic resonance (MR) images, usually needing less than 100 msec for complete acquisition; however, these images require extremely rapid switching of gradients, which may not be possible with many clinical MR units. Highly optimized gradient sets are currently available that allow two-dimensional spatial encoding to be completed in less than 20 msec for images of moderate spatial resolution. Even with extremely rapid gradient switching, a finite interval is necessary to sample each signal, resulting in a relatively long duration for spatial encoding. During this time, transverse magnetization decays owing to T2* relaxation, including decay secondary to imperfections of the main and local magnetic fields and to imperfections of the magnetic gradients themselves. The relatively long encoding period results in a large chemical shift displacement along the phase-encoding direction. Therefore, EPI sequences usually

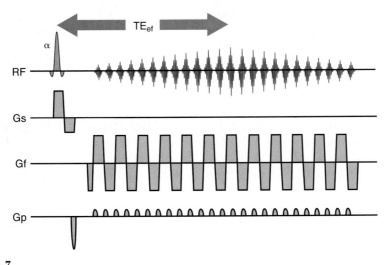

Figure 16-7
Echo planar pulse sequence, showing multiple signals created following a single excitation pulse (α). After an initial strong negative phase-encoding gradient pulse, successive weak phase-encoding gradient pulses (blips) gradually move the phase encoding toward zero, corresponding to the TE_{ef}. Further phase encoding blips incrementally increase the phase encoding.

incorporate fat suppression. Even with the best imaging systems available, the spatial resolution of single-shot echo planar images is limited by the shot duration, also referred to as the *acquisition window*. Single-shot echo planar images can be extremely T2- or T2*-weighted. As there is effectively no TR, the excitation is not repeated. This is sometimes referred to as *infinite TR*. The EPI acquisition may be preceded by a variety of preencoding pulses. If a 180° pulse is first applied, for example, the images exhibit inversion recovery contrast behavior. Magnetization transfer, chemical shift selective, flow-encoding, and other prepulses are equally easy.

The signal-to-noise ratio (SNR), spatial resolution, and reduction of some artifacts can be improved by using multishot echo planar techniques. After each excitation pulse, several, but not all, signals are obtained (Figs. 16-8 and 16-9). Thus, in contrast to single-shot techniques, there is an explicit TR. The use of multiple shots reduces the

duration of each shot, thereby reducing blurring and some other artifacts. Obtaining two or more signals for each line of k-space can also increase the SNR. Multishot images are far more sensitive to motion, however, as the overall acquisition time is longer.

T2* contrast, and artifacts from heterogeneous magnetic susceptibility, can be reduced by refocusing transverse magnetization during acquisition of the central lines of k-space. This is accomplished via a single 180° refocusing pulse timed so that the maximum refocusing occurs at the effective echo time (TE_{ef}) (Fig. 16-10). The gross contrast on these images is principally T2-weighted, rather than T2*-weighted, although susceptibility artifacts cannot be avoided entirely.

There are practical limits to the ultimate speed at which the magnetic field gradients may be switched. As the rate increases, less time is available for readout encoding of each line, so the amplitude of the gradients must be increased correspondingly (remember that the total encoding is the product of the

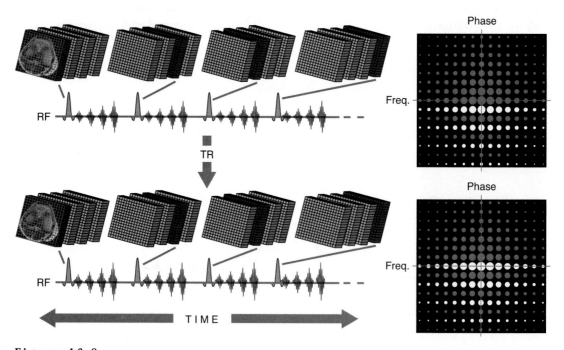

Figure 16-8

Filling of k-space in multislice, multishot echo planar techniques. In this example, four echoes follow each excitation pulse, filling four lines of k-space for a given slice. After each slice has been excited once, filling four lines of k-space for each, the slices are excited for a second time, at the TR, filling four additional lines of k-space.

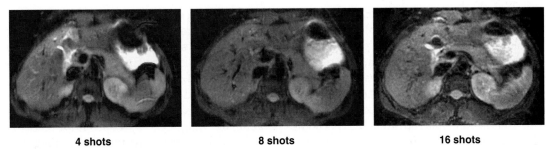

4 shots   **8 shots**   **16 shots**

Figure 16-9
Effect of the number of shots on axial echo planar images with a TR/TE$_{ef}$ ratio of 2500/60 msec. With four shots of 24 echoes each (*left*) there is substantial blurring and other artifact. Image quality improves as the acquisition is divided into a larger number of shots, such as 16 shots of six echoes each (*right*).

gradient time and the amplitude). The power required for such gradient amplifiers can be extremely large and the engineering difficult. The decreased readout period and increased gradient amplitude result in an increased bandwidth and a decrease in the SNR. More importantly, however, changing magnetic fields result in the induction of electrical currents in conductors such as the human body. Extremely high switching rates in MRI devices have been shown to induce perceptible electrical currents in patients, that can become large enough to cause pain. Commercial instruments are designed to stay safely below this operating range, but do so at a loss to the potential efficiency of echo-planar scans.

EPI methods are particularly significant when extreme imaging speed is important. Such applications include the study of rapidly moving structures such as the heart or with functional imaging of the brain (discussed in Chapter 25). The rapid acquisition time also makes single-shot EPI data relatively insensitive to gross tissue motion. As a result, diffusion-weighted imaging, whose contrast depends on microscopic motion of water molecules, is much more practical with EPI-based acquisitions.

Fast Spin Echo (Rapid Acquisition with Relaxation Enhancement, Turbo Spin Echo)

Rapid acquisition with relaxation enhancement (RARE) is the spin echo analog of EPI. Vendor-introduced terms for RARE include

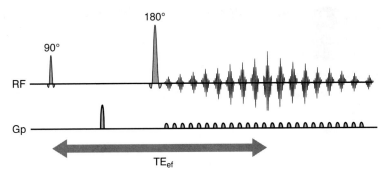

Figure 16-10
Spin echo–echo planar imaging pulse sequence. The 180° refocusing pulse occurs at half the TE$_{ef}$, refocusing the echo at this TE. Refocusing of other echoes is less complete at greater distances from the TE$_{ef}$.

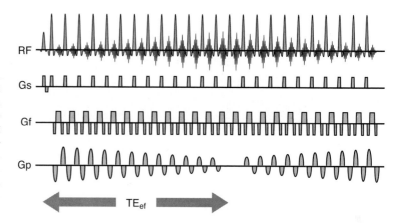

Figure 16-11
Fast spin echo pulse sequence. Multiple echoes are created following a single excitation pulse. Each echo is a spin echo refocused by a 180° refocusing pulse. The phase-encoding gradient pulse that precedes each echo has a different value, and each echo is followed by a rewinding gradient that restores phase.

fast spin echo and *turbo spin echo*. Because of wide familiarity with the term, *fast spin echo* has become an acceptable generic alternative to the less familiar term *multishot RARE*.

With fast spin echo, each raw data line is preceded by a refocusing pulse (which can be 180°, but is often less). Thus, whereas EPI involves acquisition of multiple gradient echoes per excitation pulse, fast spin echo involves acquisition of multiple spin echoes per excitation pulse. The refocusing pulses correct for magnetic field and chemical shift heterogeneity, eliminating many of the artifacts and sources of image degradation that plague EPI though they greatly increase power deposition to the subject, which can sometimes limit their use. The refocusing pulses and the slice-select gradient (Gs) pulses that accompany them add considerably to the duration of the echo train (Fig. 16-11). The refocusing pulses invert the effects of each phase-encoding pulse. It is therefore necessary to undo, and then reapply, the phase encoding with each data line, which further extends the time needed to collect each data line.

Like EPI, fast spin echo allows single-shot techniques. With the initial versions of fast spin echo the long echo train took so much time, and the effective TE was so long, that only simple fluid was depicted. Although there were some signals from tissues with short T2 relaxation times, blurring was so severe that their margins were unidentifiable. Better images are now obtained with improved implementations that use high-speed imaging gradients and partial-Fourier techniques. Examples include half-Fourier acquisition single-shot turbo spin echo (HASTE) and single-shot fast spin echo (SSFSE). With the SSFSE technique, every echo is refocused, resulting in relative insensitivity to susceptibility artifacts (Fig. 16-12). These images can be obtained in less than 0.5 second and are nearly free from visible motion-induced artifact (Fig. 16-13). Multishot fast spin echo techniques are far more common for most clinical applications (Fig. 16-14). In fact, for acquiring T2-weighted images these techniques have virtually replaced single-echo spin echo techniques in most practices.

Figure 16-12
Comparison of T2-weighted multiecho images of the brain. The multishot echo planar images (*bottom*) show mild blurring and susceptibility artifacts near the petrous air spaces (*arrows*). The images at top were acquired using a single-shot fast spin echo technique where every echo is refocused, whereas only the central echo of each echo train is refocused for echo planar images. The contrast between gray and white matter is better with echo planar imaging because of the near absence of magnetization transfer effects.

Single-Shot FSE; TE = 96 msec

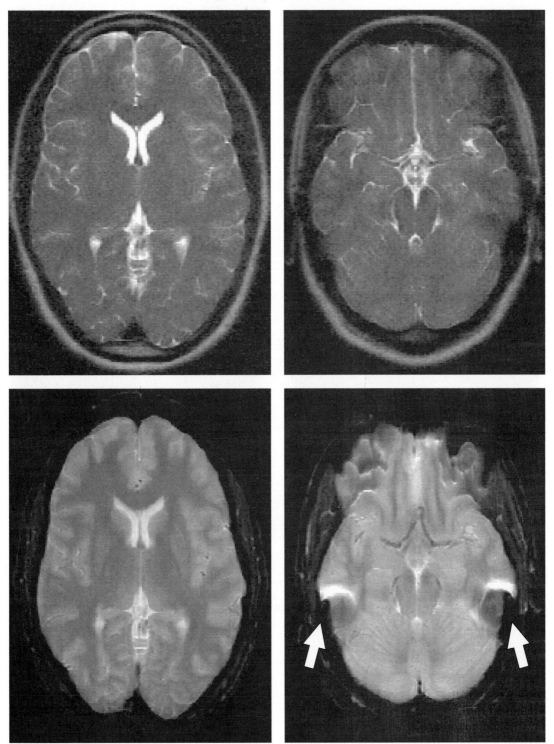

Multishot EPI; TR/TE = 3400/80

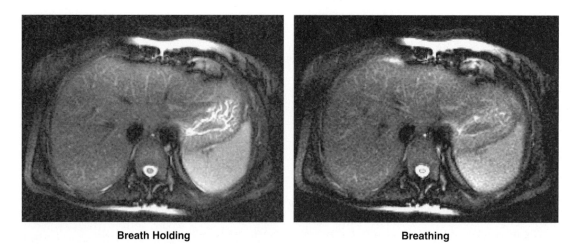

Breath Holding   **Breathing**

Figure 16-13
Single-shot fast spin echo images with a TE of 100 msec, acquired during breath holding (*left*) and during quiet breathing (*right*) show negligible artifacts even with motion.

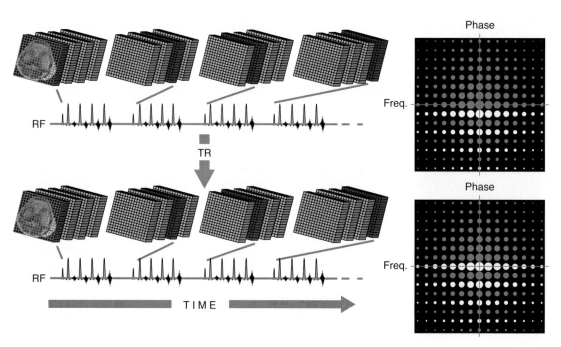

Figure 16-14
Filling of k-space by the multislice fast spin echo technique. This is similar to the filling of k-space by the multislice echo planar method (see Fig. 16-8).

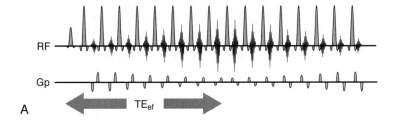

A

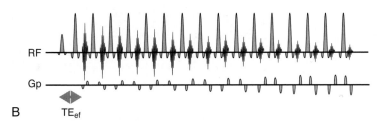

B

Figure 16-15
For a given echo train, the TE_{ef} with fast spin echo imaging can be varied by changing the order of the phase-encoding steps; the TE_{ef} is defined by the timing of zero-phase encoding. (A) TE_{ef} is defined by the middle echo in the echo train. (B) TE_{ef} is defined by the first echo.

Fast spin echo images contain several excitation pulses, each of which is followed by a train of refocusing pulses that, in turn, generate a train of spin echoes. Each of these echoes is usually free of degradation due to magnetic field and chemical shift heterogeneity. These images can have high spatial resolution and high SNR. Although fast spin echo images are subject to blurring and edge artifacts, these problems can be minimized by use of a high acquisition matrix and judicious choice of echo train length and TE_{ef} (Fig. 16-15). Generally, edge definition is sharpest with a high acquisition matrix, short echo train length, short echo train duration, and a TE_{ef} that is near the end of the echo train (Fig. 16-16).

In fast spin echo techniques, most of the time is spent applying refocusing pulses and sampling echoes. The major gain in efficiency, compared with single-echo spin echo techniques, is that during a given TE multiple echoes are acquired. This increases efficiency by a factor equal to the number of echoes obtained by the time the TE_{ef} is reached. For example, if six echoes can be obtained in 90 msec, a fast spin echo technique with an echo train of 6 and a TE_{ef} of 90 msec is six times as efficient as a

single-echo technique with a TE of 90 msec. When the echo train length increases beyond six, however, fewer image slices can be acquired if the TR remains constant. To obtain the same number of image slices using a longer echo train, it is necessary to increase the TR (Fig. 16-17). Thus, efficiency is not substantially improved once the echo train becomes longer than the TE_{ef}. Echoes acquired after the TE_{ef} contribute to image blurring but do not reduce the acquisition time of a multislice stack of images (Fig. 16-18).

There are certain situations in which the echo train should increase beyond the TE_{ef}, even though this could increase artifacts. Such situations include those in which the TR necessary to obtain the required number of image slices is shorter than the TR that would result in the desired tissue contrast (e.g., sagittal imaging of the spine) or in which a short acquisition time is essential (e.g., breath-holding imaging).

In some instances, blurring in fast spin echo images can, paradoxically, produce an appearance of edge enhancement. This is because blurring is greatest for tissues with a short T2 but minimal for those with a long T2. For example, simple fluid has crisp

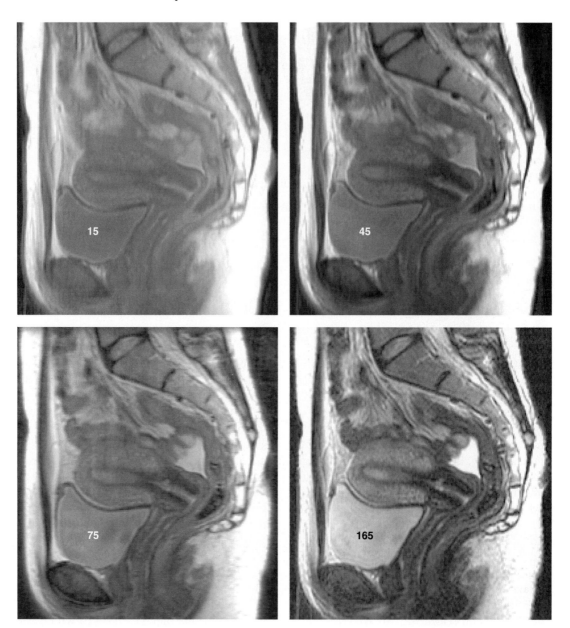

Figure 16-16
Effect of increasing the TE$_{ef}$ on sagittal fast spin echo images of the pelvis using a TR of 3000 msec and an echo train of 16. For these images, the timing of each of the 16 echoes in the train is identical, but the order of phase encoding is changed. Note that image blurring decreases and T2 weighting increases as the TE$_{ef}$ increases.

edges on long echo train images. Tissues with a short T2, however, have blurred edges. This causes some signal intensity to be mapped in adjacent pixels, increasing their apparent signal intensity. At the interface between fluid and tissues with a short T2, the short-T2 tissue's signal intensity is smeared, overlapping the signal intensity of adjacent fluid. This produces artifactual edge enhancement because the periphery of the short-T2 tissue has decreased signal intensity, whereas the margins of the

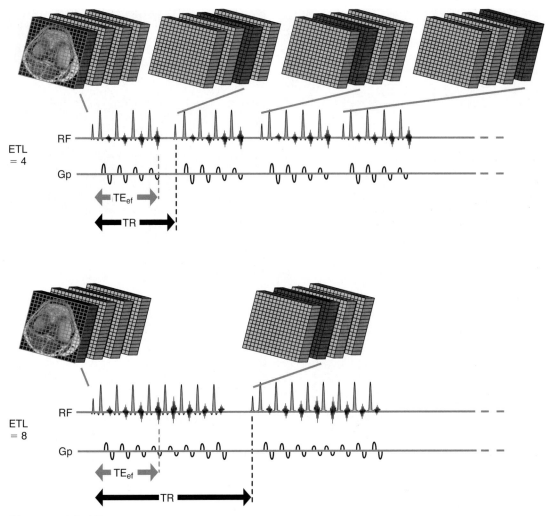

Figure 16-17

Acquisition efficiency with the multislice fast spin echo technique is not necessarily improved by increasing the echo train length (ETL) beyond that needed for a given TE_{ef}. In this example, with an ETL of 4 the TE_{ef} is defined by the last echo. With an ETL of 8 the TE_{ef} is unchanged, but only half as many image slices can be obtained during a given interval. To obtain the same number of image slices with double the ETL, the TR must be approximately doubled.

long-T2 tissue have increased signal intensity (Figs. 16-19 and 16-20).

A major determinant of efficiency with fast spin echo techniques is echo spacing (i.e., the time between echoes). If echoes are obtained rapidly, the echo train length can be long for a given echo train duration, decreasing the number of excitations that must be repeated (Fig. 16-21). Tight echo spacing also reduces many artifacts associated with fast spin echo. Therefore, minimizing echo spacing should be considered a priority when setting parameters for fast spin echo pulse sequences.

Most fast spin echo pulse sequences are implemented so as to minimize echo spacing; however, changes in bandwidth affect the duration of echo sampling and thus have a

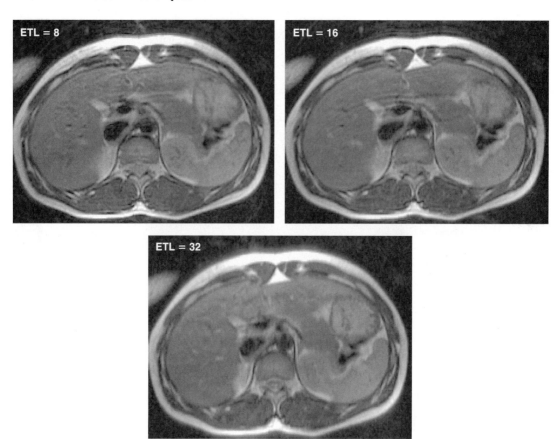

Figure 16-18
Increased blurring with increasing echo train length on axial images of the abdomen with a TR/TE$_{ef}$ ratio of 3000/100 msec.

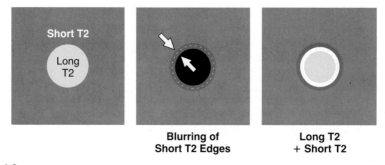

Figure 16-19
Paradoxical edge enhancement due to blurring of short-T2 tissue (e.g., brain) on fast spin echo images with a long echo train. Blurring of brain tissue causes decreased signal intensity at its margins that extends into the area occupied by a tissue with a longer T2 (e.g., fluid). The middle image depicts brain tissue with fluid omitted. The *dotted line* represents the true margin of brain tissue, and the *arrows* indicate its blurred boundary. The image at *right* depicts brain and fluid. Note the decreased signal intensity adjacent to the fluid and increased signal intensity at the edge of the fluid, the result of the summation of signal intensities from fluid and the blurred brain edge.

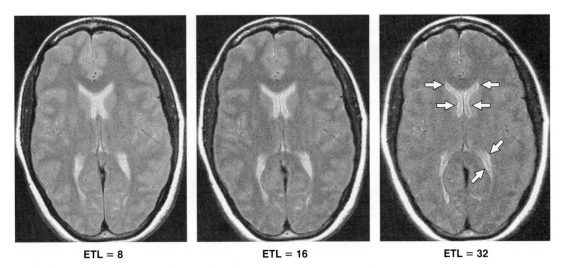

ETL = 8   ETL = 16   ETL = 32

Figure 16-20
Blurring of contrast between gray and white matter and artifactual edge enhancement of the cerebral ventricles with increasing echo train length (*arrows*).

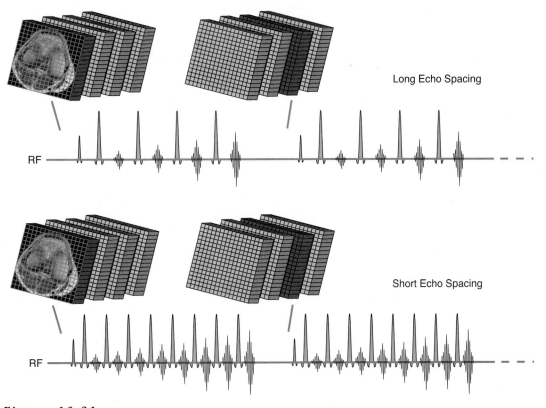

Figure 16-21
Effect of echo spacing on acquisition efficiency. With shorter echo spacing the echo train length can be increased without reducing the number of image slices obtained at a given TR.

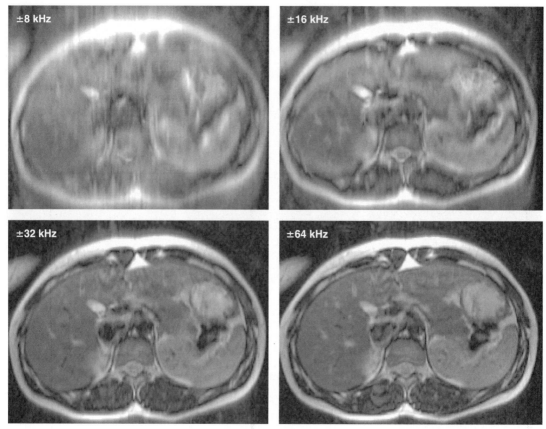

Figure 16-22

Effects of increasing the sampling bandwidth on fast spin echo 3000/100 images with an echo train of 16. With a low bandwidth the blurring artifact is severe owing to the longer echo spacing and echo train duration. Detail increases with higher bandwidth.

substantial effect on echo spacing. As the bandwidth increases, echo spacing can be decreased (Fig. 16-22). For this reason, the sampling bandwidth should be as high as possible with fast spin echo techniques unless it is limited by system hardware or the SNR. Recall that a wide bandwidth reduces the SNR.

Tissue Contrast on Fast Spin Echo Images

The principal apparent differences between contrast on fast spin echo images and conventional spin echo images with comparable TRs and TEs are that, relative to simple fluid, adipose tissue is brighter and solid tissues are darker (Fig. 16-23). These differences are the result of the more frequent application of refocusing radio pulses with fast spin echo compared with standard spin echo techniques.

The signal intensity of adipose tissue on standard spin echo T2-weighted images is lower than would be predicted from its true T2 relaxation time. This is because adipose tissue has multiple proton environments that produce many chemical shift resonances. This leads to a phenomenon known as *J coupling,* in which signal loss occurs due to interaction between different lipid

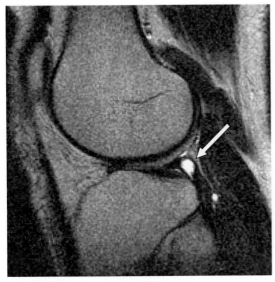

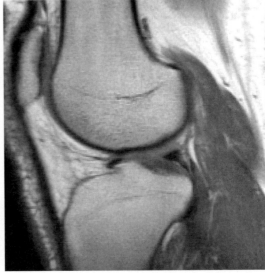

SE 2000/100   FSE 2000/105

Figure 16-23
Comparison of conventional spin echo (SE) (*left*) and fast spin echo (FSE) (*right*) T2-weighted images with similar parameters. With FSE the adipose tissue and bone marrow have higher relative signal intensity because of the higher signal intensity of lipid. Overall, the signal-to-noise ratio (SNR) and detail are higher with FSE imaging, but fluid (*arrow*) is more conspicuous with SE imaging. To depict fluid on FSE images with comparable conspicuity, a longer TE, a longer TR, driven equilibrium, fat suppression, or a combination of these factors is necessary.

resonances during the gaps between refocusing radio pulses. These gaps are large in conventional spin echo T2-weighted imaging, typically 40 msec or more. In contrast, with fast spin echo techniques, refocusing radio pulses occur much more rapidly (currently 5 to 15 msec apart), allowing less time for signal loss due to J coupling. Thus, on fast spin echo images adipose tissue has high signal intensity because the images reflect the T2 relaxation of adipose tissue more accurately than do standard spin echo T2-weighted techniques.

The relatively poor field inhomogeneity in body fat means also that as water protons diffuse through the tissue their precessional frequencies vary, and their signal becomes dephased. When the time between successive 180° pulses is kept very short, little motion occurs, and the dephasing effects are compensated. On the other hand, when the echo spacing is longer, the signal losses from diffusion are much greater. For this reason the signal intensity in physically complex tissues such as fat tends to be greater in fast spin echo sequences.

A similar effect can be seen in the apparent T2 of rapidly moving tissues, especially that of blood. With a long period between 180° pulses the tissue motion results in considerable dephasing as the blood moves from one magnetic domain to another; the measured T2 is thus extremely short. If 180° pulses are applied rapidly, as with fast spin echo imaging, the T2 of blood becomes much longer; hence, it may appear bright even on strongly T2-weighted scans.

Solid tissues have lower signal intensity using fast spin echo than on standard spin echo T2-weighted images, because magnetization transfer (MT) saturation is greater with fast spin echo. MT (see Chapter 7) involves saturation of the longitudinal magnetization of macromolecular protons such as those in protein molecules. The saturated magnetization of these macromolecular protons is transferred to water protons that are closely associated with these macromolecules. Thus, MT reduces the signal intensity of solid tissues because of their large concentrations of macromolecules. With multislice fast spin echo techniques, each refocusing radio pulse targeted to a particular image slice has the added effect of partially saturating macromolecular protons in the other imaging planes, as macromolecular protons are saturated by a wider range of RF frequencies (Fig. 16-24). The MT effects on fast spin echo

imaging can be reduced by using refocusing pulses that are less than 180°, which also reduces RF power deposition. However, substantial MT effects are unavoidable with fast spin echo imaging.

Driven Equilibrium (DRIVE; Fast Recovery)

In Chapter 14 we discussed the difference between spoiled and unspoiled gradient echo techniques. With unspoiled gradient echo techniques, transverse magnetization that does not decay between excitation pulses (because the T2 of the tissue is similar

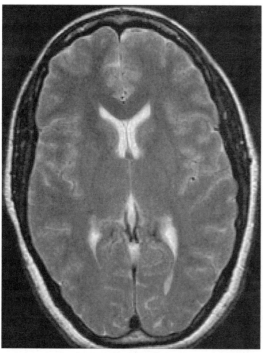 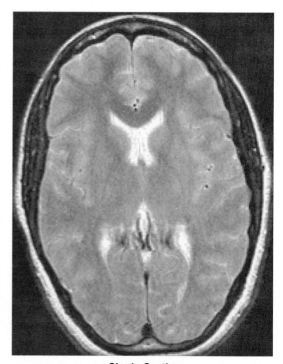

**Multisection
100% Gaps**   **Single-Section**

Figure 16-24

Effects of magnetization transfer (MT) on multislice axial fast spin echo images of the brain (TR/TE$_{ef}$ of 2000/105 msec). The images on the *left* were acquired using 100% gaps to eliminate cross-talk, but signal intensity is decreased because of MT effects. MT contrast is eliminated by using a single-slice technique (*right*). Note the higher signal intensity of brain parenchyma, especially of white matter, with the single-slice technique.

to, or longer than, the TR) is "rewound" (reverse phase-encoded), so that coherent magnetization can be returned to the longitudinal axis following successive excitation pulses. This return of nondecayed transverse magnetization to the longitudinal plane increases the signal intensity of tissues such as fluid that have a long T2.

The signal intensity of tissues with a long T2, can similarly be increased in acquisitions other than gradient echo studies. For example, T2-weighted fast spin echo pulse sequences often use TRs of 3000 msec or less; TRs such as these are comparable to or less than the T1 of free water. Because of the long T1 of free fluid, its longitudinal magnetization does not recover completely between excitation pulses. By itself, this situation causes fluid to have a lower signal intensity than if the TR were longer. However, the T2 of simple fluid may also be long enough that it is not fully decayed at the time of the next excitation pulse. If so, this residual transverse magnetization can be rewound and then returned to the longitudinal axis with a reversed 90° (–90°) pulse. This increases the signal intensity of simple fluid, as with unspoiled gradient echo techniques. This process of speeding the return of transverse magnetization to equilibrium is calle *driven equilibrium*. Vendor-specific terms for this process include DRIVE and Fast Recovery.

Gradient Recalled and Spin Echo Techniques

Gradient recalled and spin echo (GRASE) techniques are a hybrid between echo planar and fast spin echo. In echo planar imaging all echoes are gradient-refocused, whereas with fast spin echo techniques all echoes refocused by both RF and gradient echoes. With GRASE, multiple gradient echoes are acquired following each spin echo (Fig. 16-25). GRASE images thus have some of the artifacts present in echo planar images but ameliorated with fast spin echo imaging. The GRASE images are more efficient than fast spin echo images but less efficient than echo planar images (Figs. 16-26 and 16-27). Less MT contrast is present in GRASE images than in fast spin echo images because there are fewer refocusing pulses.

The major limitations of echo planar techniques relate to the length of the non-refocused echo trains. The long acquisition windows necessary to acquire the echo trains of echo planar imaging render these images subject to degradation from a heterogeneous magnetic field and chemical shift. Such artifacts can be corrected by applying 180° refocusing radio pulses. If there are fewer refocusing pulses than echoes, some

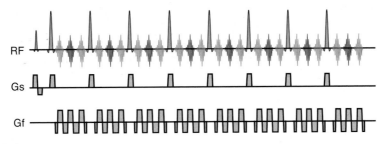

Figure 16-25
GRASE pulse sequence. In this example, there is one 180° refocusing pulse for every three echoes, producing complete refocusing for one third of the echoes and only partial refocusing for all the others. The echoes indicated in *black*, the second echo after each refocusing pulse, are spin echoes.

GRE-EPI

SE-EPI

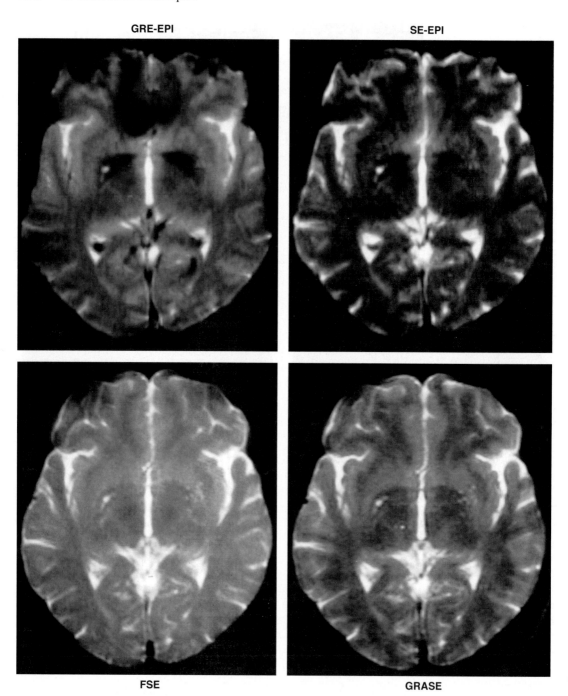

FSE

GRASE

Figure 16-26

Comparison of the axial single-shot gradient recalled and spin echo (GRASE) technique and other methods of single-shot T2-weighted images of the brain. With the gradient echo–echo planar technique (GRE-EPI) (*top left*), a susceptibility artifact from nearby bone and air has degraded the image quality. This is reduced somewhat by refocusing the echo at the center of k-space via the spin echo–echo planar technique (SE-EPI) (*top right*). The artifact is nearly eliminated by refocusing every echo using the fast spin echo (FSE) technique (*bottom left*), although magnetization transfer has reduced tissue contrast. With the GRASE technique (*bottom right*), the artifact is minimal and soft tissue contrast is preserved. (Courtesy of David A. Feinberg, M.D., Ph.D.)

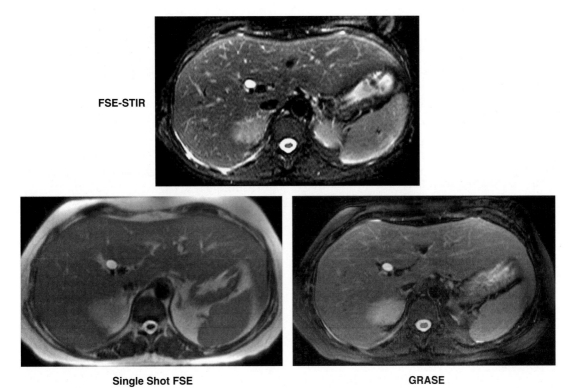

FSE-STIR

Single Shot FSE

GRASE

Figure 16-27
Comparison of the axial multishot GRASE technique and other methods of breath-holding T2-weighted images of the abdomen. With the FSE-STIR technique (*top*), additive effects of T1 and T2 differences produce strong image contrast between liver and spleen. With the single-shot FSE technique (*bottom left*), MT contrast and unsuppressed fat have reduced the conspicuousness of this contrast. With the fat-suppressed GRASE technique (*bottom right*), there is less effect from MT and the contrast is improved. (Courtesy of Neil M. Rofsky, M.D.)

of the echoes are refocused and others only partially refocused. The ratio of gradient echoes to spin echoes has been referred to as the *GRASE factor*.

At the time of this writing, clinical applications for GRASE have not been established, nor have the best methods of varying phase encoding to minimize artifacts. GRASE promises an extremely flexible platform of fast, efficient imaging, trading off efficiency for completeness of refocusing. GRASE can potentially yield a wide spectrum of control, varying the echo train length from one echo (conventional gradient echo or spin echo) to the total number of echoes (single-shot echo planar or fast spin echo imaging) and varying the GRASE factor from zero (fast spin echo) to infinity (echo planar).

▼
Essential Points to Remember

1. Two or more echoes can be acquired after each excitation pulse. If each echo is acquired using the same phase-encoding value, each may be used to provide one view for two or more images with different TEs.

2. Two or more echoes can be acquired after each excitation pulse using different phase-encoding values. These echoes can be used to fill different portions of k-space within the same image to reduce the acquisition time.

3. Images in which two or more gradient echoes are obtained per excitation pulse are referred to as *echo planar images*.

4. With echo planar imaging (EPI) techniques, the phase-encoding gradient typically is pulsed at constant strength, so that phase encoding builds up with successive pulses or "blips".

5. Images in which two or more spin echoes are obtained per excitation pulse are referred to as *fast spin echo* images, or as RARE or turbo spin echo images.

6. Compared with fast spin echo images, echo planar images are faster but have different, potentially severe artifacts and lower spatial resolution. The most problematic EPI artifacts can be addressed through the use of specialized hardware, especially with advanced gradient systems.

7. Image contrast with multiecho techniques is determined by the timing of the center of k-space within the echo train.

8. With multiecho techniques, artifacts often can be reduced by minimizing the time between echoes (the interecho interval, or echo spacing).

9. On fast spin echo images with a TR similar to, or shorter than, the TE of simple fluid, nondecayed transverse magnetization can be returned to the longitudinal axis, as with unspoiled gradient echo images. This is called *driven equilibrium*, or DRIVE, and is implemented in fast recovery fast spin echo techniques.

10. Images in which a combination of two or more gradient echoes and spin echoes are obtained per excitation pulse are referred to as *GRASE images*.

11. Echo planar, fast spin echo, or GRASE images can be obtained using single-shot techniques (only one excitation pulse) or as multishot techniques (two or more excitation pulses, each followed by the acquisition of several echoes).

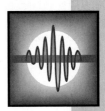

Strategies of Fast Imaging

In previous chapters we introduced the principles of magnetic resonance (MR) data acquisition and the basic building blocks of magnetic resonance imaging (MRI) pulse sequences. In later chapters, we discuss the various techniques used to obtain the sets of images desired for clinical imaging. In all instances, tradeoffs are made to generate images with satisfactory information content in the shortest amount of time. This is done to maximize patient throughput and to allow time for acquiring additional sequences. Fast imaging is also often needed to capture information about physiological events or to prevent image degradation secondary to them.

In this chapter, we review first how principles introduced in earlier chapters are implemented in various strategies to minimize the acquisition time. They included pulse sequence choices, parameter optimization, and making intelligent choices with regard to tradeoffs between anatomical coverage, the signal-to-noise ratio (SNR), spatial resolution, and the acquisition time.

In the remainder of the chapter, we discuss some recent innovations that are gradually being incorporated into clinical imaging protocols. They include several variations on filling the k-space that, alone or in combination, increase the rate at which images are generated. We also discuss parallel imaging, which uses the spatial information available from acquisitions using phased-array coils. Many of these fast imaging strategies can be used in various combinations and hybrid situations.

Conventional Strategies of Fast Imaging

Maximizing Efficiency: General Principles

In all instances, we should strive to maximize the efficiency of data acquisition, even if fast imaging is not our principal intent. Efficient data acquisition allows us to maximize the SNR or image resolution without unnecessarily prolonging the examination time. Once we have maximized the efficiency of data acquisition, we can make appropriate decisions regarding acquisition time, SNR, and spatial resolution, the three basic imaging attributes that must be balanced against each other.

In some instances we require several minutes to accumulate a large amount of data, such as in high-resolution three-dimensional data sets. The efficiency of data acquisition such as this might be higher than that of a 2-second acquisition of a single low-resolution image. We should always avoid, if possible, any intervals of time without data acquisition (dead time). This involves eliminating unnecessary pulse sequence events and the appropriate choice of parameters such as the TR and TE. Interrelationships between acquisition time, the SNR, and spatial resolution were discussed in Chapter 9. In this section, we explore how pulse sequences can be altered so more data can be acquired in less time.

Pulse Sequence Components

Some time-consuming pulse sequence components are not needed for certain applications. For example, preparatory pulses for fat suppression, flow suppression, or contrast alteration should be omitted if not required by the protocol. If they cannot be eliminated entirely, they can sometimes be applied intermittently. For example, rather than saturate fat prior to every excitation, it is often possible to saturate fat at regular intervals, such as once per 32 excitations.

Refocusing pulses, and their associated gradients, also add time to data acquisition, thereby reducing efficiency. Refocusing pulses *may* be necessary to reduce artifacts from heterogeneous chemical shift or susceptibility, as discussed in Chapter 4. If these artifacts do not present problems for a given acquisition, however, refocusing

pulses should be omitted to increase efficiency. If satisfactory image quality can be obtained, gradient echo techniques (rather than spin echo techniques) and echo planar or gradient recalled and spin echo (GRASE) techniques (rather than fast spin echo techniques) should be considered.

Repetition Time

If all other image acquisition variables are held constant, the image acquisition time is directly proportional to the TR. Therefore, the TR should be minimized whenever the resulting image characteristics are satisfactory for a given clinical application. This does not always mean that the TR should be as short as possible, however. In particular, two-dimensional (2D) multislice techniques involve exciting several image slices during a moderate to long TR, as discussed in Chapter 8. For maximizing efficiency, the critical goal is to minimize the time between excitations. For 2D multislice techniques, this means using the shortest TR *necessary to acquire the desired number of image slices*. The number of image slices excited during a given TR can be maximized by eliminating the use of preparation pulses if possible and by reducing the echo time.

Echo Time

When single-echo techniques are used, the TE should generally be the shortest possible within the constraints of the other chosen parameters and the required image contrast. If a much longer TE is desired, multiecho techniques should be considered to maintain efficiency. The goal should be continuous data acquisition, without dead time. A choice can therefore be made to minimize the TE or to accept a longer TE to improve image quality. Image quality improvements that requires a longer TE include increased spatial resolution (by increasing the number of data samples per echo) or increased SNR (by reducing the bandwidth or sampling a larger fraction of each echo).

If a longer TE is desired to achieve a particular type of image contrast or to optimize chemical shift in-phase or opposed-phase images, dead time should not be introduced unnecessarily. Rather, spatial resolution, the SNR, or both should be increased so the desired TE becomes the new "minimum" TE.

The following measures can be used to reduce the TE.

1. *Eliminate gradient moment nulling.* As discussed in Chapter 13, gradient moment nulling is used to reduce within-view phase changes due to motion. However, if the TE is sufficiently short, within-view phase changes are minimal, and gradient moment nulling is not needed. Furthermore, gradient moment nulling may *increase* motion artifacts from higher orders of motion, such as acceleration.

2. *Sample faster*, at the expense of a reduced SNR. The sampling period is decreased as the sampling bandwidth is increased. If the SNR is more than adequate, the sampling bandwidth should generally be increased. Conversely, if a longer TE is desired, one should consider reducing the sampling bandwidth to gain an increased SNR (at the cost of an increase in chemical shift and motion artifacts and possibly increased shape distortion).

3. *Obtain fewer samples.* This point was discussed in Chapter 9. The number of samples for analog-to-digital conversion is reduced using a lower spatial resolution in the frequency-encoding axis. It is also possible to reduce the number of samples without affecting spatial resolution by sampling less than a full echo. As discussed in Chapter 10, the data at the beginning and end of an echo are symmetrical, so it is not necessary to sample the entire echo. Relative to an image constructed from complete sampling of the echo, partial-echo sampling does not affect the spatial resolution; but

because there is less signal sampled, the SNR is lower.

If the resulting SNR is acceptable, partial echo sampling is generally used. Conversely, if a longer TE is desired, one should consider sampling a full echo as an alternative to reducing the sampling bandwidth; both measures increase the SNR and TE. Reducing the sampling bandwidth increases the chemical shift misregistration artifact and the signal loss due to heterogeneous susceptibility (as discussed in Chapter 4). Increasing the fraction of an echo that is sampled does not affect either of these factors.

Optimized Field of View

Imaging is most efficient when only the desired region of interest is included in the acquired image or volume; one should generally not spend time acquiring data in which one is not interested. To achieve a desired spatial resolution with a larger field of view (FOV), it is necessary to increase the image matrix, which requires additional time. Therefore, the smallest possible field of view is usually desirable. When appropriate, the FOV should be rectangular so the phase matrix resolution can be maintained while filling k-space with fewer echoes, as discussed in Chapter 7. Generally, whenever air is visible across an axis of an image, the FOV is too large in at least one axis.

Let us further consider the FOV. Increases in the FOV can be achieved in the readout axis by sampling at a higher rate without changing the gradient strength. There is no burden on imaging time, but the SNR is reduced. Such increases in the FOV can reduce wrap-around artifacts that might otherwise be present if the object being scanned is larger than the imaging FOV. Increasing the FOV in the phase-encoding direction requires either an increase in imaging time (as well as in the SNR) or a decrease in spatial resolution. Increased FOV in the slice-selection axis generally amounts to acquiring more, or thicker, slices, thereby increasing the minimum time or decreasing spatial resolution.

For many applications, a small amount of wrap-around artifact (aliasing) is acceptable, allowing tissues that are not of interest to overlap at the edges of the image. However, this must be avoided if parallel imaging (discussed later in the chapter) is used to reduce the acquisition time. With parallel imaging, uncorrected aliasing overlaps the center of the image rather than the edges.

If an image with a reduced FOV has a low SNR, there are two basic approaches for remediation. One is to increase the pixel size by using a coarser image matrix, which also reduces the acquisition time. Alternatively, one may reduce the sampling bandwidth, sample more of the echo, or acquire more signals for averaging, all of which increase the acquisition time.

Decreased Number of Averages

Sometimes increased signal averages are used to increase the signal relative to random or systematic (e.g., motion) artifacts; when this is not necessary, the number of signals averaged should be reduced to decrease the acquisition time. Because k-space is approximately symmetrical, it is not necessary to fill it completely with real data. Within a single image plane the center and one side of k-space may be filled with real data, and the other size may be filled with calculated data. With three-dimensional (3D) acquisition, the periphery of k-space may be filled with zeros to interpolate between slices (without an actual increase in resolution).

Although collection of only a fraction of the phase-encoding lines is useful for reducing the imaging time, there are cases where a better trade-off may be to collect data with the absolute minimum TE. To do so, we can take advantage of the k-space symmetry as well, this time by collecting just over half of the echo for each of the phase-encoding lines. Usually this means acquiring each line

starting near the center of k-space (with minimal gradient preencoding on the readout axis) and collecting the second half of each echo. Using extremely short echo times can reduce artifacts from field inhomogeneity, as might be caused by metal clips or implants.

Multiecho Imaging

Single-echo techniques are not efficient methods for acquiring images with a moderate or long TE. Fast spin echo or echo planar techniques should therefore be used, as discussed in Chapter 16. Optimization of multiecho T2-weighted images is discussed in Chapter 19.

For overall efficiency, single-shot and multishot techniques are similar with regard to the number of image slices obtained during a given period of time. However, there are distinct reasons to choose one over the other. Single-shot techniques tend to have less fine detail, due not only to a tendency for a low matrix, but also the necessarily variable TE of the echoes acquired, as discussed in Chapter 16. On the other hand, single-shot techniques usually have fewer motion-induced ghost artifacts. Additionally, certain edge artifacts in multishot multiecho techniques that are introduced by abrupt transitions in the filling of k-space are avoided by the continuous filling of k-space following a single excitation.

▧ Alternative Strategies of k-Space Filling

Most currently used methods fill k-space by applying frequency encoding and phase encoding sequentially; frequency encoding is accomplished during continuous application of a gradient while a signal is being sampled, whereas phase encoding is accomplished by repetitively applying a gradient pulse between signal readouts. In this manner, k-space is filled line by line, forming a cartesian (rectilinear) grid. Frequency encoding and phase encoding are not fundamentally different processes, as discussed in Chapter 7. It is possible to apply these two gradients simultaneously while sampling, filling k-space in a noncartesian manner. By varying the manner in which these gradients change strength, the k-space filling trajectories can be tailored to suit different applications.

Many of these non-cartesian methods share the feature that the center of k-space is filled more densely than the periphery.

Radial Imaging

The first MR images were reconstructed using radial k-space trajectories, but the image quality was unsatisfactory using the technology of that era. Improved gradient and radiofrequency (RF) technology has made radial and other non-cartesian methods viable options for fast imaging.

Radial imaging relies on using a combination of orthogonal gradients during readout, thereby filling k-space along diagonal lines;

there is no distinction between frequency encoding and phase encoding. These lines of k-space filling intersect in the center of k-space, so k-space is sampled more densely in the center than in the periphery (Fig. 17-1). Each line may begin in the center, so the center of k-space is filled almost immediately after excitation, reducing sensitivity to T2* and to within-view motion artifacts (Fig. 17-2). However, if radial imaging is implemented as a multishot technique, view-to-view errors can still occur. Because TR elapses between rotations however, the motion artifacts propagate radially rather than along one axis. The severity of other artifacts depends on the application. Chemical shift and susceptibility artifacts, for example, result in size-dependent blurring rather than a spatial shift.

Spiral Imaging

The most well known noncartesian method of filling k-space is spiral imaging, first described during the mid-1980s. Like radial imaging, two orthogonal gradients are

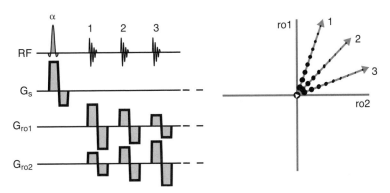

Figure 17-1

Radial imaging, implemented as a multiecho technique, is diagrammed *at left*. A radiofrequency (RF) excitation pulse α occurs during application of the slice-select gradient (G_s). Then two readout gradients, G_{ro1} and G_{ro2}, are applied simultaneously. A rephasing lobe of each gradient removes the encoding following echo sampling, so sampling the next echo begins at the center of k-space. By varying the strength of these two gradients during readout, the trajectory through k-space is altered. The k-space trajectories for these three readouts is illustrated *at right*. The k-space is filled more densely in the center than in the periphery.

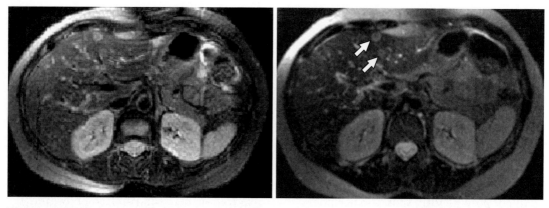

Figure 17-2
Left. Fast spin echo image obtained using two-dimensional Fourier transform (2D-FT) k-space filling. *Right.* A comparable fast spin echo image obtained using radial k-space filling shows reduced motion artifact, and somewhat better contrast. *Arrows* indicate small hepatic metastases. (From Altbach MI, Outwater EK, Trouard TP, et al: Radial fast spin-echo method for T2-weighted imaging and T2 mapping of the liver. J Magn Reson Imaging 2002;16:179–189.)

applied simultaneously. However, with spiral imaging, the gradients are oscillated during readout, producing a spiral trajectory through k-space. Data collection typically begins at the center of k-space and then curves toward its edges. Often the center of k-space is sampled more densely than the periphery, as with radial imaging (Fig. 17-3). When the center of k-space is filled first for each spiral, there is little signal decay from T2* and fewer artifacts due to motion. Under certain conditions the spiral trajectory is also self-correcting for phase errors due to motion. Usually, multiple interleaved spirals

are needed to collect enough data for an image of moderate resolution.

PROPELLER Imaging

In PROPELLER (*p*eriodically *r*otated *o*verlapping *parallel l*ines with *e*nhanced *r*econstruction) imaging, multiple sets of parallel lines (blades) in k-space are filled. The angle is then shifted, and another set of parallel lines are filled, overlapping the first in the center. This is continued until the full range of k-space is filled (Fig. 17-4).

Figure 17-3
Left. Spiral imaging, shown diagrammatically. The two readout gradients, G_{ro1} and G_{ro2}, are applied simultaneously, oscillating throughout the readout. *Right.* The k-space trajectory for two readouts.

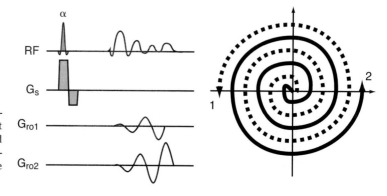

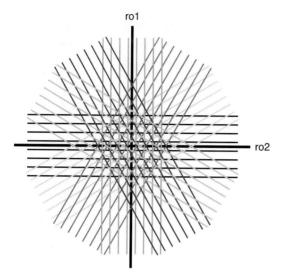

ro1

ro2

Figure 17-4
k-Space filling for PROPELLER imaging. Each "blade" consists of multiple parallel lines. Successive blades are acquired with different angles with respect to the two readout axes (ro1 and ro2) so they overlap in the center of k-space. Each blade is depicted in a different shade of gray.

Because the central region of k-space is sampled repeatedly, motion artifact is suppressed.

Common to spiral, radial, and PRO-PELLER scans is the need for special reconstruction methods, as the fast Fourier transform requires that the raw data be collected at points on a cartesian grid. Processing for noncartesian methods usually requires an interpolation step to re-grid the data. Furthermore, certain artifacts, such as chemical shift, are particularly egregious during radial and spiral imaging, and special processing steps are required to minimize them.

View Sharing

Most MRI reconstruction techniques use the acquired views to reconstruct a given image slice or volume, although the data can be shared between one or more images. This decreases the amount of data that must be newly sampled per image, thereby increasing acquisition efficiency.

One of the earliest implementations of view sharing was to increase the temporal resolution of fast MRI techniques using an approach similar to that of radiographic fluoroscopy. With the latter technique, real-time radiographic images are generated by continually replacing alternate lines in a CRT (cathode ray tracing) monitor, so that each image includes lines that were actually obtained at two different times, effectively doubling the apparent temporal resolution, although there is "temporal blurring" in that each image contains some data from the previous image. As with radiographic fluoroscopy, *MR fluoroscopy* involves intermittently refreshing some of the image data, retaining some data from the previous image but discarding the oldest data. For example, an image with 128 lines of k-space in the phase-encoding axis can be refreshed by replacing the eight oldest lines with the 8 lines most recently acquired. In this manner, 16 times as many images are generated, each different from the previous one by only 8 lines of k-space. The actual rate of data acquisition is not changed, but there is now a smooth temporal transition between images. Although this approach was first used more than a decade ago, it has only recently been widely implemented on clinical MRI units, as modern computer subsystems are now capable of extremely rapid image reconstruction.

View sharing also has been used to increase the efficiency of dual TE_{ef} fast spin echo (FSE) techniques. Standard dual TE_{ef} FSE imaging involves splitting the acquired echo train into two parts, the first used to reconstruct short TE_{ef} images and the second to reconstruct long TE_{ef} images. Views in the middle portion of the echo train, acquired with high values of the phase-encoding gradient, can be used to contribute fine detail to both images. With this technique, the center of k-space is obtained separately within each of the two echo train portions. The result is more efficient acquisition of short and long TE_{ef} images. One implementation of this method is called *sh*ared-view *a*cquisition using *r*epeated *e*choes (SHARE).

Another common use of view sharing is to double the number of portions of the cardiac cycle depicted in cine images of the heart. With extremely short TRs, multiple MR signals are obtained during a brief interval. Several of these signals (e.g., eight) can be grouped together as a cardiac segment, so several lines of k-space (views) are filled during each of these segments. Additional interpolated segments are created by combining the latter half of the views of one segment with the first half of the views of the next segment, creating a new segment that occurs between the preceding and subsequent views (Fig. 17-5).

View sharing can provide impressive reductions in imaging time. It does so, however, at the cost of complex artifacts and contrast aberrations, as the contrast or even the position of the patient may differ with its spatial encoding.

Keyhole Imaging

More recently, view sharing has been used to increase the temporal resolution of dynamic contrast-enhanced MR images, or dynamic events during functional imaging, taking advantage of the different contributions of the center and the periphery of k-space. As discussed in Chapter 8 and reinforced in later chapters, image contrast for large image features is determined by data in the center of k-space, whereas fine detail depends on data at the periphery. Therefore, a bolus of contrast agent has its greatest effects on data in the center of k-space.

A class of techniques referred to as *keyhole imaging* involves first obtaining a full sampling of k-space and then updating only the center of k-space to depict contrast enhancement once the bolus of contrast agent arrives. For example, in an image with a 256×256 matrix, the 32 central lines can be repetitively sampled as the bolus of contrast agent arrives and passes. Moreover, each of these 32 lines can be sampled more

quickly if only 32 data points (instead of 256) are frequency-encoded, thereby reducing the TE. These central 32×32 points of k-space could be used for rapid generation of images with low spatial resolution, but they would be degraded because of blurring and a truncation artifact. To improve the appearance of these images, the keyhole technique reuses the remaining reference data points from the original 256×256 image obtained before the contrast agent bolus. The result is rapid generation of new images that have the same apparent spatial resolution as the initial baseline image but depict changing image contrast with more than an eightfold improvement in the temporal resolution.

There are two major limitations to such basic keyhole imaging techniques. One is that there must be no significant anatomical motion between the baseline higher resolution images and the dynamic contrast-enhanced images. Otherwise, there would be misregistration between the contrast and the fine detail of the image, which would defeat the purpose of including the fine detail. Additionally, keyhole imaging may distort changes in the fine detail caused by the contrast agent bolus, such as enhancement of small vessels or a finely heterogeneous pattern of tissue morphology. Keyhole imaging is therefore most useful for depicting large or medium-sized vessels or bulk tissue enhancement.

These limitations of keyhole imaging may be reduced by hybrid implementations that intermittently update peripheral views. For example, the central views might be updated once per image, with only one third of the peripheral views for each image. The periphery of k-space is therefore filled in an interleaved manner (Fig. 17-6). This has been applied to 3D MR angiography (MRA) and contrast-enhanced applications using a technique called 3D *t*ime-*r*esolved *i*maging of *c*ontrast *k*inetics (3D-TRICKS) (Fig. 17-7). At the time of this writing, these newer methods have not been optimized or, in some cases, even incorporated into clinical instruments. As a consequence, image

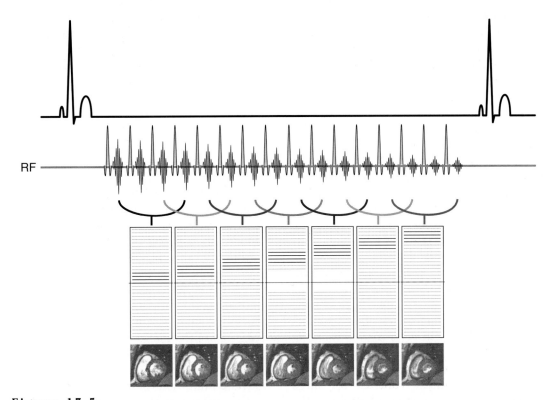

Figure 17-5
View sharing, implemented for segmented cine cardiac imaging. In this example, there are four echoes (views) per segment, providing four lines of k-space. Sampling for the first image at the left begins at the center of k-space. The next image shares two of the views from the first image and two of the views from the third image. Therefore, the 16 echoes provide data for seven cardiac phases rather than only four.

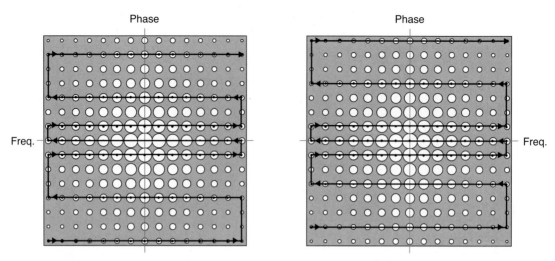

Figure 17-6
Example of a k-space trajectory that samples the center of k-space more frequently than the periphery. The first two passes through k-space are shown.

reconstruction times may be impractically long, or other features may be incomplete.

When hybrid keyhole techniques are implemented with gradient echo, spin echo, or FSE sequences, the filling of k-space by each MR signal is determined by the strength of the phase-encoding gradient. When keyhole techniques are implemented with multishot echo planar acquisitions, however, a different approach is needed. This is because with echo planar shot the phase encoding builds up cumulatively as the phase-encoding gradient is repetitively blipped. However, the density at which k-space is filled using echo planar techniques can be varied if the strength of these blips is changed. This is illustrated in Figure 17-8, where the high negative views of k-space are filled initially. Then the center of k-space is filled more densely by reducing the strength of the phase-encoding blips. Finally, the high positive views of k-space are filled less densely by increasing the strength of the gradient blips to that used for the initial high negative views. The process is repeated for the next excitation but altering the initial phase-encoding preparation so the k-space trajectory begins on a different line.

With many keyhole implementations the center of k-space is filled in stripes, so frequency-encoding resolution is maintained for the updated information. However, phase-encoded resolution depends on reusing information from the initial reference image. One novel variation is to alternate the phase and frequency axes, so updated images include new high resolution from alternate axes, and the central square is updated for every image. This approach as been called *ph*ase *r*ead *e*xchange *k*eyhole (PHREAK).

The above survey of uses of the concept of view sharing is not meant to be exhaustive, and it is anticipated that innovative combinations of these and other methods, often combined with other approaches to fast imaging, will continue to increase the rapidity and quality of fast imaging for clinical MRI.

Parallel Imaging

Acquisition time can be decreased greatly, at the expense of the SNR, by using the spatial information available when phased-array coils are used. With the standard

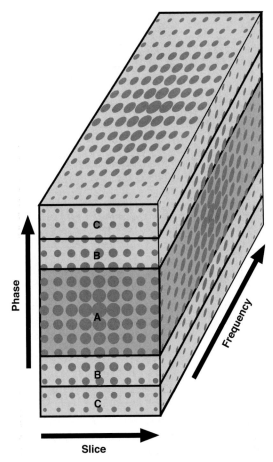

Phase

Slice

Frequency

C
B
A
B
C

Figure 17-7
The k-space segments for one implementation of 3D time-resolved imaging of contrast kinetics (3D-TRICKS). For the first image, all of k-space is sampled (C-B-A-B-C). In the next image, the views of B are re-used, along with the newly sampled B-A-B views. In the third image, the B views are reused, and C-A-C views are replaced. In this manner, temporal resolution for depicting gross contrast is doubled, while spatial resolution is maintained.

The use of phased-array coil elements to augment spatial localization is referred to generically as *parallel imaging*. The two most widely used techniques, which are similar to each other, are SENSE (*sen*sitivity *en*coding) and SMASH (*s*imultaneous *a*cquisition of *s*patial *h*armonics). A more recent hybrid that combines features of each is SPACE-RIP (*s*ensitivity *p*rofiles from an *a*rray of *c*oils for *e*ncoding and *r*econstruction *in p*arallel), which is essentially an extension of the SENSE technique for large-coil arrays.

Most current implementations of parallel imaging allow improvement of the temporal resolution by a factor of one half the number of coil elements. For 3D Fourier transform (3D-FT) acquisitions, parallel imaging can be applied in both the phase- and slice-encoding axes, allowing an improvement equal to the number of coil elements. The recent introduction of parallel imaging as a clinical technique has spurred equipment vendors to expand the number of receiver channels available for simultaneous reception and to optimize multicoil geometry for parallel imaging.

With parallel imaging the acquisition time is reduced by undersampling k-space. This reduced number of MR signals fills k-space less densely in the phase axis, which ordinarily would reduce the FOV. For example, if every other line of phase encoding were omitted, it would reduce the FOV by half (as discussed in Chapter 7). Without any form of correction, this produces severe aliasing, as a given phase change might arise from two locations, at one end of the image or the other along the phase-encoding axis. Phase-encoding ambiguity, such as this, generally results in an image degraded by a fold-over artifact. The various forms of parallel imaging use the spatial information available from a phased-array coil to resolve this ambiguity and produce an image without fold-over. SENSE, SMASH, and other forms of parallel imaging differ primarily in the mathematical model used to compensate for the missing phase-encoding values.

With SENSE, each component of the image is weighted according to the local

phased-array detectors, imaging data from two or more coil-receiver pairs are combined for each line of k-space to improve the SNR. However, the use of separate signals from different receiver coils contains potential spatial information that is not used with these standard techniques. That is, the different signal strengths from a given location detected by different coils can be used to help determine the spatial location of the signals.

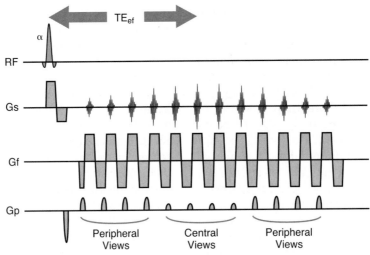

Figure 17-8
Pulse sequence diagram of a multishot echo planar implementation that samples the center of k-space more densely than the periphery. The stronger blips of the phase-encoding gradient at the beginning and end of each shot cause larger differences between the position in k-space of the peripheral lines compared to the smaller blips, which correspond to the center of k-space. If the initial negative phase-encoding gradient strength is changed, the trajectory begins at a different place, allowing interleaving of the lines in the periphery of k-space, as shown in Fig. 17-6.

sensitivity of each coil, allowing separation of aliased pixels by means of linear algebra, essentially "unwrapping" the image on a pixel-by-pixel basis (Fig. 17-9). It is generally a robust method that preserves much of the image quality, but it requires detailed coil sensitivity maps, and reconstruction times are currently long. The image quality depends on an accurate estimate of the coil sensitivity profile, which may be difficult to achieve.

The standard implementation of SMASH relies on a linear combination of component coil signals to emulate the effects of encoding gradients. Because the received signal is modulated by the strength of the

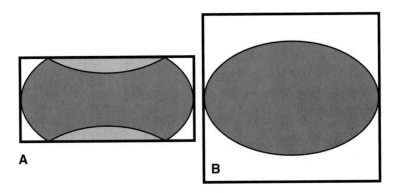

Figure 17-9
"Unwrapping" of an image using SENSE. By sampling k-space half as densely as if SENSE were not used, an image with a small field of view is obtained. (*A*) There is a severe wrap-around artifact. (*B*) SENSE is used to fill in the missing k-space lines, "unwrapping" the image.

phase-encoding gradient, as well as by the sensitivity profile of a given coil component, the spatial information received by each coil differs from that of the others, even though the gradient-induced phase change may have been the same. This allows simultaneous generation of more than one line of k-space per phase-encoding value by using the spatial harmonics that result from different signal modulations by the different coil components. Therefore, even though fewer MR signals are sampled, the density of k-space filling is maintained.

The reconstruction of an unaliased image by SENSE involves the generation of pixels to fill in the remainder of the image using pixel data from a reference image of coil sensitivity; it thus occurs in the image domain. Reconstruction by SMASH, however, occurs in the Fourier domain in that k-space is directly filled with the calculated data. Compared with SENSE, some versions of SMASH have more restrictions with regard to phased-array coil composition, imaging plane, and k-space trajectory; and they may produce more artifacts. However, SMASH generally requires only a linear sensitivity map, and reconstruction times are generally shorter than they are for SENSE. Newer variants of SMASH have allowed nonlinear coil arrays and various k-space trajectories to be used.

Parallel imaging greatly extends the flexibility of fast MR techniques. Improved temporal resolution allows greater imaging of physiological motion such as cardiac activity, improved depiction of contrast enhancement, greater anatomical coverage, and improved spatial resolution during a given interval, such as suspended respiration.

The major disadvantage of parallel imaging is its loss of the SNR when compared to simple reconstruction from multicoil arrays, as the data from the various phased-array coil elements no longer are combined for each view of k-space. The direct impact on the SNR is proportional to the square root of the improvement in temporal resolution, which is the factor by which the number of data samples is reduced. However, the impact on the SNR often appears to be less, particularly for echo train techniques.

For echo train techniques such as fast spin echo and echo planar techniques, parallel imaging can be used to generate images with comparable spatial resolution and reduced echo train length. The reduced echo train length, in turn, allows an increased number of excitations per repetition time. For example, consider a set of FSE images with an echo train length of 32 and an echo spacing of 10 msec. The duration of the entire echo train is therefore 320 msec. For many tissues the echoes toward the end of the echo train have low amplitude, resulting in blurring and a reduced SNR. Parallel imaging with a four-channel phased-array system may allow the echo train length to be reduced to 16, allowing twice as many image slices to be excited between excitation pulses if the TR is unchanged. Although there are half as many echoes sampled for each image, the duration of the echo train is reduced to 160 msec; the echoes at the end of this shorter echo train suffer far less signal decay than they would have with an echo train length of 32. Therefore, image sharpness is increased, the SNR is relatively preserved, and the contrast is more consistent. The comparison between images obtained with and without parallel imaging varies depending on the T2 of the tissues; but for many body parts, parallel imaging often improves the image quality even though data from fewer signals are applied to each image.

With SENSE, it is particularly important that the intended FOV of the final image be large enough to include all pertinent anatomy. With conventional imaging, artifacts due to aliasing result in wrap-around at the periphery of the image, which is often acceptable for clinical imaging so long as the wrap-around does not obscure the tissues of major interest. SENSE, however, involves acquiring an image with severe aliasing and then "unwrapping" the image. If the FOV is too small, the aliasing is only partially corrected. The residual aliasing remains in the center of the image, rather than at its periphery (Fig. 17-10).

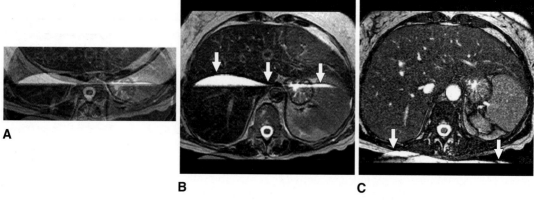

Figure 17-10

Central wrap-around artifact in an image acquired with SENSE due to an insufficient field of view. By sampling k-space half as densely as if SENSE were not used, an image with a small field of view is obtained, acquired using the single shot fast spin echo technique (TE$_{ef}$ = 200 msec) with only 51 echoes. (*A*) There is a severe wrap-around artifact. (*B*) SENSE is used to fill in the missing k-space lines, "unwrapping" the image. However, residual wrap-around artifact remains, projected over the center of the image (*arrows*). (*C*) A balanced steady-state free precession image (5/2.5/80°), acquired without SENSE, is shown for comparison, depicting typical wrap-around of anterior adipose tissue so it is projected over the posterior part of the image (*arrows*).

▼
Essential Points to Remember

1. To maximize efficiency, data should usually be acquired continually, without dead-time. The competing importance of the SNR, spatial resolution, and acquisition time should be balanced.

2. Eliminating unnecessary preparatory and refocusing pulses reduces the acquisition time.

3. Efficiency is improved, and the acquisition time is reduced, if the TE is as short as possible.

4. The TE can be reduced by avoiding gradient moment nulling, increasing the bandwidth, and reducing the resolution in the frequency-encoding axis (which reduces the number of samples measured per echo).

5. Spatial resolution in images with a given matrix is improved by using a smaller FOV.

6. If air is present across one axis of an image, the FOV is not optimized.

7. When appropriate, the FOV should be rectangular to reduce the number of phase-encoding views needed to achieve the desired spatial resolution.

8. When the SNR is adequate, the number of signals averaged should be reduced to decrease the acquisition time.

9. Single-shot techniques are not necessarily more efficient than multishot techniques for acquiring images at multiple locations, but they are less sensitive to motion-induced ghost artifacts.

10. Methods such as echo-planar imaging or spiral scanning that use the gradients at or near their maximum amplitude result in shorter encoding times.

11. Views at the periphery of k-space can be shared by one or more images to improve acquisition efficiency. Examples include dual-TE FSE, MR fluoroscopy, and keyhole imaging.

12. With parallel imaging methods, the position-dependent differences in the signals received by the elements of a phased-array surface coil can be used to generate several lines of k-space from each echo sampled, reducing the number of phase-encoding views required.

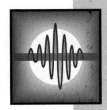

Chapter 18

T1-Weighted Pulse Sequences

Most applications of magnetic resonance imaging (MRI) involve obtaining at least one set of images emphasizing T1 differences between tissues. T1-weighted images without fat suppression are also useful for depicting adipose tissue as high signal intensity, which can help define anatomy in many body parts. Many methods are currently available for accomplishing this. In this chapter, some of the basic T1-weighted techniques introduced in the previous sections are reconsidered and put into perspective.

Spin Echo

During the first two decades of clinical MRI, the conventional spin echo technique (Fig. 18-1) was the most common method for acquiring T1-weighted images. Using the optimized spin echo technique, high-quality images with moderate T1-weighting can be obtained within a few minutes with few artifacts for much of the body. Of all techniques, T1-weighted spin echo images are perhaps the most robust and the most forgiving of hardware limitations.

Generally, the repetition time (TR) is 600 msec or less for T1-weighted images. As field strength decreases, shorter TRs are needed. One limitation that results is that only a few image slices can be acquired per TR. With modern software, however, this limitation is not significant because several sets of images can be programmed simultaneously and acquired sequentially. For example, two sets of images with a TR of 300 msec can be acquired as simply and as rapidly as one set of images with a TR of 600 msec, whereas the T1 contrast of the former is superior (Fig. 18-2).

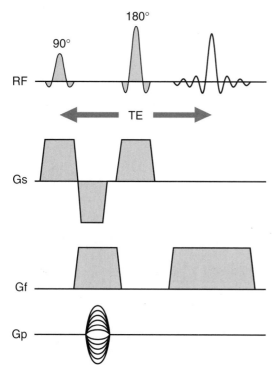

Figure 18-1
Standard spin echo pulse sequence for T1-weighted spin echo images.

do not contain refocusing radio pulses. This introduces additional T2 contrast and permits fewer image slices per TR. Thus, the two major limitations of the spin echo technique for acquisition of T1-weighted images are contamination by inclusion of T2 contrast and a long acquisition time. For both of these reasons, gradient echo images with minimized TE are becoming more popular for T1-weighted imaging. For applications where some inclusion of T2 contrast is acceptable or even desirable, and where minimized acquisition time is not essential, the spin echo technique remains attractive for generating T1-weighted images. An example is much of musculoskeletal imaging, where an acquisition time of several minutes is often acceptable and where inclusion of some T2 contrast facilitates recognition of menisci, tendons, and ligaments on "T1-weighted" images.

Inversion Recovery

Inversion recovery techniques can be used to achieve stronger, more flexible T1 contrast on spin echo images than can be achieved using the conventional spin echo technique. As discussed in Chapter 12, spin echo inversion recovery images are acquired by preceding each excitation pulse with an inversion pulse (Fig. 18-4).

On conventional T1-weighted images, tissues with a short T1 are depicted as having high signal intensity. Heavily T1-weighted images with this appearance can be obtained by applying an excitation pulse at a time after inversion (TI) so a tissue with a long TE is nulled; tissues with shorter T1 relaxation times have higher signal intensity because they have passed their null point. The use of an inversion pulse does not decrease the contribution of T2 contrast due to the TE; rather, it improves the dynamic range of T1 contrast and thus exaggerates depiction of T1 contrast

The echo time (TE) is at least as critical a factor as the TR for maximizing contrast in T1-weighted spin echo images. Quite simply: the shorter, the better. During the TE, transverse magnetization decays depending on the T2, reducing the signal-to-noise ratio (SNR) but, more importantly, introducing T2 contrast. Because T2 contrast works in opposition to T1 contrast for most tissue comparisons, T2 contrast is generally undesirable on T1-weighted images. T2 contrast can be minimized by using the shortest possible TE (Fig. 18-3).

Because a certain amount of time is required to produce a refocusing radio pulse and its associated imaging gradients, spin echo techniques require a longer TE than comparable gradient echo techniques, which

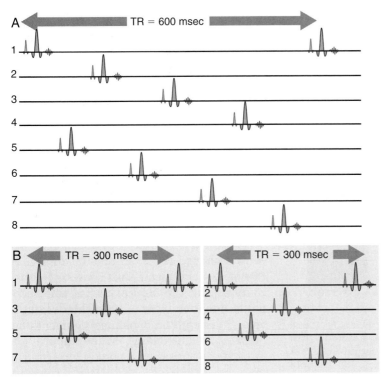

Figure 18-2
(A) Eight image slices are acquired in a single spin echo acquisition with a TR of 600 msec. (B) Four images are acquired in each of two interleaved spin echo acquisitions with a TR of 300 msec, each of which is acquired in half the time because of the shorter TR. The result is improved T1-weighting without increasing the total acquisition time.

beyond that depicted on standard spin echo T1-weighted images.

Inversion recovery spin echo images have stronger T1-weighted contrast than do comparable conventional spin echo images, but the acquisition time is increased considerably and the SNR is usually lower. Given the wide choice of currently available techniques, a technique with a lower SNR and longer acquisition time is rarely preferred. Therefore, the inversion recovery technique is rarely used to obtain spin echo images with "conventional" T1 contrast (short T1 depicted as high signal intensity).

The spin echo inversion recovery technique is often used to obtain inverse T1-weighted contrast, where tissues with a long T1 have high signal intensity, for short TI inversion recovery (STIR) images. These images are often substituted for fat-suppressed T2-weighted images, particularly at lower field strengths.

Multislice Spoiled Gradient Echo

As discussed in Chapter 14, T1-weighting is achieved on gradient echo techniques by spoiling the transverse magnetization prior to each excitation pulse, either by gradient-induced dephasing or inherent dephasing within the excitation pulses themselves. Multislice spoiled gradient echo images are acquired in a manner similar to that used for multislice spin echo images but without the refocusing pulses and their associated imaging gradients. The greater simplicity of gradient echo techniques, compared with spin echo techniques, allows the use of shorter TEs. As the TE is reduced, more image slices can be obtained for a given TR, improving efficiency. Therefore, with appropriate hardware and software, multislice

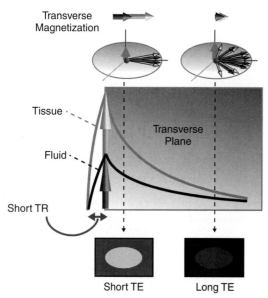

Figure 18-3

Degradation of T1 contrast by a long TE in a pulse sequence with short TR. Tissue with a short T1 (*light arrow*) recovers more longitudinal magnetization than does fluid with a long T1 (*dark arrow*). *Top.* Decay of transverse magnetization for tissue and fluid is indicated by spreading, respectively, of *light arrows* and *dark arrows. Bottom.* Contrast between fluid (*dark rectangle*) and tissue (*light oval*) is indicated. With a short TE, tissue has high signal intensity, so the image is T1-weighted. With a long TE, transverse magnetization has decayed faster for tissue, so there is less contrast.

spoiled gradient echo images can have equivalent or better T1 contrast and a higher SNR per unit time than comparable spin echo images. The reduced acquisition time can be used to allow breath holding or dynamic scanning after the injection of contrast material (Fig. 18-5).

Artifacts caused by magnetic field heterogeneity can limit some gradient echo images. However, this is not a significant problem with most gradient echo images optimized for T1 contrast because their short TEs and high sampling bandwidth reduce the severity of these artifacts.

As the TE is changed on spoiled gradient echo images, signal intensity oscillates owing to chemical shift heterogeneity, complicating the clinical use of this technique for obtaining T1-weighted images (see T1-Weighted Chemical Shift Pulse Sequences). Depending on the application, fat–water in-phase or opposed-phase images may be preferred, and tissue contrast can be significantly different. Fat–water effects must be carefully considered when choosing the TE for T1-weighted gradient echo images.

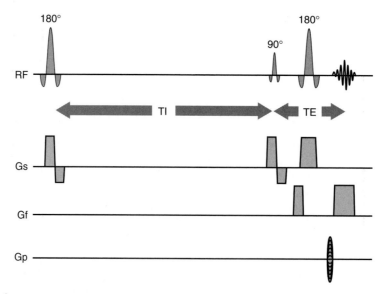

Figure 18-4

Spin echo inversion recovery pulse sequence. A 180° inversion radio pulse inverts magnetization for the selected slice, defined by Gs. Following TI, a 90° excitation pulse creates transverse magnetization, which is refocused by a 180° refocusing pulse and detected at TE.

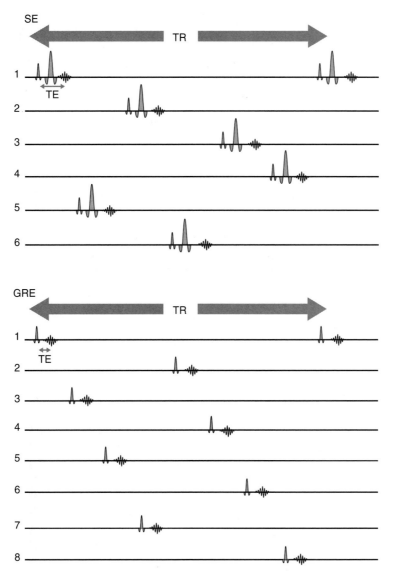

Figure 18-5
Comparison of spin echo (SE) and gradient echo (GRE) techniques. The absence of refocusing pulses in gradient echo techniques allows the use of a shorter TE than with spin echo techniques and thus allows acquisition of more image slices during a given TR.

Single-Slice Spoiled Gradient Echo

Single-slice spoiled gradient echo images can be acquired within 1 second or less. However, acquisition of these images is not more *efficient* than acquisition of multislice images with a longer TR but

comparable TE because for a given number of image slices the same number of excitation pulses are applied and the same number of echoes are sampled. The principal difference between these techniques is that with the multislice technique a stack of several slices is acquired in an interleaved manner during a particular interval, whereas with the single-slice technique several images are acquired separately and sequentially over the same interval (Fig. 18-6).

If the goal is to acquire a set of images during a specified interval, the multislice technique is generally preferred. Multislice techniques allow a longer TR and larger flip angle, producing a greater SNR per unit of time. However, if the goal is to obtain images rapidly with little motion artifact or rapidly during several phases of a physiological event (e.g., dynamic motion or perfusion with a contrast agent), the single-slice technique is preferred. Although overall efficiency is comparable with the two techniques, temporal resolution can be much better with single-slice methods, especially if only one or a few images are obtained.

Magnetization-Prepared Gradient Echo

Inversion recovery–prepared gradient echo techniques (see Chapter 14) can generate

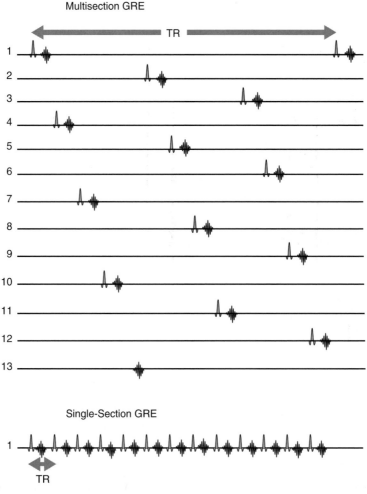

Multisection GRE

Single-Section GRE

Figure 18-6
Comparison of multislice and single-slice gradient echo techniques. In this example, 13 slices are obtained during a comparable interval with each technique; however, acquisitions are interleaved with the multislice technique and sequential with the single-slice technique, and the TR is much longer with the multislice technique.

rapid images with heavy T1-weighting. The SNR of magnetization-prepared gradient echo images is less than that of multislice spoiled gradient echo techniques. Factors that contribute to a low SNR in these sequences include the reduced signal intensity inherent in all inversion recovery techniques (see Chapter 11) as well as the short TR and small flip angles of rapid gradient echo images. The strong, flexible T1-weighted contrast obtainable, however, makes these techniques interesting in situations in which an acceptable SNR is possible, as with large voxel sizes or the use of specialized local receiver coils.

Three-Dimensional Spoiled Gradient Echo

The popularity of three-dimensional (3D) spoiled gradient echo imaging has continued to increase over the past several years. Compared with two-dimensional (2D) techniques, 3D techniques allow the use of thinner slices at higher SNRs. Typically, TR, TE, and the flip angle are similar for 2D single-slice and 3D acquisition techniques. However, the SNR is much higher with 3D techniques because each view during the entire acquisition contributes signal to every image in the entire volume. In contrast, with 2D single-slice techniques, each view contributes signal only to a given slice. For example, acquisition of a 3D volume with 32 partitions (slices) has 32 times as many views contributing signal as does a 2D acquisition with a similar matrix and number of signal averages. This large number of sampled views also leads to increased averaging of ghost artifacts secondary to repetitive motion such as pulsation, rendering these techniques particularly well suited for magnetic resonance (MR) angiography.

Not only are there no gaps between image slices with 3D techniques but image slices can overlap each other. This is accomplished by filling in the periphery of

3D k-space with zeros (zero-filling) in the slice-encoding axis. As discussed in earlier chapters, the periphery of k-space is used to encode fine detail. In the slice-encoding axis, detail defines the images' slices, so extending k-space farther into the periphery of this axis produces a larger number of image slices at finer increments. Because the zeros do not contribute real information, the actual spatial resolution in the slice-encoding axis is less than the increment between slices, so the effect is comparable to the generation of overlapping image slices. This allows for smoother paging of images during viewing and smoother 3D reconstruction from the data set.

One potential source of artifact in 3D Fourier acquired images that is not a problem with 2D acquisitions is truncation artifact in the slice-encoding axis. As discusssed later in Chapter 26, ring-down artifact results from truncation of reconstructed data when spatial resolution is not sufficient to encode high contrast borders. The result is a ring-down that gradually decreases over several pixels from the high contrast border. The artifact is minimized by increasing the spatial resolution in the axis of the high contrast border. For 3D Fourier techniques, truncation artifacts are most severe when thick image slices are acquired. Thick image slices have more edge artifacts with 3D than with 2D acquisition. However, the image quality of 3D Fourier images increases as slice thickness decreases. Thus, 3D techniques are best applied to acquire thin image slices. With the extremely short TRs and TEs that are possible with modern MRI equipment, the utility of 3D spoiled gradient echo images compared with 2D techniques has continued to improve.

Another artifact unique to 3D Fourier techniques is wrap-around (aliasing) artifact in the slice axis. This is not a problem with 2D Fourier techniques, as slices are *selected* by applying a slice-select gradient during excitation. With 3D Fourier techniques, however, slices are *encoded* by phase-encoding, as discussed in Chapter 8. The range of encoded slices is represented by phase shifts with a

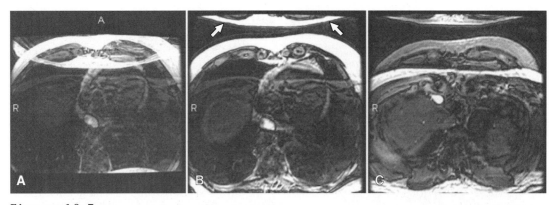

Figure 18-7

Wrap-around artifact in both the phase-encoding and slice-encoding axes with the three-dimensional (3D) Fourier gradient echo technique. (A) Axial image from the top slice in a 3D volume at the level of the heart and hepatic dome is degraded by a wrap-around artifact. (B) The field of view in the phase-encoding axis is increased, so posterior tissues that wrap-around to the front (*arrows*) no longer overlap anterior body tissues. However, the image is still degraded by wrap-around in the slice-encoding axis, so tissues from the mid-abdomen, at the bottom of the 3D volume, are included. (C) Image at the bottom of the 3D volume shows mid-abdominal anatomy degraded by a wrap-around artifact from tissue just superior to that shown in (B).

range of 360°, and shifts outside this range are encoded ambiguously. For example, a phase shift of 5° is indistinguishable from a phase shift of 365°. The result is that slices beyond one end of the 3D volume overlap slices at the other (Fig. 18-7).

T1-Weighted Chemical Shift Pulse Sequences

Because of the short T1 of methylene (CH_2) protons, most biological lipids contribute more signal intensity on T1-weighted images than would be expected from their proton density alone. As a result, T1-weighted images are sensitive to the presence of lipids owing to their short T1. Thus, chemical shift techniques often have greater impact on T1-weighted images than on other images. This is true of both fat-suppressed images and fat–water opposed-phase images.

Fat suppression, whether by saturation, selective inversion, or spatial-spectral excitation (see Chapter 15), can be used to reduce artifacts and optimize the dynamic range on T1-weighted images for special applications. Perhaps the greatest use of fat suppression on T1-weighted images is for improving the conspicuousness of enhancing tissue after administration of gadolinium chelates. If surrounding adipose tissue has high signal intensity, mild enhancement may be subtle. Fat suppression can also increase the conspicuousness of hemorrhage or of subtle contrast in musculoskeletal structures (e.g., menisci) or within tissues with high signal intensity such as hepatic or pancreatic parenchyma.

Even if fat-suppressed T1-weighted images are obtained, additional T1-weighted images without fat suppression are often important. It is on these images that fat planes and fatty bone marrow are depicted with the greatest clarity, providing important anatomical detail of many body parts.

In addition to improving the intensity of contrast between certain tissues, chemical shift techniques are useful for sensitive, specific identification of lipid in tissues. Definitive identification of lipid is accomplished best by comparing in-phase T1-weighted images with either fat-suppressed images or opposed-phase images. The choice between these two techniques depends on the relative tissue concentration of lipid.

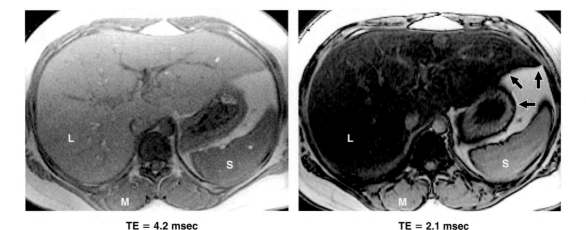

TE = 4.2 msec   TE = 2.1 msec

Figure 18-8
Fatty infiltration of the liver depicted using gradient echo in-phase (TE 4.2 msec) and opposed-phase (TE 2.1 msec) images at 1.5 T. (Although these TE values are less optimal than 2.25 and 4.50 msec, they are close enough to be effective.) On the in-phase image (*left*), liver (L) has higher signal intensity than spleen (S) or skeletal muscle (M). With the opposed-phase technique, liver has markedly low signal intensity owing to destructive interference between comparable amounts of water and lipid magnetization. There has been little change in the signal intensity of adipose tissue, most of which is due to lipid magnetization. The *black arrows* (*right*) indicate signal voids at fat–water interfaces secondary to inclusion of water and lipid in these voxels.

For tissues whose MR signal originates principally from lipid, the high signal intensity of fat must be distinguished from other high–signal intensity sources (e.g., hemorrhage, flow, contrast enhancement). Fat saturation techniques can change the signal intensity of fat on T1-weighted images most dramatically, converting it from high to low signal intensity.

In contrast, the effect of fat saturation pulses on tissues with minimal fat, such as mildly fatty liver or adrenal adenoma, may be barely noticeable. For definitive identification of small quantities of lipid, comparison of in-phase and opposed-phase images is best (Fig. 18-8). This is because a small quantity of lipid signal interferes destructively with and removes from the image an equivalent amount of water signal. The opposed-phase effect is therefore double the effect of fat saturation on tissues with small amounts of lipid. Water suppression can also be effective; if water is completely saturated, any visible signal indicates lipid. In clinical practice, however, water-suppression techniques are particularly vulnerable to artifact;

it may be difficult to distinguish minimally fatty tissue from artifactual signal. Figure 18-9 explains the effects on relative signal intensity of partially fatty tissues of various chemical shift techniques.

One potential pitfall of determining the lipid content by comparing in-phase to opposed-phase gradient echo images is related to their use of different TEs; in most situations the TE of the in-phase image is double that of the opposed-phase image. The difference in TEs is inversely proportional to the magnetic field strength. At 0.3 T, 1.5 T, and 3.0 T, opposed-phase and in-phase TEs are about 11.5 and 23 msec, 2.25 and 4.5 msec, and 1.15 and 2.3 msec, respectively. At lower field strength, in-phase gradient echo images therefore have a stronger component of T2*-weighted contrast than do in-phase images at higher field strength.

An alternative to the exclusive use of gradient echo images for comparing in-phase and opposed-phase T1-weighted images is to compare opposed-phase gradient echo images to conventional spin echo images of identical TE. So long as the refocusing pulse occurs at

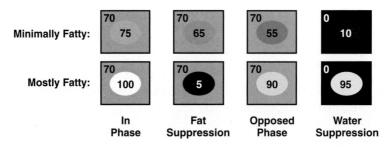

Figure 18-9

Contrast between water (*boxes*) and minimally fatty (*top ovals;* 65 signal units from water and 10 from fat) or mostly fatty (*bottom ovals;* five signal units from water and 95 from fat) tissues on T1-weighted images with a variety of chemical shift techniques. *Numbers* indicate arbitrary signal intensity units. Mostly fatty tissues (*bottom*) have short T1 and, therefore, more signal intensity on in-phase T1-weighted images. With fat suppression, the signal intensity is markedly reduced for mostly fatty tissues but is only minimally affected for minimally fatty tissues (*top*). On opposed-phase images, the signal intensity reduction is greater for minimally fatty tissues but less for mostly fatty tissues compared with that due to fat suppression. With water suppression, all remaining signal intensity is from fat, which is much greater for mostly fatty tissues.

one half the TE, spin echo images are always in phase, regardless of the TE. For example, at 0.3 T the gradient echo and spin echo images with TEs of 11 msec can be compared. Although spin echo images have less sensitivity to susceptibility effects than do gradient echo images, the use of identical TEs reduces the differences in T2-weighting between the two techniques.

Another alternative technique is the use of spin echo opposed-phase images. Conventional spin echo images are always in phase because the refocusing pulse occurs at the center of the TE. If it is moved away from the center of the echo time by an amount equal to the lowest opposed-phase TE (e.g., by 11 msec at 0.3 T or by 2.25 msec at 1.5 T), opposed-phase spin echo images are obtained. These images can be created as a separate acquisition or as part of a double echo spin technique.

▼
Essential Points to Remember

1. The spin echo technique is useful for obtaining images with moderate T1 contrast and less artifact than many other techniques. There is more experience with the spin echo technique than with any other technique for obtaining T1 contrast.

2. For T1-weighting, regardless of the method, T1 contrast is maximal if the TE is minimized.

3. Inversion recovery spin echo techniques can be used to achieve strong, flexible T1 contrast, but the acquisition time is long and the SNR per unit of time is low.

4. Multislice spoiled gradient echo techniques allow acquisition of moderately T1-weighted images with high efficiency and high SNR per unit of time. It is important to recognize that the phases of fat and water magnetizations are commonly opposed to each other on these images.

5. Single-slice spoiled gradient echo techniques have efficiency similar to that of multislice techniques but with a lower SNR and less contrast; however, they are less sensitive to motion and have greater temporal resolution.

6. Inversion recovery magnetization-prepared gradient echo images have strong, flexible T1 contrast but low SNR and spatial resolution.

7. Three-dimensional gradient echo techniques with a short TR and low flip angle allow acquisition of thin, contiguous or overlapping slices with a high SNR.

8. Because of the high signal intensity of fat on T1-weighted images, chemical shift techniques are usually most useful when applied with T1-weighted pulse sequences.

9. T1-weighted images without fat suppression are most useful for depicting anatomy based on the high signal intensity of fat planes or fatty marrow.

10. Fat saturation is useful for decreasing artifacts due to fat and for improving the conspicuousness of subtle changes in nonfatty high-signal tissues.

11. Definitive identification of tissue lipid is accomplished best by comparing in-phase T1-weighted images with either fat-suppressed or opposed-phase images.

12. Fat suppression is most useful for identifying tissues that contain principally fat, whereas fat–water opposed-phase images are most useful for depicting small quantities of lipid.

13. The difference between the TEs of in-phase and opposed-phase gradient echo images is inversely proportional to the magnetic field strength.

Chapter **19**

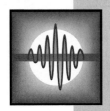

T2-Weighted Pulse Sequences

Nearly all clinical imaging protocols involve obtaining at least one T2-weighted pulse sequence. In this chapter we review some of the techniques used to show T2 differences between tissues and to consider their relative advantages and disadvantages.

Spin Echo Techniques

Like T1-weighted images, T2-weighted images were obtained principally via the spin echo (SE) technique during the first decade of widespread clinical magnetic resonance imaging (MRI). T2-weighted SE images provide acceptable T2 contrast for most tissues. The signal-to-noise ratio (SNR) per unit time is much lower for T2-weighted than for T1-weighted SE images, however, because of the unproductive dead time

during the echo time (TE). This is because there is no data acquisition during the TE interval prior to readout. Although strong T2 weighting with the conventional SE technique is possible, the number of image slices that can be acquired per TR decreases further with a longer TE. Therefore, there is a practical limit to the TE that can be tolerated in clinical practice before unacceptably low anatomical coverage and long acquisition times are reached (Fig. 19-1).

One benefit of the conventional SE technique for obtaining T2-weighted images is that one or more additional echoes can be obtained to generate other images with an identical TR but a lower TE without taking any more time. Two images, acquired during the same period of time using the double-echo SE technique, can be used to calculate T2 values or T2 images. In clinical practice, these images are usually compared visually to gain an impression of a tissue's T2 (Fig. 19-2). Until recently, the principal

249

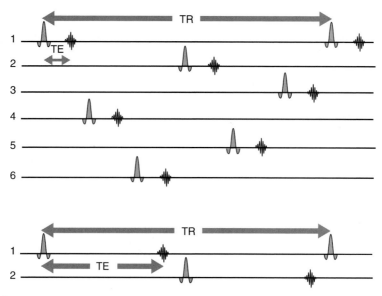

Figure 19-1
Effect of TE on efficiency. With a short-TE spin echo technique (*top*), more slices can be acquired for a given TR than with long-TE spin echo techniques (*bottom*).

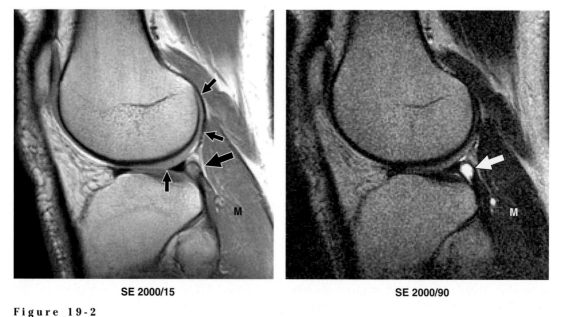

SE 2000/15   SE 2000/90

Figure 19-2
Comparison of first and second echo images regarding the inference of tissue T2. With the spin echo 2000/15 technique (*left*), articular cartilage (*small arrows*), synovial fluid (*large arrow*), and muscle (M) are all isointense. By comparing these two images, it becomes clear that articular cartilage has a T2 intermediate between the high T2 of synovial fluid and the low T2 of muscle.

reason for the long survival of T2-weighted SE images in clinical practice, despite their relative inefficiency, was the lack of acceptable alternatives.

Gradient Echo Techniques

Gradient echo images with a moderate TE depict T2* contrast. In some situations, such as certain spinal or musculoskeletal applications, these images resemble T2-weighted images. However, compared with similar images with a short TE, gradient echo images with a long TE are less efficient and have a lower SNR and more artifacts. In clinical practice it is often difficult to obtain sufficient T2* contrast without introducing unacceptable levels of image degradation (Fig. 19-3).

For some applications, T2*-weighted images can be quite useful, as they are sensitive to heterogeneous susceptibility.

These images can have a short TR, allowing thin-slice acquisition by a three-dimensional (3D) Fourier transform technique. Bone trabeculae decrease the magnetic field in their immediate vicinity, creating heterogeneous susceptibility. The resulting signal intensity loss near bone can make it more visible (Fig. 19-4). Bone marrow is obscured on T2*-weighted images; SE or fast SE images (or gradient echo images with a short TE) are needed for its evolution. Tissue iron increases the magnetic field in its vicinity, also creating heterogeneous susceptibility. T2*-weighted images therefore show iron sensitively (Fig. 19-5).

Steady-State Free Precession

Heavily T2-weighted gradient echo images can be obtained by sampling the spin

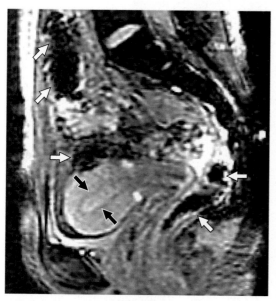

GRE 80/34/20°

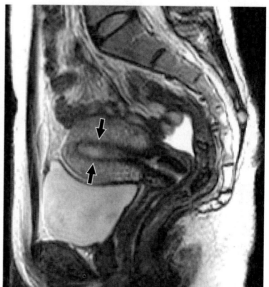

FSE 3000/165

Figure 19-3

Comparison of T2* and T2 contrast. With the gradient echo (GRE) 80/34/20° technique (*left*), there is moderate contrast between the uterine zones (*black arrows*), but the T2* contrast has caused prominent loss of signal intensity near bowel gas (*white arrows*) and in bone marrow. With the fast spin echo (FSE) 3000/165 technique, there is more contrast between uterine zones and better image quality.

FSE 2000/29　　　　　　　　　　　　　　　FSE 2000/87

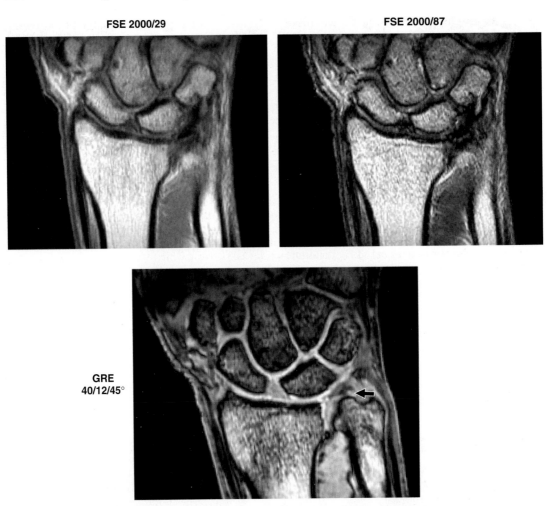

GRE
40/12/45°

Figure 19-4
Comparison of fast spin echo (FSE) and three-dimensional (3D) Fourier transform gradient echo (GRE) 40/12/45° images. The 3D gradient echo technique allows acquisition of contiguous 1.2-mm slices, less than half the thickness of the fast spin echo images. Additionally, bone structures are defined more clearly, as is the triangular fibrocartilage complex (*arrow*).

echoes, rather than the gradient echoes, that result from repeated application of radio pulses (see Chapter 14). On these images the TE is approximately twice the TR. Because the echo cannot be sampled during application of a radiofrequency (RF) pulse, it is sampled shortly before the RF pulse, at which time it is not completely refocused (the time of complete refocusing of the spin echo occurs *during* the next excitation pulse). Such images therefore include both T2 and T2* contrast. Owing to a short TR, a small flip angle, and degradation due to magnetic field heterogeneity, T2-weighted steady-state free precession images tend to have a low SNR and substantial artifacts. The SNR is increased and the artifacts decreased, however, if 3D acquisition is used, but the image quality is still generally lower than with fast SE (Fig. 19-6).

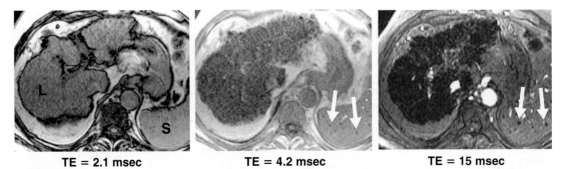

TE = 2.1 msec   TE = 4.2 msec   TE = 15 msec

Figure 19-5
Gradient echo images in a patient with preclinical idiopathic hemochromatosis show increasing sensitivity to iron with increasing TE, because of increasing $T2^*$ weighting. With a TE of 2.1 msec (*left*), liver (L) is slightly less intense than spleen (S). At a TE of 4.2 msec (*middle*), the liver is seen to consist of numerous low signal intensity nodules. At a TE of 15 msec (*right*), the liver has markedly decreased signal intensity relative to spleen, muscle, and other tissues. Low signal intensity iron-containing nodules in the spleen (*arrows*) become visible at 4.2 msec and appear larger at 15 msec because of "blooming."

Although not used by most clinicians, 3D steady-state free precession techniques have aroused some interest as a way of rapidly obtaining 3D T2-weighted images. In fact, this technique might have become more popular had not fast SE been introduced into clinical practice just as T2-weighted steady-state free precession techniques were being developed.

More recently, balanced steady-state free precession [fast imaging with steady-state precession (true-FISP), fast imaging employing steady-state acquisition (FIESTA), balanced fast field echo] sequences have been implemented. These techniques are discussed in Chapter 14. Balance steady-state free precession images are T2/T1-weighted and therefore depict tissues with a long T2 as high signal intensity. Desirable attributes include fast acquisition time, high SNR, and insensitivity to motion artifact. However, T2 contrast is usually depicted with greater clarity and less ambiguity on T2-weighted fast SE images (Fig. 19-7).

Vendor-specific terminology has contributed to confusion between various types of steady-state free precession images. Therefore, some review of the differences between these techniques is appropriate here.

1. Early implementation of unspoiled gradient echo techniques, such as *g*radient *r*ecalled *a*cquisition in the *s*teady *s*tate (GRASS) and FISP, had T2/T1 contrast, but the steady state was not fully maintained, and some signal was lost.
2. Reducing the TR, and balancing all gradient effects, allowed nearly complete recovery of both the spin echo and free induction decay, as well as more accurate T2/T1 contrast, with less signal loss; this revised sequence was therefore referred to by some as "true FISP." Other vendor terms are FIESTA and balanced fast field echo.

Multishot Fast Spin Echo Techniques

Within a few years of its introduction into clinical practice, multishot fast SE became the method of choice for T2-weighted

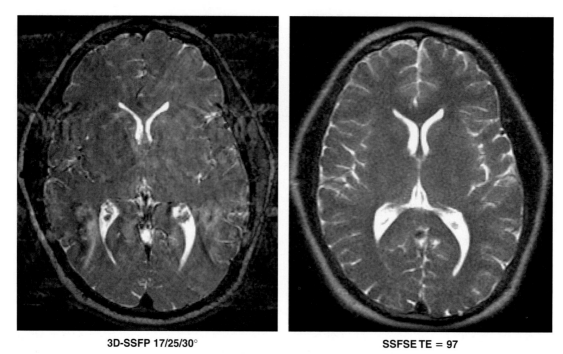

3D-SSFP 17/25/30°   **SSFSE TE = 97**

Figure 19-6
Three-dimensional steady-state free precession (3D-SSFP) 17/25/30° technique allows rapid acquisition of T2-weighted images (*left*), although the image quality may be poor. A single-shot fast spin echo image is shown for comparison (*right*).

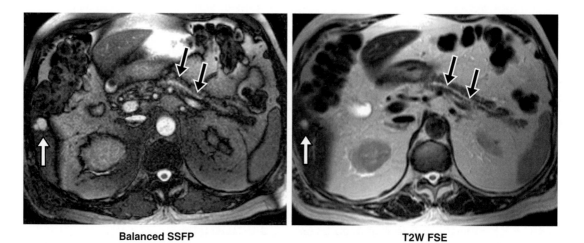

Balanced SSFP   **T2W FSE**

Figure 19-7
Left. Balanced steady-state free precession image (TR/TE/flip angle 4/2/60°) shows a cavernous hemangioma (*white arrow*) and the pancreatic duct (*black arrows*) as bright because their T2/T1 ratio is high. Note that fluid in blood vessels also has high signal intensity regardless of the velocity and direction of blood flow. *Right*. A T2-weighted fast spin echo image is shown for comparison.

imaging of most body parts. It is a modified SE technique that corrects the most glaring disadvantage of conventional SE imaging for generating T2 contrast: inefficiency (Fig. 19-8).

The conventional SE technique is inefficient for generating T2 contrast because the echo time (approximately 100 msec for most applications) is essentially unproductive dead time, except for the generation of a second, less heavily T2-weighted image. Fast SE improves efficiency by acquiring data throughout the effective TE (TE_{ef}). If the echoes are acquired rapidly enough (i.e., if echo spacing is minimized) and the echo train is just long enough to allow acquisition of enough echoes to fill the TE_{ef}, fast SE images resemble SE images. For a given acquisition matrix, fast SE images are more blurry than comparable SE images; however, the added efficiency of multishot fast SE permits the use of a greater acquisition matrix, allowing generation of images with crisp edge definition.

For most applications, fast SE is preferable to standard SE for T2-weighted images because of its greater efficiency and flexibility. There are more user-selectable options with fast SE techniques, however, and they must be selected carefully for optimal clinical

effectiveness. One of the most fundamental differences between these two classes of T2-weighted techniques is that with standard T2-weighted images a second set of images of identical TRs and shorter TEs can be obtained without increasing the acquisition time. With fast SE, a subset of the echo train can be designated to create a first echo image, but this practice increases the acquisition time in direct proportion to the number of echoes that are not used to form the T2-weighted images. Thus, the use of a dual-echo technique is a virtual "free lunch" with standard SE techniques but not with fast SE.

The first step toward choosing a fast SE protocol for clinical imaging is to decide whether an image with a long TR and a short TE_{ef} both are necessary. If not, the fast SE acquisition time can be reduced significantly by assigning all echoes to a single T2-weighted image. For most applications outside of the central nervous and musculoskeletal systems, images with a long TR and a short TE have little clinical importance and can be eliminated.

If an image with a long TR and a short TE_{ef} is considered important, the next step is to determine if both this image, and its corresponding T2-weighted image, can be

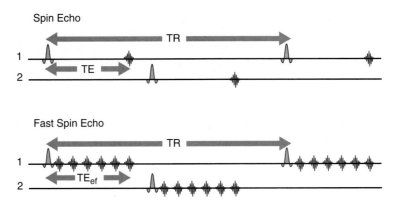

Figure 19-8
Fast spin echo techniques reduce the acquisition time dramatically compared with the conventional spin echo technique by acquiring several echoes during the effective TE.

optimized within the constraints of a dual-echo fast SE pulse sequence. For most currently available implementations of fast SE, the TR, acquisition matrix, and number of signal averages must be identical for the two images. In many situations, images with a long TR and a short TE can be optimized best by a second acquisition rather than as a component accompanying the T2-weighted images. Images with a long TR and a short TE (commonly referred to as *proton density-weighted* images but more appropriately as *intermediate-weighted images*) are considered in more detail in Chapter 20.

Fast SE allows a greater range of practical choices than does standard SE with regard to the familiar parameters of TR and TE$_{ef}$. With standard SE, the TR is usually set as the minimum needed to ensure acquisition of sufficient image slices; increasing the TR beyond this increases the acquisition time proportionally. As the TE increases, there is less time available to excite additional image slices; increasing the TE decreases the number of image slices that can be acquired during a given TR. Thus, increasing the TE often leads to an increased TR and therefore to an increased acquisition time. Choosing the TR and TE for standard SE images is often a compromise between the desired tissue contrast and constraints on the acquisition time.

With fast SE, both TR and TE$_{ef}$ can be increased without increasing the acquisition time by making appropriate increases in the number of echoes in the echo train (echo train length). For example, an echo train length of 32 allows one to choose a TE of 300 msec or longer without imposing any penalty on the acquisition time. Heavily T2-weighted images, with a TR of more than 10,000 msec and a TE$_{ef}$ of more than 300 msec can therefore be obtained within a few minutes with fast SE but not with standard SE.

As the echo train length increases, the time available for additional image slices per TR decreases. In contrast to standard SE techniques, however, the longer time required for a longer TR is balanced by the smaller number of excitation radio pulses needed; because each echo train is longer, fewer trains are needed. In practice, the acquisition time changes little, if at all, as the TR increases along with the echo train length so the same number of image slices can be acquired (Fig. 19-9).

Once the desired TE$_{ef}$ is chosen for multishot fast SE, many other parameters are easier to choose. Generally, the echo train length should be as short as possible, so long as the desired TE$_{ef}$ is one of these echoes and the echo spacing is kept as short as possible. Increasing the echo train length beyond what is needed to accommodate the desired TE$_{ef}$ has little or no effect on acquisition time, as the TR usually must be increased as well, but the longer TE$_{ef}$ leads to increased image blurring and other artifacts. The TR is generally chosen as the minimum needed to accommodate the echo train length and number of image slices needed. Blurring and artifacts are minimized if the acquisition matrix is large, preferably at least 256×256, and if the field of view is kept as small as possible, within the constraints of the SNR and anatomical coverage.

The increased signal intensity of adipose tissue on fast SE images, due to decreased J-coupling (see Chapter 16), can be either an advantage or a disadvantage depending on the clinical application. High signal intensity of adipose tissue, comparable to that typically present on T1-weighted SE images, allows clear depiction of fat planes; however, high signal intensity lesions, such as bone marrow edema, may become less conspicuous; and artifacts caused by moving fat increase when adipose tissue is made brighter (Fig. 19-10). The signal intensity of moving fat can be reduced by preceding each radio excitation pulse with a fat-saturation pulse or with an inversion pulse and short inversion time (TI) chosen to null the signal intensity of adipose tissue. Alternatively, artifact due to moving fat can be eliminated by acquiring images during suspended respiration.

Reduced signal intensity of solid tissue, relative to fat or fluid, as a result of

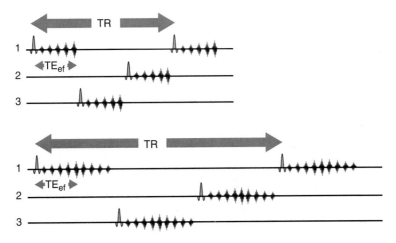

Figure 19-9
Relationship of the TR and the echo train. If the echo train is increased beyond the TE_{ef} (*bottom*), the TR must be increased to allow sufficient time for acquisition of a given number of image slices. Overall acquisition time for a given number of image slices is not necessarily changed by increasing the echo train beyond the TE_{ef}.

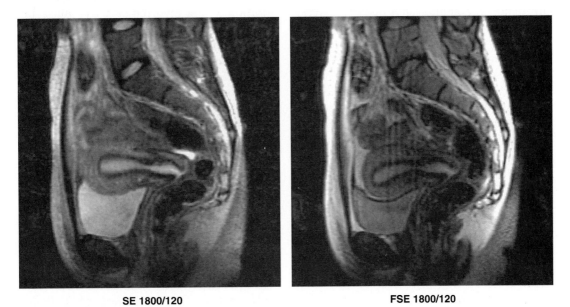

SE 1800/120   FSE 1800/120

Figure 19-10
Effect of high signal intensity of adipose tissue on motion-induced artifact. Sagittal T2-weighted images of the pelvis without fat suppression, using identical TR and TE. The increased signal intensity of adipose tissue with fast spin echo (*right*) has led to increased motion artifact and decreased conspicuousness of the high signal intensity of urine, endometrium, and peritoneal fluid posterior to the cervix.

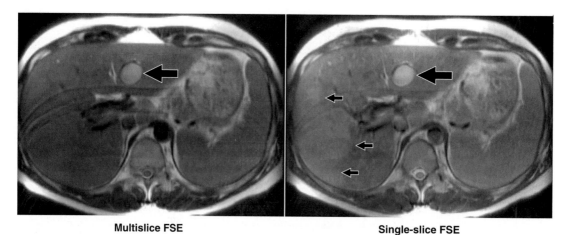

Multislice FSE   Single-slice FSE

Figure 19-11

Left. Magnetization transfer effects with the multislice fast spin echo technique have obscured a large hepatocellular carcinoma. A simple cyst (*large arrow*) is extremely conspicuous. *Right.* The identical pulse sequence was repeated but with acquisition of only one image. The conspicuousness of the cyst is unchanged, but the hepatocellular carcinoma is now visible (*small arrows*).

magnetization transfer (MT) is more difficult to prevent on multishot fast SE images. MT is helpful for depicting fluids, such as cerebrospinal fluid, synovial fluid, or fluid in cysts or ducts; however, MT can also reduce tissue contrast between solid tissues (e.g., between hepatic parenchyma and solid malignant tumor) (Fig. 19-11). The decreased contrast is often more than compensated for by increased spatial resolution and SNR, which is made possible by the added efficiency of fast SE, allowing more signal averaging and a larger acquisition matrix.

Fast Spin Echo–Inversion Recovery

Attractive features of short TI inversion recovery (STIR) include nulling of the fat signal and synergistic T1 and T2 contrast. The major deficiencies of STIR—low SNR and long acquisition times—can be addressed by using a fast SE rather than a single-echo SE pulse sequence following the inversion pulse (Fig. 19-12).

In fast SE STIR, the longitudinal magnetization is first inverted by a 180° pulse, followed by a delay (the TI) before the 90° excitation pulse, just as with conventional SE STIR. However, with fast SE STIR, a train of echoes follows each excitation pulse. Just as fast SE requires fewer TRs than SE to acquire a given amount of data, fast SE STIR requires fewer TIs as well. For example, a fast SE STIR technique with an echo train of 16 requires only one inversion pulse, and therefore only one TI, per 16 echoes. Fast SE STIR is thus far more efficient than conventional SE STIR.

Spin echo STIR techniques usually use relatively short TEs (e.g., 30 msec or less) because long TEs decrease the SNR and decrease the number of image slices that can be acquired per TR. With fast SE STIR, however, a longer TE_{ef} is practical. The SNR can be maintained because the increased efficiency of fast SE STIR allows more signal averages. Further, there is no time penalty when using a longer TE_{ef} with fast SE techniques, including fast SE STIR, as long as the echo train is long enough to cover the TE_{ef}. If a long TE_{ef} is used, fast SE STIR images are truly T2-weighted in addition to

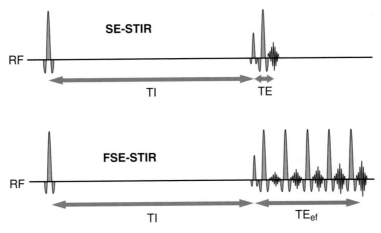

Figure 19-12
Compared with the conventional spin echo short TI inversion recovery (SE STIR) technique (*top*), more echoes are obtained per inversion pulse with fast spin echo (FSE STIR) (*bottom*). Fewer inversion pulses are therefore necessary.

the T1 contrast inherent in STIR techniques. T2-weighted STIR images are easy to distinguish visually from STIR images with a shorter TE. Because of its short T2, muscle appears dark on T2-weighted images. STIR images with a TE of 30 msec or less depict muscle as having moderate signal intensity.

In summary, there are two major advantages of fast SE STIR techniques compared to standard SE STIR. One is that there is far less dead time with fast SE STIR, so it is much more efficient than standard SE STIR. The other is that T2-weighted STIR is practical with fast SE STIR but not with standard SE STIR. With modern MRI systems, fast SE therefore is used for virtually all STIR acquisitions.

Fast SE (without an inversion pulse) is more efficient than fast SE STIR. This is because there is often no data acquisition during the TI. Compared with fast SE without an inversion pulse, fast SE STIR involves spending more time to acquire less signal. Compared with T2-weighted fast SE STIR, fat-suppressed fast SE produces similar images with greater SNR per unit of time. It is therefore a more efficient alternative to T2-weighted fast SE STIR.

The relative inefficiency of fast SE STIR should be considered along with its advantages, which include generally more reliable fat suppression and additive T1 and T2 contrast (see Chapter 15). The increased efficiency of fast SE techniques renders practical the use of extremely long TIs, allowing nulling of the fluid signal on fluid-attenuated inversion recovery (FLAIR) images.

Single-Shot Fast Spin Echo (HASTE) Techniques

Generally, fast SE image quality is best if the echo train is no longer than necessary to fill the TE_{ef} with echoes, because longer echo, trains tend to increase blurring and other artifacts. However, there are benefits that result when *all* echoes are obtained in one train.

Single-shot techniques can be used if the acquisition time must be minimized. Several concurrent strategies are available. Data sampling should be as fast as possible, which can be accomplished using high receiver bandwidth and rapid switching of gradients. Measures to reduce the amount of data needed for image reconstruction further decrease the duration of the echo train. These include partial sampling of each echo and half-Fourier reconstruction, which together allow acquisition of only slightly more than 50% of k-space and interpolation of the remainder. The echo train can be reduced even further by using parallel imaging techniques, so two or more lines of k-space can be filled for each echo.

Single-shot fast SE has no TR, as the excitation pulse is not repeated. This is sometimes referred to as infinite TR. The lack of a repetition removes T1-weighting. Motion-induced ghost artifact is far less severe on single-shot images, which can often be acquired in less than half a second. Additional benefits include the lack of abrupt transitions in the filling of k-space and therefore the absence of certain edge and ghost artifacts that may be more conspicuous on multishot images. Another advantage of single-shot fast SE over multishot fast SE is reduced MT contrast. This occurs because only one image slice is excited during any given period. However, rapid acquisition of nearby image slices can produce MT contrast.

Although single-shot fast SE generally has little motion artifact and is often particularly effective for depicting fluid, motion of fluid in large collections through a slice may result in signal voids, probably from time-of-flight effects. A similar appearance of heterogeneous signal intensity within moving fluid collections may be seen on fast single-slice 2D-FT gradient echo images. The intrinsic averaging of motion effects in multishot FSE (and gradient echo) images tends to mitigate this effect (Fig. 19-13).

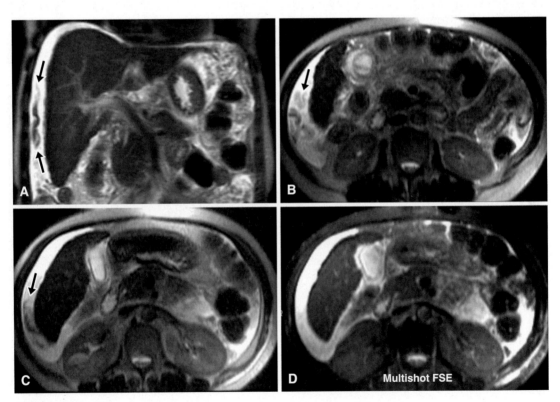

Figure 19-13
Irregular signal loss due to the motion of ascites is seen in coronal (A) and axial (B, C) single-shot fast SE images. A comparable multishot fast SE image (D) depicts the ascites with homogeneous high signal intensity.

The major limitations of single-shot fast SE are a low SNR and blurring of tissues with short or intermediate T2. As with multishot fast SE, image contrast depends on the phase-encoding order. If the last echo is chosen to provide data for the center of k-space (i.e., the TE$_{ef}$ is extremely long),

images consist almost entirely of signal from free fluid. These fluid-dominant "hydrograms" can be obtained as contiguous thin slices that may be combined in a maximum intensity projection (MIP), or a projection image may be obtained directly as a thick slab (Fig. 19-14). Typical image attributes

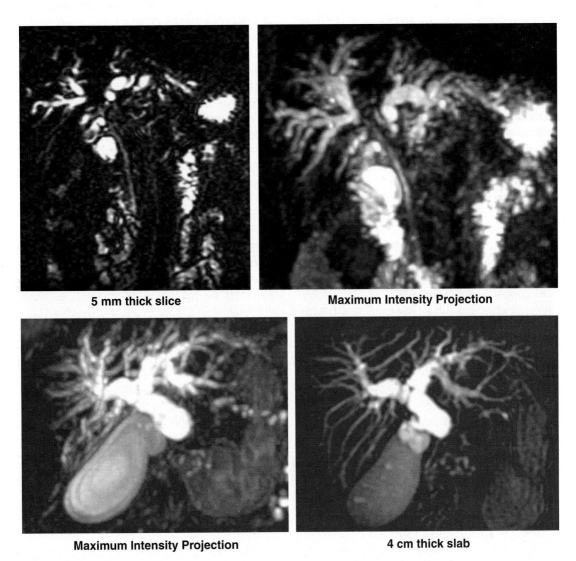

5 mm thick slice

Maximum Intensity Projection

Maximum Intensity Projection

4 cm thick slab

Figure 19-14

Single-shot fast spin echo images with a TE$_{ef}$ of more than 700 msec. Fluid is depicted clearly. *Top.* Contiguous 5 mm thick coronal slices (*left*) were obtained during a single breath hold, forming a maximum intensity projection (MIP) "MR cholangiogram" (*right*) in a patient with an obstructing cholangiocarcinoma at the confluence of the left and right bile ducts. *Bottom.* A similar technique was used in a patient with an obstructing pancreatic carcinoma to generate the MIP image (*left*). Because of unsuccessful breath holding, the individual thin slices were acquired at slightly different positions, resulting in a misregistration artifact. A 4 cm thick slab was then acquired in about 1 second, producing a superior image (*right*).

Table 19-1 ■ ATTRIBUTES OF THE SINGLE-SHOT TECHNIQUE RELATIVE TO MULTISHOT FAST SPIN ECHO TECHNIQUES

Image Attribute	Comparison to Multishot Techniques
Anatomical coverage	Slightly better
Signal-to-noise	Usually lower
Motion artifact	Less
Edge sharpness	Less
Tissue contrast	Usually less
Suitability for long TE	Better

of single-shot fast SE, compared to multishot fast SE, are presented in Table 19-1.

The edge sharpness of single-shot fast SE images can be greatly improved by using parallel imaging techniques such as sensitivity-encoding (SENSE) or simultaneous acquisition of spatial harmonics (SMASH) (see Chapter 17). Parallel imaging involves using spatial information from a phased-array coil acquisition to reduce the number of MR signals needed to reconstruct an image with a given spatial resolution. For example, consider a single-shot fast SE image with an effective TE of 200 msec, an echo train of 100, and echo spacing of 4 msec. The total duration of this echo train is 400 msec. The echoes acquired during the end of the echo train, which contribute to the fine detail, have negligible signal intensity, particularly for soft tissues such as muscle, liver, and liver lesions, among others, as the T2 of these tissues is less than 100 msec. If parallel imaging is used to reduce the echo train from 100 to 50 echoes, the echo train duration is now 200 msec, and the fine detail is provided by echoes that have a TE of less than 200 msec. Although the use of parallel imaging often leads to a lower SNR, because fewer echoes are sampled there may be minimal impact in this setting. This is because the echoes that are eliminated—those with a TE of more than 200 msec—had negligible soft tissue signal intensity compared with the echoes with TEs of less than 200 msec that are retained. The net

result of the use of parallel imaging on single-shot techniques therefore is reduced acquisition time, improved edge sharpness, and retained SNR.

Echo Planar Imaging and Gradient Echo and Spin Echo Techniques

Echo planar imaging was implemented initially as a single-shot technique. This form of echo planar imaging is useful principally for maximizing temporal resolution, which is helpful for cardiac imaging and monitoring of other processes that exhibit rapid physiological variation, such as with functional neuroimaging. Single-shot echo planar T2-weighted techniques have the added advantage of having an "infinite" TR, which eliminates T1 contrast. They have the disadvantage of requiring an extremely long echo train, during which there is no RF refocusing except at the central echo. Artifacts can thus be far more intrusive than with single-shot fast SE.

Multishot echo planar techniques have a much shorter echo train length, which leads to less severe susceptibility artifacts than with the single-shot echo planar technique. Although multishot techniques do not have infinite TR, they can be obtained with TRs of more than 5000 msec, allowing for nearly complete recovery of longitudinal magnetization. However susceptibility, eddy current, and chemical shift artifacts can still occur; and as with other techniques acquired over several seconds or more, multishot echo planar images are extremely sensitive to motion.

Although long, or infinite, TR reduces or eliminates T1 contrast, T1-weighted images can be acquired with the echo planar technique. By preceding each excitation pulse with an inversion pulse, inversion recovery images can be obtained, as they can with fast SE techniques (Fig. 19-15; Table 19-1).

Single-Shot FSE

TE$_{ef}$ = 62 | TE$_{ef}$/TI = 62/2500

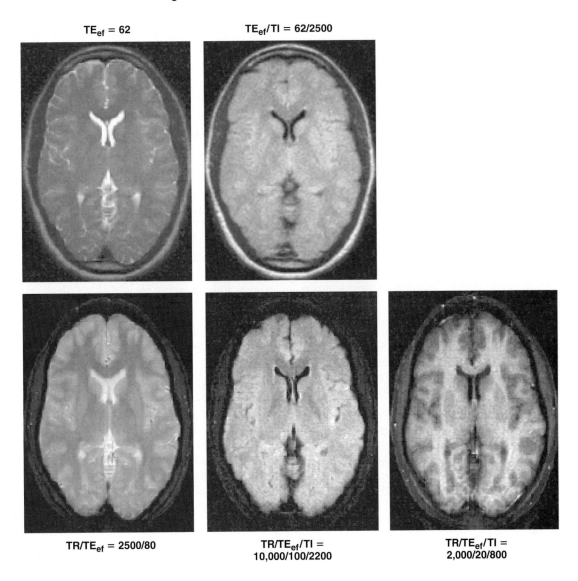

TR/TE$_{ef}$ = 2500/80 | TR/TE$_{ef}$/TI = 10,000/100/2200 | TR/TE$_{ef}$/TI = 2,000/20/800

Multishot Echo Planar

Figure 19-15

Axial images of the brain using single-shot fast spin echo and multishot spin echo–echo planar techniques. *Top.* Images with a TE$_{ef}$ of 62 msec are compared without (*left*) and with (*right*) the use of a single inversion pulse with a TI of 2500 msec. With a TI of this length, the fluid signal is nulled [fluid-attenuated inversion recovery (FLAIR)]. *Bottom.* Echo planar images are compared without an inversion pulse (*left*), with a TI of 2200 msec (FLAIR), a short TE$_{ef}$ (20 msec), and a TI of 800 msec, producing T1-weighted images. FSE, fast spin echo.

The gradient echo and spin echo (GRASE) technique can be used to produce T2-weighted images with efficiency intermediate between that of the fast SE and echo planar techniques (see Chapter 13). Artifacts, however, may degrade the images. GRASE currently is not widely available, and its role in clinical imaging has not yet been defined.

▼
Essential Points to Remember

1. Although T2-weighted SE images may be diagnostically useful, their acquisition is highly inefficient owing to substantial dead time during the long TE.

2. T2- or T2*-weighted gradient echo and steady-state free precession images tend to have significant artifacts due to magnetic field heterogeneity.

3. Fast SE images have fewer artifacts than gradient echo and steady-state free precession images and can be acquired more efficiently than standard SE images.

4. Fast SE images tend to be blurrier than standard SE images and may have more artifacts. This can be compensated for by larger higher acquisition matrices.

5. The high signal intensity of adipose tissue on fast SE images, if considered undesirable, can be reduced by using fat-saturation or inversion recovery techniques.

6. Fast SE images have more MT contrast than do standard SE images. This causes solid tissues to lose more signal intensity than fat or fluid, increasing the conspicuousness of fluid but reducing some forms of tissue contrast.

7. Dual TE_{ef} fast SE techniques require more acquisition time than single TE_{ef} fast SE images.

8. With multishot fast SE, the choice of the TE_{ef} should be based on the desired tissue contrast. The echo train should be long enough to accommodate this TE_{ef} but otherwise should generally be as short as possible to reduce artifacts and blurring. Echo spacing should be minimized.

9. Once the TE_{ef} and echo train are chosen, the TR should generally be selected to allow adequate anatomical coverage.

10. Echo planar and GRASE images can be acquired in less time than standard SE or fast SE images, but they may have more artifacts.

11. Single-shot echo planar images can show physiological phenomena with greater temporal resolution than multishot techniques, but they usually have lower spatial resolution and more artifacts.

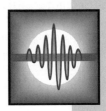

Intermediate-Weighted
Pulse Sequences

Early clinical magnetic resonance imaging (MRI) protocols almost invariably included spin echo images with the following combinations of TRs and TEs: (1) short TR and short TE (T1-weighted); (2) long TR and long TE (T2-weighted); and (3) long TR and short TE. The latter is referred to commonly as being *proton density-weighted*. In this chapter we discuss contrast on this image, and explain why *intermediate-weighted* is a more appropriate description for such images. We then describe attributes of these images that lend them clinical importance and review the pulse sequences that can be used to obtain this type of contrast.

Definition

T1 contrast is usually achieved by using a TR short enough that the longitudinal

magnetization of some tissues does not relax completely between excitations. T2 contrast arises from the use of a TE long enough that substantial decay of transverse magnetization of some tissues occurs. In other words, both T1 contrast and T2 contrast depend on achieving lower signal intensity of some tissues than would occur solely from their proton density. If the longitudinal magnetization of all tissues is allowed to recover completely between excitations (infinitely long TR, small flip angle, or both), and if no transverse magnetization is allowed to decay (zero TE), T1 contrast and T2 contrast both could be eliminated. Tissue contrast would thus be dominated by other contrast mechanisms, such as proton density, chemical shift, and magnetization transfer.

Full recovery of longitudinal magnetization of all tissues can be ensured by using a single-shot technique or an extremely long TR (e.g., 10,000 msec). Decay of transverse magnetization can be prevented if the transverse magnetization is measured as soon as it is created, with a TE of 0 msec. Even though pulse sequences have been introduced clinically with a TE of less than 2 msec, there is some decay of transverse magnetization of some tissues and therefore at least some T2 or T2* contrast.

The term *proton density-weighting* suggests that proton density contrast is in fact the dominant contrast mechanism in the image; however, this usually is not true. Many so-called proton density-weighted images have a TR that is too short or a TE that is too long to eliminate T1 and T2 contrast. Tissue contrast on these images commonly includes a combination of T1 and T2 contrast in addition to other effects such as chemical shift and magnetization transfer.

To indicate that T1 contrast and T2 contrast are present, images with a long TR and a short TE have been referred to as *balanced,* but this term also is misleading because it suggests that the effect of T1 differences on tissue contrast is equal to that of T2 differences. There is no basis for this assumption, however, because depending on the pulse sequence and pair of tissues either T1 or T2 contrast may dominate.

One term that does not include any incorrect assumptions is *intermediate-weighted.* In all situations, contrast on an image that might be called *proton density-weighted* is intermediate between that of a T1-weighted image and a T2-weighted one. Therefore, we recommend use of this term in place of the more popular but less appropriate term *proton density-weighted.*

Attributes for Clinical Use

Intermediate-weighted images usually have a higher overall signal-to-noise ratio than comparable T1-weighted or T2-weighted pulse sequences because longitudinal recovery is maximized and transverse decay is minimized. In fact, most other pulse sequences can be thought of as modifications of intermediate-weighted images, decreasing the signal of some tissues to achieve the desired contrast. For example, decreasing the TR causes reduced signal intensity of tissues with a long T1, creating T1-weighting. Similarly, increasing the TE causes reduced signal intensity of tissues with a long T2, creating T2-weighting. Preceding each excitation pulse in an intermediate-weighted pulse sequence with an inversion pulse creates an inversion recovery pulse sequence.

Clinically, intermediate-weighted images are particularly useful for depicting structures with low signal intensity (e.g., bone, fibrous tissue, air) contrasted with a background of soft tissues or fluid with higher signal intensity. These tissues are often best seen if intermediate-weighted images are acquired using a high-resolution technique, taking advantage of their typically high SNR. Intermediate-weighted images are useful for imaging the brain, vertebral column, and musculoskeletal system. They provide a useful combination of mild T1 and T2 contrast (Fig. 20-1).

Spin Echo Techniques

A spin echo technique is generally the best method for obtaining intermediate-weighted images. During the first decade of clinical MRI use, intermediate-weighted images were obtained routinely as the first echo of a dual-echo spin echo sequence. In this manner, intermediate-weighted and T2-weighted images were collected together during the acquisition time necessary for T2-weighted images alone. If a spin echo technique is used to obtain T2-weighted images, sampling the first echo with a short TE is certainly the most efficient way to provide additional images with intermediate-weighting. When intermediate-weighted images are acquired simultaneously with T2-weighted spin echo images, the TR, acquisition matrix, section thickness, and

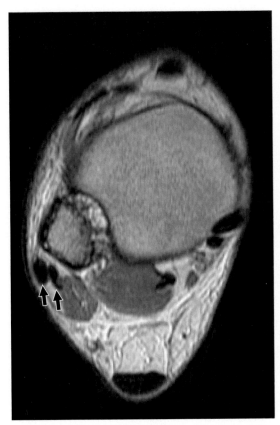 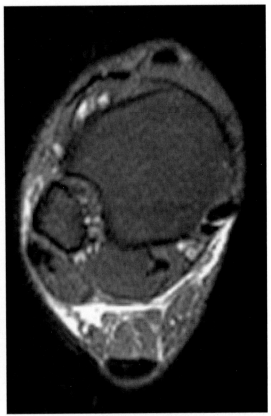

FSE 4433/40   FatSat FSE 3817/72

Figure 20-1
Left. Axial intermediate-weighted fast spin echo (FSE) 4433/40 image of the ankle TE_{ef} of 40 msec is long enough for tendons to be depicted as signal voids but short enough for muscle to have much higher signal intensity. A shorter echo train length (four), and a larger matrix (512 × 256) were used than for the fat-saturated T2-weighted FSE 3817/72 image. *Right.* Separate acquisition of intermediate- and T2-weighted images allows separate optimization of parameters for each. *Arrows* in the left image indicate the peroneus longus and brevis tendons, which are depicted more clearly than in the right image. High-signal perimuscular edema is shown better in the right image.

many other parameters are identical for the two images (Fig. 20-2).

Fast Spin Echo Versus Spin Echo Techniques

For most applications, the fast spin echo (FSE) method has replaced spin echo sequences as the preferred technique for acquiring T2-weighted images. Acquisition of intermediate-weighted images in addition to T2-weighted images with the FSE technique takes substantially longer than acquisition of T2-weighted images alone. Therefore, concurrent acquisition of intermediate-weighted and T2-weighted images by the dual-echo FSE technique is not the only method that should be considered.

If intermediate-weighted and T2-weighted images are acquired together as part of a dual-echo pulse sequence, parameters such

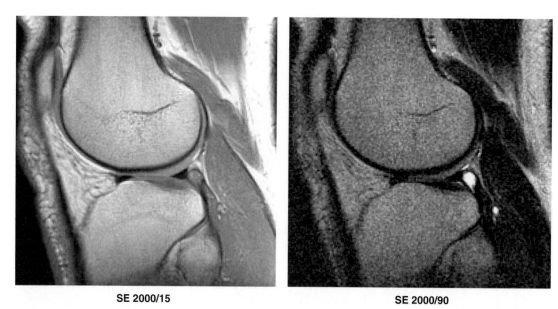

SE 2000/15   SE 2000/90

Figure 20-2
Double spin echo sagittal images of the knee. The intermediate-weighted image (*left*) depicts anatomical detail with a high signal-to-noise ratio (SNR) and no additional time for acquisition than the T2-weighted image (*right*), which is needed to depict fluid. The TR, matrix, and other parameters are identical.

as the TR, acquisition matrix, and number of signal averages must generally be identical, even though the *optimal* parameters may not be identical for the two images. Acquisition of two independent sets of images should be considered so intermediate-weighted and T2-weighted images can be optimized separately. The two most attractive techniques for acquiring intermediate-weighted images are the multishot FSE and spin echo (SE) techniques. They are compared next.

Blurring with the FSE technique is most severe when the effective TE (TE_{ef}) is short, because of the rapid changes in transverse magnetization between successive echoes that occur at a short TE_{ef}. Because the high spatial resolution of intermediate-weighted images is one of their most important attributes, it is especially important to eliminate any source of blurring. For this reason, intermediate-weighted images should generally be acquired using the standard

SE technique (Fig. 20-3). Alternatively, intermediate-weighted FSE images with mild T2-weighting (e.g., TE_{ef} between 30 and 40 msec) and a short echo train may be useful, particularly for musculoskeletal imaging.

The principal advantage of the FSE over the SE technique for acquiring images with a long TE is that with the FSE method the TE_{ef} is not dead time that decreases the efficiency of data acquisition. With short TE/TE_{ef} imaging, however, the efficiency of data acquisition is similar with the FSE and SE techniques; as the echo train increases above one, fewer excitations are needed, but fewer slices can be excited between excitations. The SE technique remains attractive for acquiring intermediate images, even if it is no longer a "free lunch" associated with acquisition of T2-weighted images.

T2-weighted images require a long TR to reduce contributions from T1 contrast. Because there are no data acquisitions

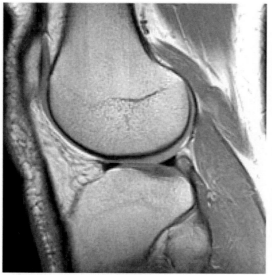

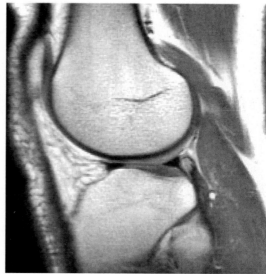

SE 2000/15   FSE 2000/15

Figure 20-3
Image detail on sagittal 2000/15 images is slightly superior with the spin echo technique (*left*) than with the fast spin echo technique (*right*).

during the long TEs used for T2-weighted SE acquisitions, a long TR often is needed to ensure adequate anatomical coverage. For intermediate-weighted images, it may not be necessary to use a TR as long as that needed for T2-weighted images. Thus, dual SE techniques may require a longer TR than is necessary to produce satisfactory intermediate-weighted images.

Optimizing Independent Acquisition of Intermediate-Weighted Images

Intermediate-weighted images usually are used to provide clear definition of high-contrast structures (e.g., bone, ligaments) rather than to depict subtle tissue contrast.

Under these circumstances, mild residual T1 contrast will not greatly compromise the value of such scans. For example, whereas a TR of 4 sec may be necessary for adequate slice coverage when TE is as long as 100 msec (for strongly T2 weighted studies), the short TE intermediate weighted image might be able to cover the same volume with a TR of only 1200 msec, while still retaining high SNR and good contrast behavior. Clarity of lesions and anatomy on such images is more important than the purity of the contrast. The use of an "intermediate" TR may show the desired anatomy in a shorter time (Figs. 20-4 and 20-5).

Other parameters may also be optimized separately when intermediate-weighted images are acquired independently. Because of their inherently high SNR, intermediate-weighted pulse sequences can often be obtained with smaller voxel size—and therefore with higher spatial resolution—than can T2-weighted images.

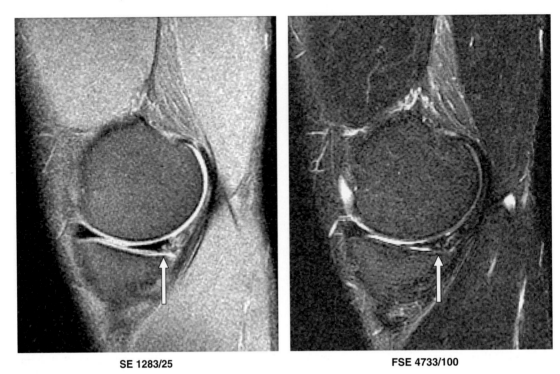

SE 1283/25   FSE 4733/100

Figure 20-4
Separate optimization of intermediate-weighted spin echo (*left*) and T2-weighted fast spin echo (*right*) images of the knee, both with fat suppression. For the intermediate-weighted images, a TR of 1283 msec was long enough for coverage of the entire knee. *Arrows* indicate a tear of the posterior horn of the medial meniscus.

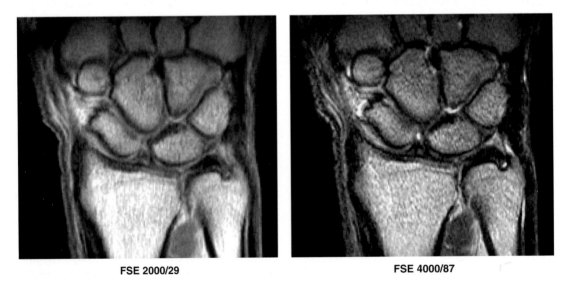

FSE 2000/29   FSE 4000/87

Figure 20-5
Separate optimization of intermediate-weighted (*left*) and T2-weighted (*right*) fast spin echo images of the wrist. With a shorter TE_{ef} and a short echo train, the intermediate-weighted image shows ligaments of the wrist more clearly. The shorter echo train allowed adequate coverage with a TR half that used for the T2-weighted image.

If other parameters are left unchanged, either the echo train length or the TR must be doubled to change from a single TE_{ef} to a dual-TE_{ef} multishot FSE acquisition. Doubling the TR reduces contributions from T1 contrast, which is usually desirable with the FSE technique. Increasing the echo train length, however, generally increases blurring and the severity of artifacts.

If a dual-TE_{ef} multishot FSE pulse sequence is changed to a single-TE_{ef} sequence, the acquisition time of the T2-weighted pulse sequence can be decreased by approximately 50%. In most instances the acquisition time is reduced by lowering the TR, thereby introducing some potentially unwanted T1 contrast. In some instances the unwanted T1 contrast introduced by reducing the TR may reduce the utility of the images. In these cases, using a dual-TE_{ef} FSE technique may be advisable. For example, sagittal coverage of the spine might be accomplished using a dual-TE_{ef} technique with a TR of 2500 msec. Reducing the TR to 1250 msec for a single-TE_{ef} acquisition is unlikely to yield satisfactory T2-weighted images. One alternative is to double the echo train length rather than to reduce the TR, possibly exacerbating blurring and artifacts. Alternatively, the best choice in this situation might be to use a dual-TE_{ef} multishot FSE technique, even though the intermediate-weighted image may have poor quality as compared to an image obtained with the standard SE technique. Essentially, the choice here is whether to prioritize optimization of the T2-weighted or the intermediate-weighted images. The other set of images should then be tailored to avoid unduly prolonging the total examination time.

Gradient Echo Techniques

The gradient echo technique can be used to obtain intermediate-weighted pulse sequences, although it is more difficult to remove T2* contrast or chemical shift effects. For these reasons the gradient echo sequences are not often used to obtain intermediate-weighted images unless three-dimensional Fourier transform (3D-FT) images with intermediate-weighting are desired. For some applications, balanced steady-state free precession images [e.g., fast imaging with steady-state precession (true FISP), fast imaging employing steady-state acquisition (FIESTA), balanced fast field echo] may depict the desired anatomy owing to the inherently high SNR of these sequences, although these images have substantial T2-weighting.

To reduce T1 contrast on intermediate-weighted gradient echo images with intermediate TR (e.g., <800 msec) or short TR (e.g., <50 msec) the excitation flip angle can be reduced. Reducing the excitation flip angle decreases the saturation resulting from each excitation radio pulse and thus reduces the time needed for complete recovery of longitudinal magnetization after excitation. The use of increasingly shorter TRs demands correspondingly smaller flip angles, especially if T1 contrast is not desired.

To reduce the contribution of T2* to the contrast, the TE must be minimized. This may be difficult if chemical shift effects are not desired. To eliminate chemical shift effects, the TE must be chosen such that fat and water signals are in-phase. The shortest TE that yields such in-phase images is approximately 2.25 msec at 3.0 T, 4.5 msec at 1.5 T, and 22 msec at 0.3 T. Opposed-phase images with shorter TEs can be achieved at these field strengths, respectively, with TEs of 1.10, 2.25, and 11.00 msec. Shorter TEs have milder chemical shift effects.

For some applications, complete elimination of T2* contrast on intermediate-weighted images may not be desirable. For example, fibrocartilage and tendons are depicted best by ensuring that they have low signal intensity. If the TE is too short these tissues may be obscured (Fig. 20-6).

TE = 4.2   **TE = 8.4**

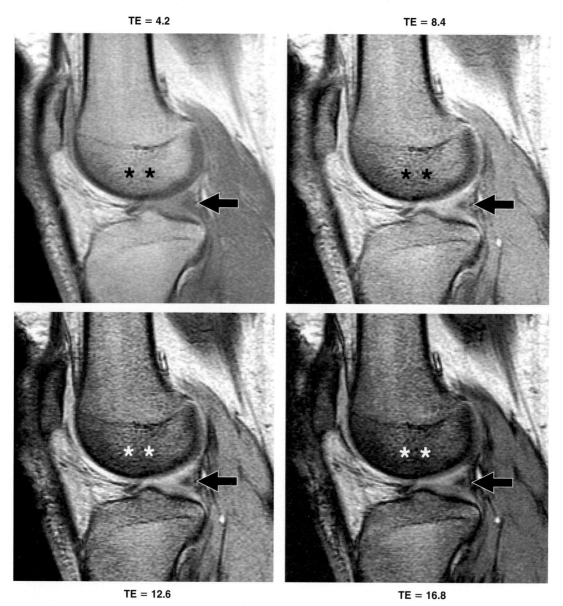

TE = 12.6   **TE = 16.8**

Figure 20-6
Effects of increasing the echo time (TE) on clarity of fibrocartilage and trabecular bone. In-phase spoiled gradient echo images show the posterior horn of the lateral meniscus (*arrow*) with increasing clarity as the TE increases. In addition, note the decreasing signal intensity of the distal femoral epiphysis (**) owing to increasing susceptibility contrast from bone trabeculae.

▼
Essential Points to Remember

1. Both T1 and T2 contrast can be reduced by using both a long TR and a short TE. Other contrast mechanisms, such as proton density, chemical shift, and magnetization transfer then become more conspicuous.

2. The term *proton density-weighting* is misleading because proton density is not necessarily the most important source of contrast on these images. A preferable expression is *intermediate-weighting*.

3. Intermediate-weighted images tend to have a high SNR and to show low-signal structures (e.g., bone, ligaments) with high anatomical detail.

4. The spin echo technique allows efficient acquisition of high-quality intermediate-weighted images, whether as a separate acquisition or along with T2-weighted images as part of a dual-TE technique.

5. The image quality of intermediate-weighted images is usually better with the standard spin echo technique than with the fast spin echo technique because the former produces less blurring and fewer artifacts.

6. When acquired independently, it is possible to optimize the T2 and intermediate contrast images separately, using standard SE for the intermediate contrast studies, and fast spin echo for the T2-weighted scans.

7. Intermediate-weighted images can be obtained using the gradient echo technique with a small flip angle and short TE, but additional contrast due to T2* and chemical shift differences is more difficult to eliminate than with the spin echo technique.

8. With gradient echo acquisition, T1 contrast can be minimized, even with a relatively short TR, if the excitation flip angle is reduced.

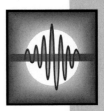

Intravenous Water-Soluble Contrast Agents

Current clinical magnetic resonance imaging (MRI) techniques are based entirely on measuring signals from protons. The active components of most MRI contrast agents contain no protons and thus are not detected directly during the magnetic resonance (MR) measurement process; however, the contrast agents act by shortening the relaxation time of water protons that are close to the contrast agent. Therefore, MRI contrast agents act by a mechanism different from that of contrast agents for all other modalities.

Most contrast agents reduce both T1 and T2 relaxation, but some affect one more than they do the other. The effect of contrast agents depends on their biodistribution as well as on pulse sequence parameters.

In this chapter and the next, we consider a variety of contrast agents, classified principally by their biodistribution and tissue effects. Relevant compartments to consider include the intravascular space, which can be subdivided into arterial-capillary and venous spaces; the interstitial space; the reticuloendothelial system; and the parenchymal cells of various organs. Some contrast agents principally affect one of these compartments, whereas others are distributed to two or more of them. Figure 21-1 depicts the relevant compartments in the hepatic parenchyma, as an example of the biodistribution of various MRI contrast agents.

In this chapter we restrict our discussion to water-soluble contrast agents. They include contrast agents that are distributed throughout the extracellular space as well as some that are taken up by some parenchymal cells. Chapter 22 includes discussions of particulate and blood pool agents, oral agents, and the contrast agent nomenclature in general.

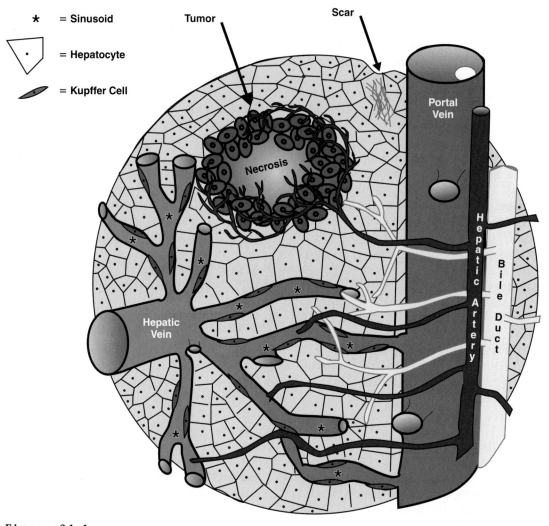

Figure 21-1
Compartments within the liver serve as an example for biodistribution of various MRI contrast agents. The hepatic vascular supply comes principally via the portal vein, whereas the hepatic artery supplies about one third of the material being perfused. These vessels drain into hepatic sinusoids, the abundance of which gives the liver a large blood volume. Kupffer cells are reticuloendothelial cells that line the walls of hepatic sinusoids. Tumors tend to have an abundant arterial supply, whereas scars are hypovascular. Both tumors and scars have large interstitial spaces. Hepatocytes produce bile, which is excreted into bile ducts.

Extracellular Paramagnetic Agents

The extracellular space consists of the sum of the intravascular and interstitial spaces. Currently available chelates of gadolinium (e.g., gadopentetate dimeglumine, gadoteridol, gadoversetamide, gadodiamide) are considered extracellular space agents. Materials such as these are distributed initially within the intravascular space and diffuse rapidly throughout the extracellular (vascular plus interstitial) space, much as water-soluble iodinated contrast agents do.

Although these agents have been described as "nonspecific," they are highly specific for enhancing the extracellular space of perfused tissues. They can also be quite specific and versatile for enhancing specific portions of the extracellular space if proper attention is directed toward choosing the pulse sequence and timing of the image acquisition relative to contrast agent administration.

Immediately after intravenous injection these agents traverse the pulmonary circulation. They are then distributed throughout systemic arteries, followed by distribution throughout the vascular space. Within seconds, substantial amounts of contrast material diffuse across capillaries into the interstitial space of tissues outside the central nervous system (CNS) and across renal glomeruli into the urinary collecting system. One can consider three basic phases of vascular and tissue enhancement following administration of extracellular space agents: arterial, blood pool, and extracellular phases. There are also transitional phases between these basic phases.

Arterial Phase

If the image data for the center of k-space are acquired during the first pass of contrast agent through the arterial system, arteriographic images can be obtained. Although two-dimensional Fourier transform (2D-FT) techniques may be used for these gadolinium-enhanced arteriograms, 3D-FT techniques are preferable for acquiring thin, contiguous sections that can be used to generate projection images via maximum intensity projection (MIP) or other algorithms (Fig. 21-2).

Images obtained during the arterial phase are also useful for depicting tissue perfusion. Only images captured during this phase can be used to judge a tissue's vascularity; images obtained at a later phase are affected by the contrast agent in the venous and capillary systems and tissue interstitium (Figs. 21-3 and 21-4).

Arterial phase images are acquired best using pulse sequences that allow completion of imaging within 30 seconds or less. Suitable techniques include single-slice or multislice 2D-FT spoiled gradient echo images or three-dimensional (3D)-FT spoiled gradient echo images with a very short repetition time (TR). Preparation pulses, such as for fat suppression or inversion recovery, can improve tissue enhancement, but they increase the acquisition time. The contrast agent must be injected rapidly (e.g., about 2 ml per second), by hand or machine. The contrast agent bolus should be followed by a rapid flush of approximately 10 to 30 ml of saline or other solution to clear the intravenous tubing and peripheral veins of contrast agent.

The arterial phase is the most technically difficult one to image. The window of opportunity for this phase—between the initial arrival of contrast material in arteries and the filling of veins—is usually no longer than 20 seconds. Signs of a successful acquisition of arterial-phase images include intense enhancement of arteries and little or no enhancement of veins. In the abdomen, arterial phase images are characterized by intense, approximately equivalent enhancement of pancreas, spleen, and renal cortex; marked heterogeneity of the spleen; near absence of renal medullary enhancement; and minimal enhancement of liver parenchyma. Although contrast material is often visible in major portal vein branches on good arterial phase images of the liver, there is little if any contrast material in microscopic portal branches or hepatic sinusoids and none in the hepatic veins (except the major central hepatic veins in some patients with tricuspid regurgitation) (Figs. 21-5 and 21-6).

Early arterial phase images are best for depicting arteries, and later arterial phase images are better for depicting hypervascular tissues. Faster imaging techniques, such as those using parallel imaging (see Chapter 17), now allow acquisition of consecutive early and later arterial phase images within a 20 second interval, referred to as *double arterial phase imaging*. It remains to be seen, however, whether the increased efficiency of techniques such as parallel

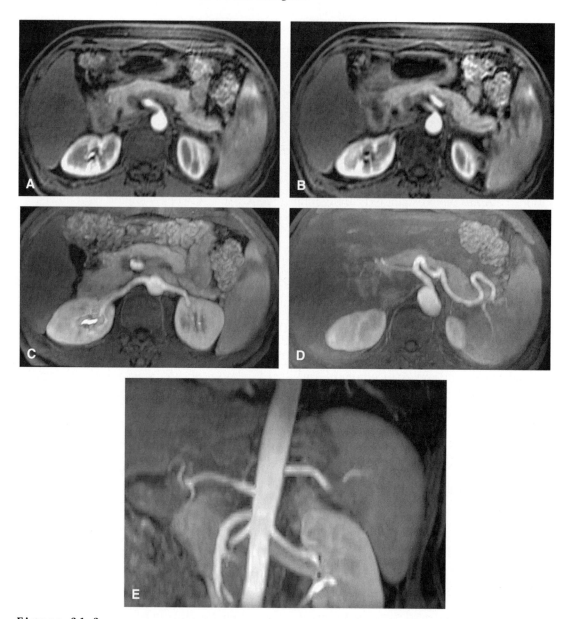

Figure 21-2

(*A, B*) Axial fat-suppressed 6.5/2.1/20° three-dimensional (3D) gradient echo images obtained immediately after a bolus of gadolinium chelate (0.1 mmol/kg), with 2.5 mm thickness, depicting enhancement of soft tissue and arteries. (*C, D*) Axial maximum intensity projection (MIP) images are created from the source images at, respectively, the renal artery and celiac axis levels. (*E*) Oblique coronal reconstruction shows these vessels in a magnetic resonance angiography image.

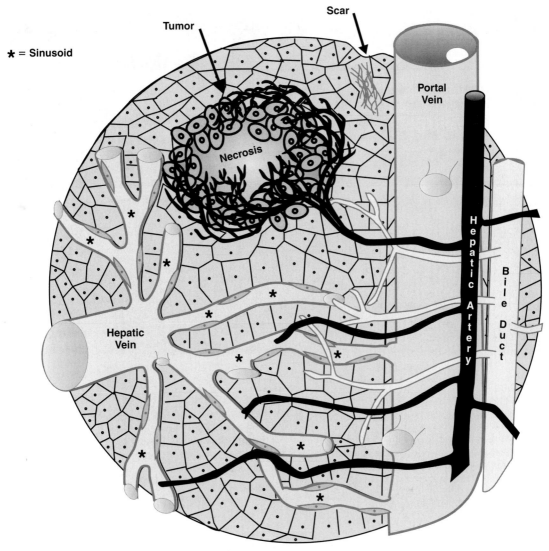

* = Sinusoid

Tumor

Scar

Necrosis

Portal Vein

Hepatic Artery

Bile Duct

Hepatic Vein

Figure 21-3
Early arterial phase of hepatic enhancement. *Dark shades* indicate arterial enhancement. There is no enhancement of portal veins, sinusoids (*), or hepatic veins. Intense enhancement of the tumor is due to its abundant arterial supply.

imaging are best applied to improving temporal resolution (e.g., double arterial phase imaging) or spatial resolution (higher matrix, thinner slices, or both).

Blood Pool Phase

Less than a minute after intravenous injection, contrast material typically is distributed throughout the body's blood vessels. At this time, the distribution of extracellular space contrast agents most closely approximates the blood pool, although some diffusion into the interstitial space and renal tubules has occurred. Throughout much of the body, tumors are depicted best during this phase owing to the small blood pool of skeletal muscle (Fig. 21-7).

In the abdomen, the blood pool phase is usually referred to as the *portal venous phase,* although arteries and parenchymal

Unenhanced   **Arterial**

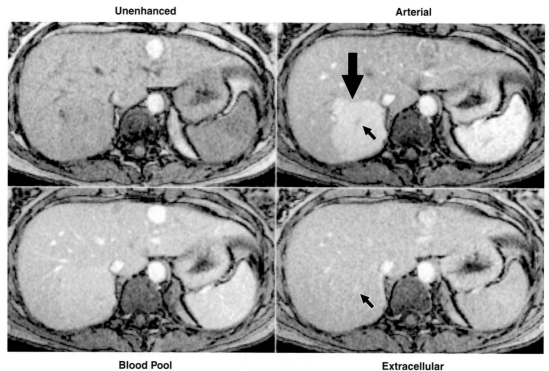

Blood Pool   **Extracellular**

Figure 21-4
Hypervascular hepatic focal nodular hyperplasia (*large arrow*), which is depicted best on T1-weighted spoiled gradient echo 122/2.3/90° images during the arterial phase after injection of gadolinium chelate. The mass is subtle during later phases because the size of its blood pool and extracellular space are similar to those of the liver. *Small arrows* indicate a central scar that is hyperintense only during the extracellular phase because it has a larger extracellular space than the rest of the tumor even though it is less vascular. Although portal veins are enhanced during the arterial phase image, hepatic sinusoids and hepatic veins are not.

tissues are enhanced prominently during this phase as well. Although hypervascular tissues such as the pancreas enhance maximally during the arterial phase, the blood pool phase is the phase of maximal hepatic enhancement (Fig. 21-6); approximately two thirds of blood flow to normal livers is supplied by the portal circulation, which arrives 20 to 30 seconds after the hepatic arterial flow (Fig. 21-8). Because of the large volume of blood in hepatic sinusoids, even many moderately hypervascular malignancies are less intense than liver on these images. Contrast between liver and hypovascular lesions is maximal on blood pool phase images (Fig. 21-9). Hypervascular lesions may be obscured on these images, however, because

their blood pool is similar to that of hepatic parenchyma (Fig. 21-10).

Extracellular Phase

Extracellular phase images are acquired at least 2 minutes after injection of contrast material. By this time, contrast material has diffused widely across capillary walls into the interstitium of most tissues, although there is still substantial contrast agent in the vessels (Fig. 21-11). Capillaries in the CNS and the testes are not permeable to contrast agents, unlike capillaries throughout the rest of the body. Interstitial contrast enhancement is particularly prominent in

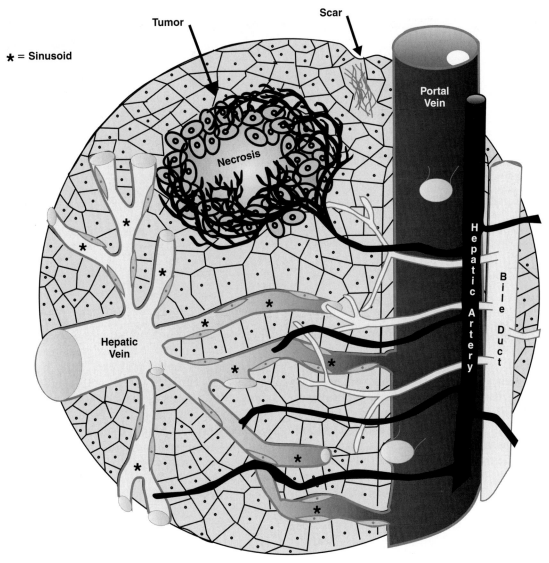

Figure 21-5
Late arterial phase. Although there is some enhancement of the portal vein and its major branches, the sinusoids (∗) and hepatic veins are not yet enhanced.

edematous tissues such as neoplasms and areas of inflammation. Fibrous tissue typically has a large interstitial space. Therefore, fibrous tissue is much enhanced on extracellular phase images, although it is usually extremely hypovascular. Many metastases have large interstitial spaces and are therefore hyperintense on extracellular phase images (Fig. 21-12).

In addition to diffusing across tissue capillary walls, extracellular space contrast agents diffuse across glomerular walls into renal tubules, within which they are concentrated as water is reabsorbed. Current extracellular space MRI contrast agents are eliminated entirely by renal excretion. Owing to the concentration of extracellular space agents in the renal parenchyma and

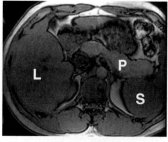 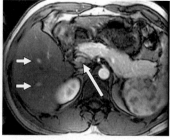 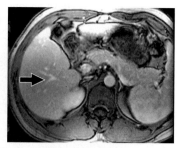

Unenhanced   **Arterial Phase**   **Blood Pool Phase**

Figure 21-6
Axial images of the abdomen obtained before (*left*) and during the arterial (*center*) and blood pool (*right*) phases after bolus injection of gadolinium chelate. The liver (L) enhances little during the arterial phase, whereas the pancreas (P) and spleen (S) enhance intensely. There is some contrast material in the main portal vein (*long white arrow*) and its major branches (*short white arrows*). Contrast material has filled hepatic sinusoids during the blood pool phase, causing the liver to become isointense with pancreas and spleen. *Black arrow* indicates an enhanced hepatic vein.

collecting system, these agents are highly effective for enhancing kidneys and the urinary tract.

Because the extracellular phase of enhancement changes little over several minutes, fast scanning techniques are less important than they are for acquiring arterial or blood pool phase images. Frequently, extracellular phase images are obtained with suppression of the lipid signal intensity, even with MRI systems where fat suppression is not practical for faster imaging. Interstitial enhancement is particularly conspicuous on these images. Note that if fat is nulled via inversion recovery with a short inversion time (STIR) enhancing tissue is also nulled because of its short T1 relaxation time. Therefore, the STIR technique is not recommended after administration of T1-shortening contrast agents.

Brain and testicular capillaries are not permeable to gadolinium chelates, which is the basis for most clinical use of contrast agents for imaging the CNS (Fig. 21-13). Enhancement of the brain is minimal, owing entirely to enhancement of the blood pool. Tumors and injured brain parenchyma enhance much more because of the enhancement of their interstitial spaces. Depiction on postcontrast images of brain lesions as high—signal-intensity entities is best if at least a few minutes is allowed to elapse after injecting the contrast agent. This interval allows the contrast agent to diffuse into the interstitium of diseased tissue while the blood pool contrast agent concentration decreases.

Extracellular phase images are helpful for documenting enhancement of solid masses, allowing them to be distinguished from cysts. Careful comparison to adjacent tissues, visually or quantitatively, may be necessary (Fig. 21-14).

Tissue-Directed Paramagnetic Agents

Gadolinium Chelates

Attachment of a suitable structure to an extracellular gadolinium chelate may allow it to be transported across cell membranes. Compounds such as these have been developed most often for preferentially enhancing hepatocytes (Fig. 21-15). Hepatocyte-directed paramagnetic agents that have been tested in humans include gadobenate dimeglumine

T1-GRE Unenhanced

T1-SE Unenhanced

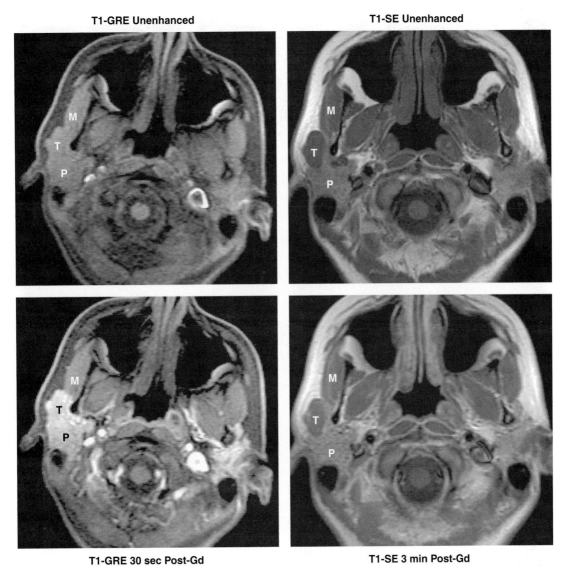

T1-GRE 30 sec Post-Gd

T1-SE 3 min Post-Gd

Figure 21-7
Hypervascular parotid tumor (T) at the anterior edge of the parotid gland (P) is isointense with skeletal muscle (M) on unenhanced images (*top left, top right*) and during the extracellular phase (*bottom right*). Contrast with muscle is greatest during the vascular phase (*bottom left*). The parotid gland is hyperintense compared with tumor on T1-spin echo images before and after contrast agent administration, owing to fat content; fat is suppressed on the gradient echo images.

(formerly Gd-BOPTA) and gadoxetic acid disodium (formerly Gd-EOB-DTPA).

Like other gadolinium chelates, these tissue-directed chelates diffuse across non-CNS capillaries and renal glomeruli, accumulating in interstitial spaces and urine. Unlike extracellular space chelates, however, tissue-directed gadolinium chelates have dual excretory pathways, being eliminated by both renal and hepatobiliary routes. In this respect, the biodistribution of these agents resembles that of iodinated radiographic contrast agents more than that of extracellular space gadolinium chelates

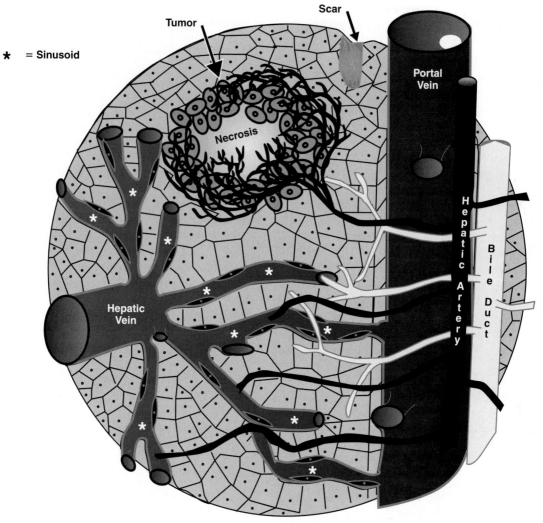

Figure 21-8

Blood pool (portal venous) phase. All blood vessels, including arteries, veins, and hepatic sinusoids (∗), are filled with contrast material. Necrotic tumor and scar have small blood pools and thus are relatively unenhanced.

because iodinated agents also have a dual excretory pathway. However, both gadobenate dimeglumine and gadoxetic acid disodium have higher biliary/renal excretion ratios than do iodinated radiographic contrast agents.

The proportion of renal versus hepatobiliary elimination depends on the particular contrast agent and on the patient's relative renal and hepatobiliary function. Five to ten minutes after intravenous administration substantial contrast agent has been distributed throughout the vascular and interstitial spaces and in hepatocytes. On later images (i.e., after 30 minutes or more) the contrast agent is cleared from the extracellular space and is then present principally in hepatocytes, bile ducts, and proximal small bowel (owing to its biliary excretion) and in the urinary collecting system (Fig. 21-16).

Unenhanced **Arterial Phase**

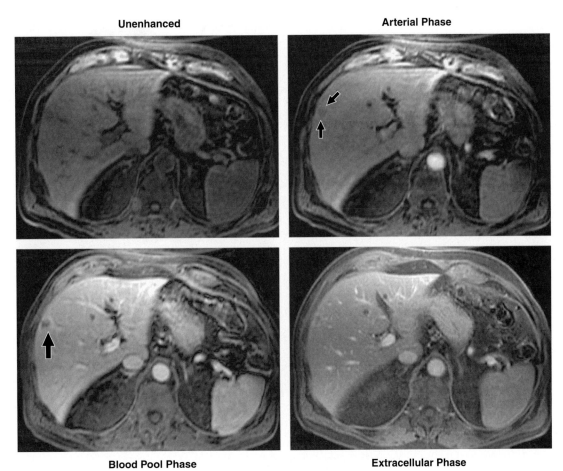

Blood Pool Phase **Extracellular Phase**

Figure 21-9
Hypovascular hepatic metastasis from colonic carcinoma depicted best on blood pool (portal venous) phase images (T1-weighted gradient echo images with fat saturation). The lesion is subtle on unenhanced image (*top left*). During the arterial phase (*top right*), there is subtle rim enhancement (*arrows*). The lesion is best seen during the blood pool phase (*arrow, bottom left*) and is subtle during the extracelluar phase.

Manganese-Based Compound

Manganese (Mn^{2+}), like gadolinium (Gd^{3+}), is strongly paramagnetic. Although manganese is an important component of a normal human diet and plays an important role in several cellular functions, free manganese is toxic if injected directly into the bloodstream. Manganese is tolerated better if it is complexed to a molecule that facilitates binding to plasma proteins. Protein binding occurs after oral ingestion of manganese and after in vivo decomplexation of some manganese chelates. In the body, manganese is located principally within mitochondria, where it is involved in cell respiration. Manganese is eliminated by biliary and intestinal secretion.

Thus far, the only parenteral manganese compound tested in humans is mangafodipir trisodium (formerly Mn-DPDP). Although mangafodipir trisodium was designed to be extracted primarily by hepatocytes, manganese appears to be delivered to several

Unenhanced

Arterial

Blood Pool

Extracellular

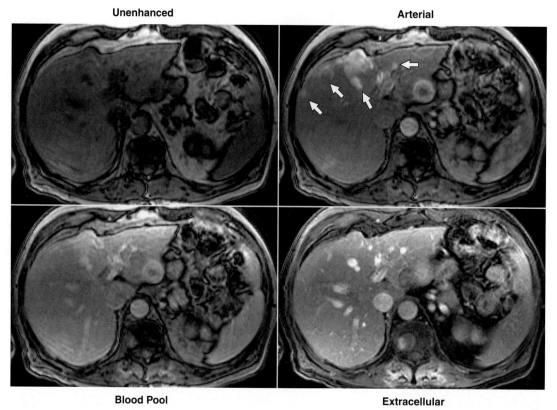

Figure 21-10
Hypervascular metastases (*arrows*) are best depicted during the arterial phase after injection of gadolinium chelate. During later phases the lesions are subtle or obscured.

tissues with active aerobic metabolism, including pancreas, renal cortex, gastrointestinal mucosa, myocardium, and the adrenal glands (Fig. 21-17). Thus, mangafodipir trisodium appears to be more of a metabolic contrast agent than are other current contrast agents; however, clinical testing in humans as well as U.S. Food and Drug Administration (FDA) approval has thus far been restricted to the diagnosis of liver lesions.

Contrast Agent Nomenclature

The most precise term for a contrast agent or any other chemical substance is the name established by the International Union of Pure and Applied Chemistry (IUPAC). The systematic chemical name indicates unambiguously the exact structure of the contrast agent; unfortunately, such names often consume several lines of text and are virtually unpronounceable. For these reasons, the systematic chemical name is rarely used in clinical practice and generally appears in the radiology literature only during the early stages of contrast agent development. For example, the first gadolinium chelate approved for human use has the chemical name 1-deoxy-1-(methylamino)-D-glucitol dihydrogen [*N*,*N*-bis[2-[bis(carboxymethyl)amino]ethyl]-glycinato-(5-)]-gadolinate (2-)(2:1).

To facilitate dissemination of information, a pharmaceutical company usually derives an abbreviated name or company code name

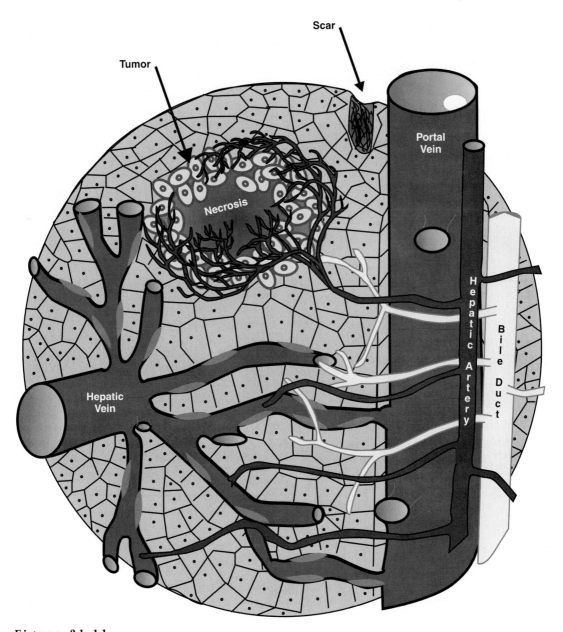

Figure 21-11
Extracellular phase. The entire extracellular space, including the vascular and interstitial compartments, is enhanced. Many tumors and scars have a large interstitial space and thus are hyperintense during this phase. Whereas complete necrosis remains unenhanced, partial necrosis may eventually enhance intensely; if there are some intact blood vessels, the large interstitial space enhances.

Unenhanced **Arterial Phase**

Blood Pool Phase **Extracellular Phase**

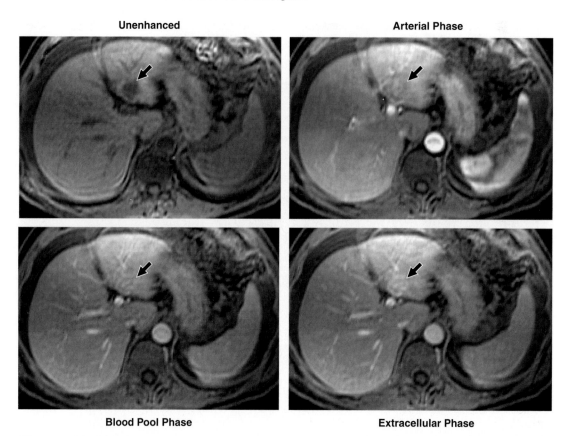

Figure 21-12
Hypervascular liver lesion (*arrows*), obscured on arterial and on blood pool (portal venous) phase images, is depicted as hyperintense during the extracellular phase because of its large interstitial space.

for a new contrast agent. Thus, 1-deoxy-1-(methylamino)-D-glucitol dihydrogen [N,N-bis[2-[bis(carboxymethyl)amino]ethyl]-glycinato(5-)]gadolinate (2-)(2:1) has been referred to as gadolinium–diethylenetri-amine pentaacetic acid, or, still shorter, Gd-DTPA. This term, although now obsolete, is still commonly used.

During early investigation of a contrast agent in humans, an official U.S. Adopted Name (USAN) is assigned to a contrast agent. The USAN is an agent's official generic name. Once this occurs, the abbreviated name introduced by the pharmaceutical company should no longer be used. Thus, the agent formerly known as

Gd-DTPA should now be referred to as *gadopentetate dimeglumine*. These generic names are usually used in other countries as well.

As the development of an agent continues, a pharmaceutical company creates a brand name for marketing. While applying to the United States Patent and Trademark Office for an official trademark, the superscript symbol "TM" is applied (e.g., Magnevist™). Once the brand name is officially registered in the United States and other countries, the symbol changes to "®" (e.g., Magnevist®). Table 21-1 lists the generic and commercial names of several currently used intravenous MRI contrast agents.

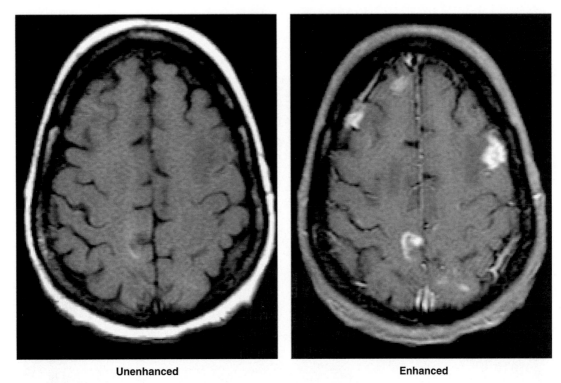

Unenhanced   **Enhanced**

Figure 21-13
Enhancement of intracranial metastases. After administration of gadolinium chelate (*right*), there is little enhancement of brain parenchyma owing to the blood-brain barrier. Contrast material had diffused into the interstitium of the metastases, causing intense enhancement of them.

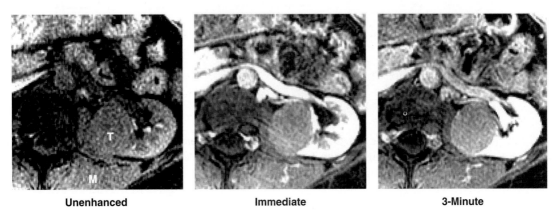

Unenhanced   **Immediate**   **3-Minute**

Figure 21-14
Hypovascular renal carcinoid tumor (T) with subtle enhancement. The tumor is slightly less intense than skeletal muscle (M) before administration of contrast agent (*left*), isointense during the vascular phase (*center*), and slightly hyperintense during the extracellular phase (*right*). A cyst would be less intense than skeletal muscle during these phases owing to greater enhancement of skeletal muscle relative to that of the cyst.

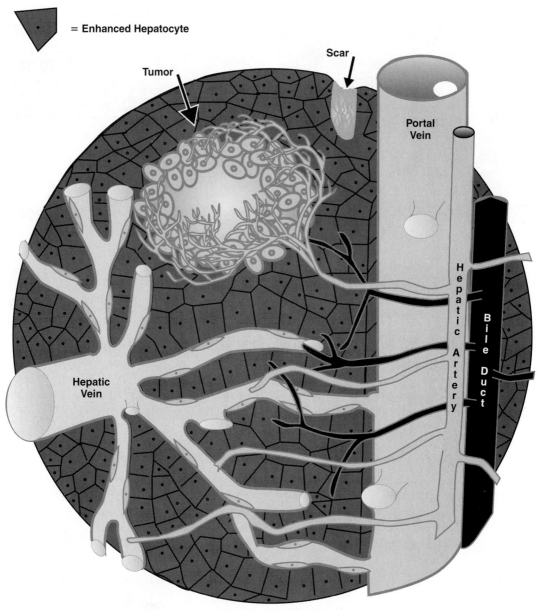

Figure 21-15
Enhancement of hepatocytes and bile ducts by hepatocyte-directed contrast material.

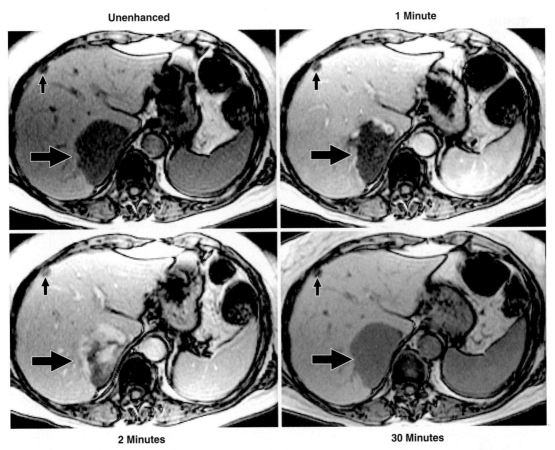

Unenhanced **1 Minute**

2 Minutes **30 Minutes**

Figure 21-16
Unenhanced, 1-minute, 2-minute, and 30-minute T1-weighted gradient echo images following injection of gadobenate dimeglumine. The 1-minute and 2-minute images show typical progressive enhancement of a cavernous hemangioma (*large arrows*) and no enhancement of a cyst (*small arrows*). By 30 minutes, contrast agent has been cleared from the blood pool but remains within hepatocytes.

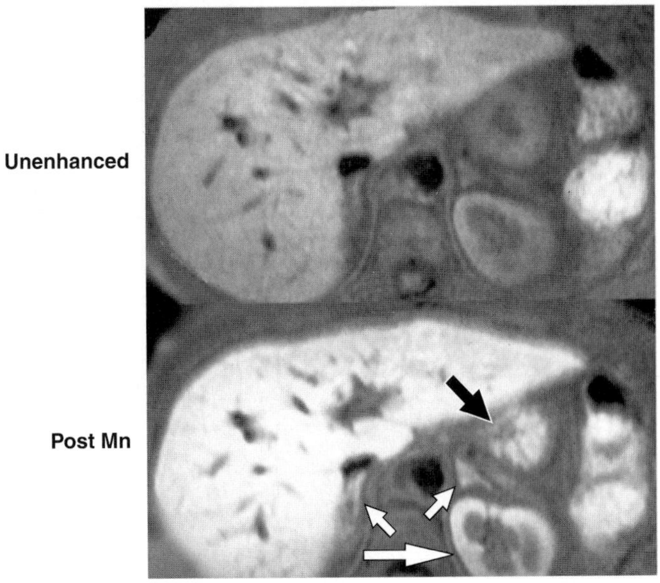

Unenhanced

Figure 21-17
Fat-suppressed T1-weighted spin echo images before (*top*) and after (*bottom*) intravenous injection of mangafodipir trisodium. In addition to the liver, there is prominent enhancement of the renal cortex (*large white arrow*), adrenal glands (*small white arrows*), and gastric wall (*black arrow*).

Post Mn

Table 21-1 ■ NAMES AND VENDORS OF INTRAVENOUS CONTRAST AGENTS, BY CLASSIFICATION

Generic (IUP) Name	Commercial Name	Vendor	Other Terms
Gadolinium Chelates, Extracellular			
Gadopentetate dimeglumine	Magnevist	Berlex Laboratories; Wayne, NJ, USA	Gadolinium diethylenetriaminepentaacetic acid dimeglumine (Gd-DTPA)
Gadoterate meglumine	Dotarem	Laboratoire Guerbet; Aulnay-sous-Bois, France	Gadolinium tetraazacyclododecanetetraacetic acid meglumine (Gd-DOTA)
Gadoteridol	ProHance	Bracco Diagnostics; Milan, Italy	Gd-HP-DO3A
Gadodiamide	Omniscan	Nycomed AS; Oslo, Norway	Gadolinium diethylenetriaminepentaacetic acid bis (methylamide) (Gd-DTPA-BMA)
Gadobutrol	Gadovist	Berlex Laboratories; Wayne, NJ, USA	Gd-DO3A-butantriol
Gadoversetamide	Optimark	Mallinckrodt Medical, St. Louis, MO, USA	MP-1177/10
Gadolinium Chelates: Biliary Excretion			
Gadoxetic acid, disodium	Eovist	Berlex Laboratories; Wayne, NJ, USA	Gadolinium ethoxybenzyl diethylenetriaminepentaacetic acid (Gd-EOB-DTPA)
Gadobenate dimeglumine	MultiHance	Bracco Diagnostics; Milan, Italy	Gadolinium benzyloxypropionictetraacetate (Gd-BOPTA/Dimeg)
Manganese Agents			
Mangafodipir trisodium	Teslascan	Nycomed AS; Oslo, Norway	Manganese dipyridoxyl diphosphate (Mn-DPDP)
Iron Oxide Particles			
Ferumoxides*	Feridex I.V.	Berlex Laboratories; Wayne, NJ, USA	AMI-25
Ferrixan*	Resovist	Schering AG; Berlin, Germany	SH U 555 A
Ferumoxtran*	Combidex	Advanced Magnetics; Cambridge, MA, USA	Code 7227; BMS 180549; AMI-227

*For iron oxide agents marketed or tested in the United States and by a different name in other nations, only the United States vendor is listed.

Modified from Mitchell DG. MR imaging contrast agents: What's in a name? J Magn Reson Imaging 1997;7:1–7.

▼
Essential Points to Remember

1. Current chelates of gadolinium are extracellular space agents. They are distributed throughout the vascular space and diffuse across capillary walls into the interstitial space, except in the CNS and testes.

2. Extracellular space MRI contrast agents are eliminated entirely by renal excretion.

3. Images for which the center of k-space is acquired within approximately 30 seconds after injection of an MRI contrast agent depict the arterial anatomy and vascularity.

4. Images acquired approximately 1 minute after injection of the MRI contrast agent depict the blood pool. In the abdomen these images are often referred to as portal venous phase images.

5. Images acquired more than 3 minutes after injection of an extracellular space agent depict enhancement of the entire extracellular (vascular plus interstitial) space. This includes enhancement of fibrous tissue, edema, and partial necrosis.

6. Gadolinium chelates can be attached to a structure that causes them to be transported across cell (e.g., hepatocyte) membranes. Hepatocyte-directed gadolinium chelates are excreted by both renal and biliary mechanisms.

7. Mangafodipir trisodium (Mn-DPDP) is rapidly decomplexed. The released manganese is transported to mitochondria within aerobically active tissues throughout the body (e.g., pancreas, renal cortex, adrenal glands, gastrointestinal mucosa). Excretion is primarily biliary and intestinal.

8. Contrast agents initially are given an abbreviated chemical name or a company code name. When an official generic name is given, it should be used in place of the older name. For example, the agents formerly known as Gd-DTPA and Mn-DPDP are now called, respectively, *gadopentetate dimeglumine* and *mangafodipir trisodium*.

Chapter **22**

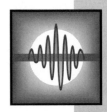

Particulate and Oral Contrast Agents

Particulate Agents

Polysaccharide-coated superparamagnetic iron oxide particles, often referred to as SPIOs, can be designed to have various properties. These particles contain a crystalline core composed of ferrous (Fe^{2+}) ions, ferric (Fe^{3+}) ions, and oxygen, coated with dextran or some other polysaccharide. Most of these particles measure between 4 and 10 nm, and their biological behavior is altered by their polysaccharide coating.

The blood half-life and distribution to different organs of the reticuloendothelial system change with effective particle or cluster size. One particulate iron oxide agent, ferumoxide (also referred to as Feridex or AMI-25), has a thin, incomplete dextran coating that causes individual particles to form polycrystalline aggregates. These aggregates behave in solution or within cells as

large particles. A different agent, ferumoxtran (also referred to as Combidex or AMI 227), contains a thicker, more complete coating, which causes these particles to remain as separate, small monocrystals in solution. Large particles or aggregates accumulate rapidly in reticuloendothelial cells of the liver and spleen (Fig. 22-1), whereas small particles remain in circulation longer and are taken up more avidly by lymph nodes.

Iron oxide polycrystalline aggregates with an average diameter of approximately 50 to 200 nm (e.g., ferumoxides) are phagocytosed rapidly by reticuloendothelial cells and are cleared from the blood in an hour or less. Iron oxide particles such as these are far more effective for T2 and T2* enhancement than for T1 enhancement. Therefore, the major use of SPIOs is for reducing the signal intensity of targeted tissues on T2-weighted or T2*-weighted images (Fig. 22-2).

Although SPIO agents may be defined by and used based on their inclusion of

295

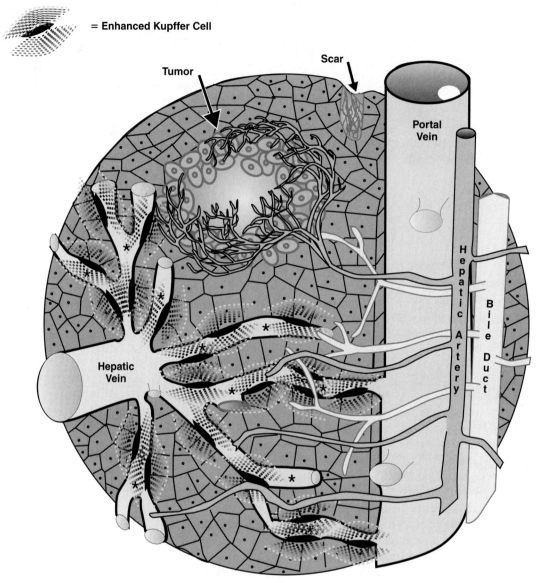

= Enhanced Kupffer Cell

Figure 22-1
Enhancement by iron oxide particles of Kupffer cells of the liver. The powerful effect of the superparamagnetic particles extends far beyond the Kupffer cells themselves.

relatively large particles, small particles are typically included as well. In fact, there is a wide range of particle sizes present in most preparations. The large particles are cleared from the blood rapidly, whereas the small particles persist longer in the blood pool, being filtered more slowly by the reticuloendothelial and lymphatic system (Fig. 22-3). Small particles, with greater T1 relaxivity and less T2* relaxivity than large particles exhibit, predominate on later images and therefore increase the signal intensity of the blood pool on images with a sufficiently short TE (Fig. 22-4). This is depicted as a T1-enhancing blood-pool effect, similar to that described in the next section.

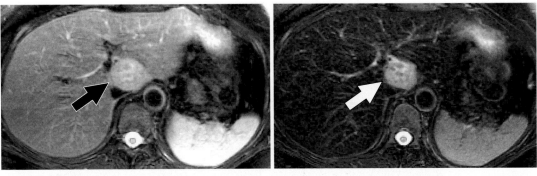

Figure 22-2
T2-weighted fast spin echo 3000/96 images before (*left*) and 10 minutes after (*right*) intravenous administration of iron oxide particles (ferrixan) show greater conspicuousness of a colonic metastasis (*arrows*) owing to decreased signal intensity of the liver. The spleen also has slightly decreased signal intensity.

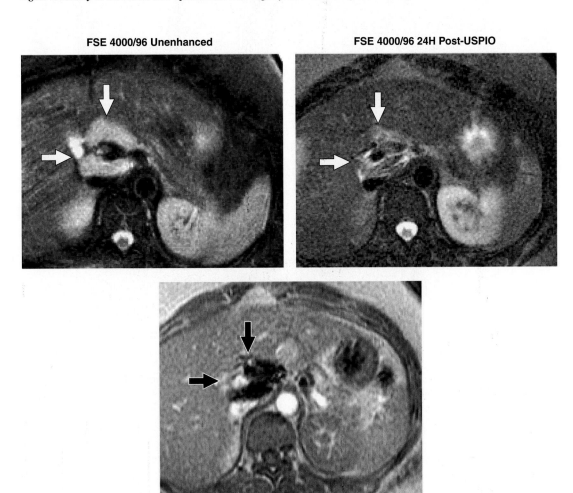

Figure 22-3
Concentration of ultrasmall iron oxide particles within hyperplastic inflammatory lymph nodes (*arrows*), 24 hours after the dose on the T2-weighted fast spin echo (FSE) 4000/96 image (*top right*) and the gradient echo (GRE) 120/4.2/90° image (*bottom*).

Reticuloendothelial contrast agents can also be created by incorporating a paramagnetic or superparamagnetic material in hollow structures with surrounding lipid bilayers (i.e., liposomes). These magnetic resonance imaging (MRI) contrast agents have not been studied in humans.

Blood Pool Agents

As the effective particle size decreases, the efficiency of phagocytosis by macrophages and reticuloendothelial cells is reduced. Therefore, small particles remain longer in the blood. Eventually, these particles

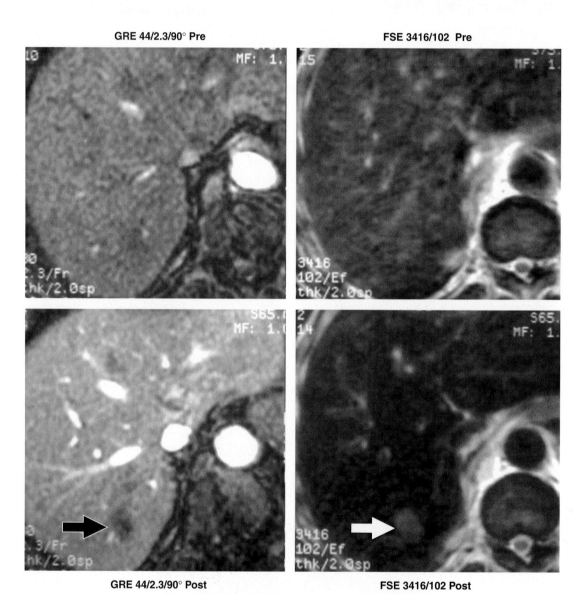

GRE 44/2.3/90° Pre   **FSE 3416/102 Pre**

GRE 44/2.3/90° Post   **FSE 3416/102 Post**

Figure 22-4
Blood pool effects of USPIO (ferumoxtran), increasing the signal intensity on T1-weighted images (*left*) and decreasing the signal intensity on T2-weighted images (*right*). On T1-weighted images (*bottom left*) the hepatic parenchyma and vessels have increased signal intensity, thereby increasing the visibility of a metastasis (*arrow*). On T2-weighted images (*bottom right*), the hepatic parenchyma and vessels have decreased signal intensity, again increasing the visibility of the metastasis (*arrow*).

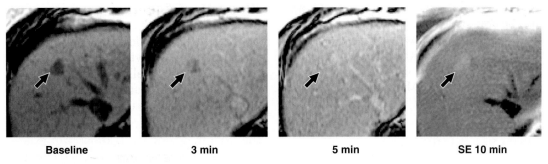

| Baseline | 3 min | 5 min | SE 10 min |

Figure 22-5

T1-enhancing effects of iron oxide particles (ferrixan), increasing the intensity of a cavernous hemangioma (*arrow*) and hepatic vessels relative to the hepatic parenchyma. Enhancement of blood vessels and the hemangioma is more apparent at 5 minutes than at 3 minutes because larger particles have been cleared from the blood pool by this time.

degrade or are phagocytosed at a slow rate by macrophages, particularly by those in lymph nodes (Fig. 22-3). These ultrasmall superparamagnetic iron oxide agents are sometimes referred to as USPIOs.

Small iron oxide monocrystals such as ferumoxtran facilitate T2 relaxation less efficiently than do large particles. These particles reduce both T1 and T2 substantially and by comparable magnitudes, increasing the signal intensity on T1-weighted images and decreasing it on T2-weighted images (Figs. 22-4 and 22-5).

Paramagnetic blood pool contrast agents have also been created by attaching paramagnetic material such as gadolinium diethylenetriamine pentaacetic acid (Gd-DTPA) to larger molecules, such as albumin or polylysine. A recently developed small molecular agent, so far referred to as MS-325, binds to blood proteins immediately after being injected as a bolus, becoming a blood pool agent.

Blood pool contrast agents are effective for enhancing blood vessels, demonstrating perfusion dynamics on rapid sequential images, and enhancing organs with large blood spaces such as the liver and spleen. In fact, the success of the portal phase for hepatic imaging after administration of extracellular agents such as iodinated contrast material for computed tomography (CT) and gadolinium chelates for MRI, is based on blood pool principles. In other words, the reason the liver enhances more than most tumors during the portal phase is that its blood pool is larger than that of most tumors. In fact, the portal phase after administration of extracellular space agents is contaminated somewhat by leakage of the contrast material into the interstitial space of tumors. It must be emphasized that the use of a blood pool agent results in enhancement that is much different from that seen on delayed images after administration of an extracellular space agent. Delayed images are defined by the type of contrast agent administered: blood pool phase images for blood pool agents and extracellular phase images for extracellular space agents.

Oral Agents

A variety of oral contrast agents have been investigated for improved delineation of bowel. They can be divided into those that have (1) low signal intensity on all pulse sequences (proton displacement or T2 shortening), (2) high signal intensity on all pulse sequence (T1 shortening), (3) high signal intensity on T1-weighted and low signal intensity on T2-weighted images (T1 and T2 shortening), and (4) low signal intensity on T1-weighted images and high signal intensity on T2-weighted images (water-based).

Low-Low Intensity

The principal advantage of reducing the signal intensity of bowel on all pulse sequences is that artifacts from moving bowel can be eliminated. This may be particularly desirable on T2-weighted images, where artifact from bowel motion may be particularly pronounced. Additionally, distinction between bowel and high-signal-intensity masses or fluid collections can be accentuated if the bowel signal intensity is reduced. On T1-weighted images, however, masses and fluid collections usually have low signal intensity, making it difficult to distinguish them from low-signal-intensity bowel.

The signal intensity in bowel can be reduced by displacing the bowel contents with a material that contains no protons, such as air. Air can be administered by intubating the small bowel or rectum. This method has not found widespread acceptance, principally because of patient discomfort. Additionally, susceptibility artifacts from air degrade T2*-weighted gradient echo images and echo planar images.

Bowel contents can also be displaced with perfluorocarbons. These agents do not contain protons, but they have the same susceptibility as water and thus do not cause artifacts. The first oral MRI contrast agent approved for clinical use was a perfluorocarbon formulation, perflubron (Imagent), but it was prohibitively expensive and was withdrawn from the market. Concentrated high-density barium sulfate, such as is used for upper gastrointestinal imaging or barium enema, also displaces the bowel contents, although it is less effective than perfluorocarbons.

The signal intensity of bowel can be reduced on all pulse sequences by administering SPIOs. A high enough concentration of these agents can shorten the T2 and T2* enough to eliminate signal from bowel even on so-called T1-weighted images. The major disadvantage of using SPIOs as a bowel agent is the resulting distortion of the local magnetic field, which can exacerbate artifacts. Fat-suppression techniques are particularly vulnerable to magnetic field distortions.

Clays, such as kaolin and attapulgite (both are used in formulations of Kaopectate) and bentonite, restrict the motion of water, shortening the T1 and T2 relaxation times. The T2 shortening is profound enough to eliminate signal from bowel on SE images with a TE of 20 msec or more. Therefore, clay agents have been described as reducing the signal intensity on all pulse sequences; however, T1-weighted gradient echo images with a TE of less than 3 msec have little T2 contrast and therefore depict clay in bowel contents as high signal intensity owing to their short T1 (Fig. 22-6).

High-High Intensity

Paramagnetic materials can reduce the T1 relaxation time and therefore increase the signal intensity of bowel contents on T1-weighted images. If the concentration of the paramagnetic material is low enough, the effects on the T2 relaxation time are minimal, and the signal intensity of bowel contents remains high on T2-weighted images.

Many nutritional supplements or foods have been used as oral contrast agents owing to their high fat content or inclusion of paramagnetic materials such as manganese. Contrast agents that produce high signal intensity of bowel may be useful for depicting the low signal intensity of the bowel wall, but the images are rendered more sensitive to degradation by motion.

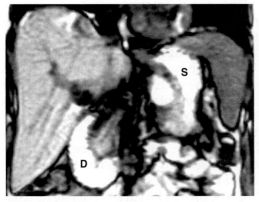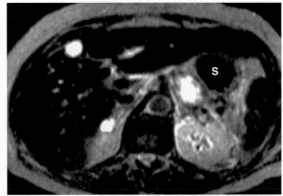

Figure 22-6
Intraluminal clay in Kaopectate causes high signal intensity on the coronal T1-weighted gradient echo 101/2.3/90° image (*left*) and low intensity on the T2-weighted spin echo 2500/100 image (*right*). A hemorrhagic pancreatic pseudocyst medial to the stomach has high signal intensity on both images. S, stomach; D, duodenum.

High-Low Intensity

Some materials shorten both T1 and T2 relaxation times enough that bowel contents have high signal intensity on T1-weighted images and low signal intensity on T2-weighted images. Examples of this type of agent include clay, gadolinium chelates in high concentrations, and compounds of manganese (Fig. 22-7). Manganese is present in high concentrations in some foods, such as bananas and blueberries.

The major appeal of a high-low agent is that the resulting signal intensity of bowel on all pulse sequences is different from those of tumors and simple fluid collections, which tend to have low signal intensity on T1-weighted images and high signal intensity on T2-weighted images. However, some T2-weighted pulse sequences (e.g., fast spin echo) may depict bowel more clearly if its contents have high signal intensity, so this form of contrast is not necessarily desirable for every application. Although the reduction of bowel signal intensity may improve depiction of biliary and pancreatic ducts on magnetic resonance cholangiopancreatography (MRCP),

the location of the duodenum on these images may be obscured.

Low-High Intensity

The least expensive, most widely available, and best understood oral contrast agent used for MRI is water. It can be used to mark bowel as low signal intensity on T1-weighted images and high signal intensity on T2-weighted images. Compounds that contain water, such as barium sulfate, have been used to produce similar effects.

Dilute suspensions of barium sulfate or dilute solutions of iodinated contrast material, such as that used for CT, are particularly useful for low-high MRI oral contrast enhancement. Whereas water is rapidly absorbed from the proximal small bowel and is therefore ineffective for enhancing distal bowel, contrast agents formulated for CT contain osmotic agents that hold water within the bowel lumen. More concentrated barium sulfate suspensions, such as that used for upper gastrointestinal imaging or barium enema, cause low signal intensity on

GRE 120/2.3/90° Pre   FSE 4000/102 Pre

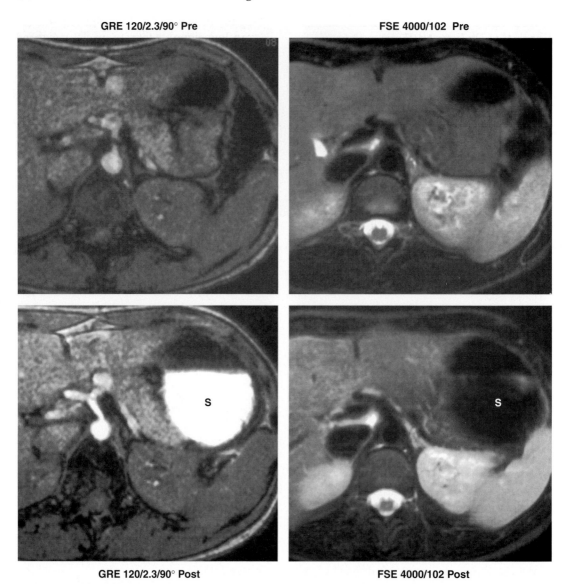

GRE 120/2.3/90° Post   FSE 4000/102 Post

Figure 22-7
Manganese-based oral contrast agent that enhances T1 and T2. Axial T1-weighted gradient echo (GRE) (*left*) and T2-weighted fast spin echo (FSE) (*right*) images before (*top*) and after (*bottom*) oral administration of LumenHance. Contrast agent in the stomach (S) has high signal intensity on T1-weighted images (*bottom left*) and low signal intensity on T2-weighted images (*bottom right*).

T1-weighted images and intermediate intensity on T2-weighted images.

Low-high agents are useful for delineating the pancreas, which has relatively high signal intensity on T1-weighted images and intermediate signal intensity on T2-weighted images. However, bowel may be difficult to distinguish from simple fluid collections and tumors, and high bowel signal intensity can intensify motion artifacts.

Essential Points to Remember

1. Iron oxide particles are taken up by reticuloendothelial cells. Large particles (i.e., 50 to 200 nm) are taken up rapidly. These agents preferentially enhance T2 and T2*, reducing the signal intensity on T2-weighted and T2*-weighted images.

2. Small iron oxide particles, which are taken up more slowly, have a much longer half-life in blood and are concentrated in lymph nodes. These agents enhance T1, T2, and T2*, causing high signal intensity on T1-weighted images and low signal intensity on T2-weighted images.

3. Oral agents that displace protons or have a very short T2 have low signal intensity on all pulse sequences.

4. Oral agents that have strong T1 enhancement and mild T2 enhancement have high signal intensity on most pulse sequences.

5. Oral agents with strong T1 and T2 enhancement have high signal intensity on T1-weighted images and low signal intensity on T2-weighted ones.

Chapter 23

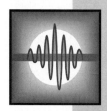

Contrast-Enhanced Magnetic Resonance Angiography

Intravenous injection of a paramagnetic agent increases the signal intensity of blood. With a sufficient dose, blood has higher signal intensity than other tissues on T1-weighted images so long as mechanisms that reduce the signal intensity of flowing blood are avoided. If the concentration of the paramagnetic agent is sufficiently high, longitudinal magnetization recovers fast enough to minimize saturation by previous excitation pulses. If an extremely short repetition time (TR) is used, the only tissue that has substantial recovery of longitudinal magnetization between excitations is contrast-enhanced blood.

In this chapter we consider optimization of the magnetic resonance (MR) angiography (MRA) pulse sequence parameters and contrast agent administration. We also explore recent improvements in the overall effectiveness of contrast-enhanced MRA as a comprehensive examination.

MRA Pulse Sequence Parameters

Contrast-enhanced MRA is usually based on three-dimensional Fourier transform (3D-FT) gradient echo techniques (Fig. 23-1). The use of 3D-FT ensures a high signal-to-noise ratio (SNR) and contiguous or overlapping image slices. The use of the shortest possible TE maximizes phase coherence, maintaining intravascular signal intensity without needing gradient moment nulling. The use of minimal TE also allows efficient image acquisition.

The TR should also be as short as possible. A short TR ensures near-complete saturation of background tissue so it does not obscure vessels of interest. The use of a short TR also maximizes the efficiency of data acquisition, generating sufficient images with

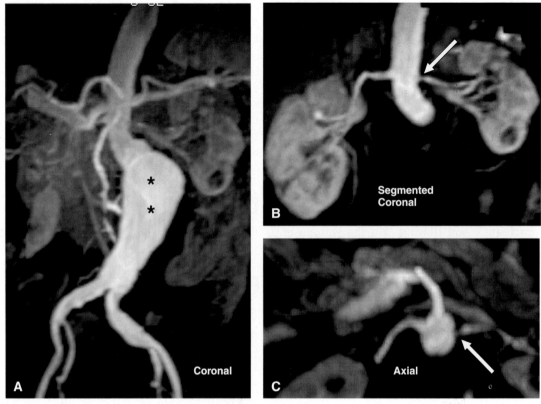

Figure 23-1

Maximum intensity projection (MIP) projections based on a coronal three-dimensional gradient echo (3D-GRE) 7/2.2/50° acquisition during the first-pass arterial phase of a 30-cc injection of gadolinium chelate. (A) Coronal projection shows an aortic aneurysm (*asterisks*). The renal arteries are obscured by overlying vessels. (B) Segmented coronal projection based on a limited portion of the data, excluding the anterior tissues and vessels that obscured the renal arteries in (A). (C) Axial projection. *Arrows* in (B) and (C) indicate left renal artery stenosis.

small voxels in the shortest possible time. A short acquisition time is important not only to ensure patient throughput and reduce motion-induced artifact, it also allows acquisition of images during a period of maximal contrast agent concentration in the blood. For longer acquisitions, a higher dose of the contrast agent is needed to produce a comparable concentration for the more extended period of time.

The flip angle should be high enough for the background tissue to remain sufficiently saturated that it has low signal intensity. The optimal flip angle for contrast-enhanced 3D-FT MRA is usually between 30° and 60°, although lower flip angles are sometimes

necessary to keep specific absorption rates within allowable limits. As the TR becomes shorter, the optimum flip angle also decreases.

The background tissue with the shortest T1, and therefore the highest potential signal intensity, is fat. There are essentially three measures that may be used, singly or in combination, to ensure that enhanced vessels have higher signal intensity than fat. One is to inject contrast agent at a sufficiently high dose and rate that the T1 of blood becomes much less than that of adipose tissue. Injection of 30 cc or more, at 2 cc/sec, can accomplish this in most patients.

Fat signal can be reduced further using fat suppression via saturation or selective inversion techniques, as described in Chapter 15. However, fat suppression adds time to the acquisition. If fat suppression is segmented (so there is only one suppression pulse per several excitation pulses), the acquisition time might be prolonged by only a few seconds. Another limitation of fat suppression is that the magnetic field may vary over a large field of view, so fat suppression at the edges of the field may be suboptimal. Even worse, the fat suppression pulse may also saturate water within blood vessels, including upstream blood flowing into the volume of interest.

Adipose and other background signal intensity can be reduced by subtracting unenhanced images from enhanced images. This is a highly effective technique unless there has been a change in the anatomical position between these image sets. Subtraction is most consistently reliable in the pelvis and extremities. Motion-induced misregistration can be reduced by inserting the intravenous catheter prior to beginning the MRA examination and obtaining the unenhanced images immediately before injecting the contrast agent. Variations in breath holding can be reduced by using end-expiration and a monitoring mechanism to maintain a consistent position of the diaphragm.

Data Acquisition and Contrast Agent Injection

Contrast agent should be administered so the bolus is maximally present within the vessels of interest during acquisition of the weakest phase-encoded views (the center of k-space). For a full-Fourier sequential acquisition (where the high negative views are acquired first and the high positive views last), the center of k-space is acquired during the midpoint of the acquisition, when the intravascular paramagnetic concentration

should be maximal. For centric or half-Fourier acquisitions, where the center of k-space is acquired at or near the beginning of the acquisition, the paramagnetic concentration should be maximal at the beginning of the acquisition. If the center of k-space is acquired before the intravascular paramagnetic concentration is high enough, high signal intensity may be restricted to the edges of the vessel, corresponding to enhancement of edge detail only (Figs. 23-2 and 23-3).

The above description of the centric view order only partly describes the filling of k-space in three dimensions, as during 3D-FT MRA. That is, a given plane in k-space

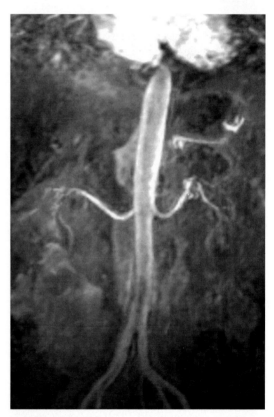

Figure 23-2
Coronal MIP projection of a coronal 3D-GRE 11/2.3/60° set of images acquired too early relative to the bolus of gadolinium chelate. Enhancement peaked after the central views of k-space were obtained, so the signal magnitude was greater for the peripheral views. This caused higher signal intensity of fine detail, resulting in greater signal intensity of the edges of the aorta and of the renal arteries than of the aortic lumen.

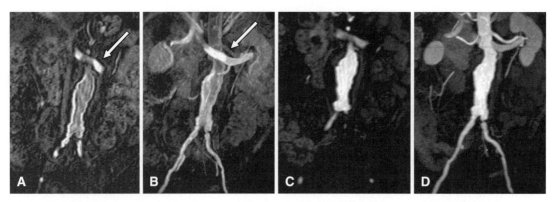

Figure 23-3
Source (*A*) and MIP (*B*) images were obtained too late, so only the periphery of the aorta is adequately enhanced. The iliac arteries at the bottom of (*B*) are well enhanced, as is the left renal vein (*arrow*). The same patient was reexamined, at which time the source (*C*) and MIP (*D*) images showed optimal timing.

can be filled using centric order, but this does not necessarily ensure that the center of 3D k-space is completely filled before any peripheral k-space data are acquired.

The most precise timing of peak enhancement relative to a rapid bolus of contrast material can be achieved if k-space is filled using *elliptical centric order*. This is shown in Figure 23-4. First, a line through the center

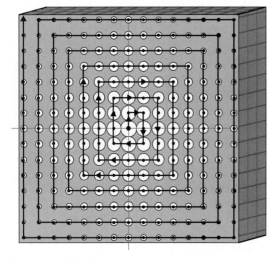

Figure 23-4
Elliptical centric filling of k-space in three dimensions. Each *black dot* represents a line, seen on end, through a cubic representation of k-space. Filling of k-space begins in the center, circling around, so successive views are farther and farther toward the periphery.

of k-space is filled, followed by a line near the center. Rather than continuing linearly toward the periphery of k-space, the third line is filled adjacent to the second, in a different direction. The fourth line filled is also near the first, again in a different direction. Filling of k-space continues in this manner, circling around the center, so successive views are farther and farther toward the periphery.

If the acquisition time is short enough, it is best to have a high blood concentration of contrast agent throughout the image acquisition, so the blood signal is high for the peripheral views of k-space as well as for the central views. Although the peripheral views do not contribute to the overall contrast of the image, they provide fine detail. Therefore, depiction of small vessels and sharp delineation of stenosis improves if the blood signal is high when the peripheral views of k-space are acquired.

The choice of the contrast agent dose for MRA represents a compromise between quality and cost. Although the package insert for some of the gadolinium chelate contrast agents indicate that they are approved for clinical use only at doses of 0.1 mmol/kg, existing data indicate that they can be safely used in most patients at doses up to 0.3 mmol/kg. Higher doses may also be safe, but there is less clinical experience at these doses.

Injection of higher doses at faster injection rates generally improves image quality and consistency but also increases the cost of the examination. The use of lower doses reduces examination costs at the expense of lower contrast between vessels and background and stronger dependence on precise timing. However, images obtained using lower doses may be sufficient for diagnostic use. When the MRA image is obtained during suspended respiration at about 25 seconds or less, satisfactory image quality can usually be obtained using about 30 cc, or approximately 0.2 mmol/kg. For some applications, rapid image acquisitions using 20-cc injections are also satisfactory.

Timing Bolus Technique

Although "guestimation" (beginning image acquisition about 20 seconds after injecting the contrast agent and the 20-cc flush) is effective in about 85% of patients, the quality is more reproducible if bolus timing is individualized to each patient. Effective methods include automated triggering, fluoroscopic triggering, or the use of a timing bolus.

The least technology-dependent method for determining the delay between injection and scanning involves obtaining a series of images immediately after injecting a 2-cc test bolus followed by a 20-cc flush. The size of the syringe should be the same as that used for injecting the bolus of gadolinium chelate, and the speed of injection should be as identical as possible. Consistent timing is ensured if a power injector is used, although hand injection may also yield satisfactory results.

If the contrast agent injection and image acquisition have approximately the same duration, the delay between the bolus injection and its arrival in the aorta can be used to determine the scan delay. However, if the duration of the contrast agent injection is substantially different from that of image acquisition, these durations should be considered for deriving the optimum delay.

If the injection duration increases, the beginning of image acquisition should be delayed; and if the image acquisition duration increases, it should begin sooner.

The optimum delay between the onset of injection and the beginning of image acquisition can be calculated using the following formula.

$$\text{Scan delay} = \text{contrast travel time} + (\text{injection duration} - \text{acquisition duration})/2$$

The ideal technique for bolus timing, if available, is an axial single-slice technique that provides dark blood, such as nonselective inversion recovery prepared gradient echo (see Chapter 15) or a spoiled gradient echo (GRE) image with superior and inferior saturation pulses (Fig. 23-5).

If this is not available, a single 20-cm sagittal spoiled GRE slice can be repeatedly obtained at a rate of about one per second, centered over the largest target vessel, such as the aorta (Fig. 23-6). Gadolinium chelate (2 cc) should be injected, followed immediately by a 20-cc flush. Image acquisition should begin when the flush is initiated. Breath holding is not necessary.

The vessel of interest has low signal intensity on all of these images until the 2-cc bolus of gadolinium arrives, at which point there is a noticeable increase in signal intensity. The time after the beginning of the GRE acquisition is the delay between the injection and its arrival in the vessel. Because branches distal to this point are of interest, an additional delay of a few seconds should be included.

Triggering Image Acquisition Relative to Contrast Agent Administration

Methods of triggering imaging acquisition to a bolus of contrast agent that do not

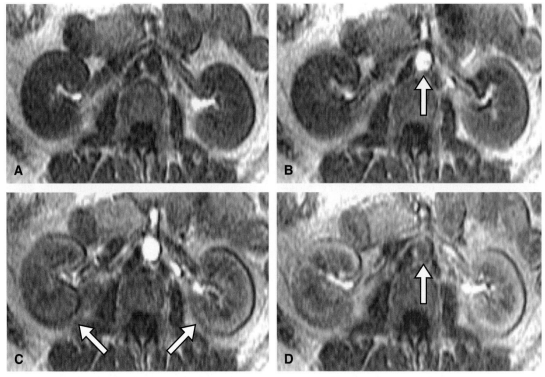

Figure 23-5
Axial T1-weighted single-slice gradient echo images with superior and inferior saturation pulses used as a timing bolus sequence. (*A*) Unenhanced image. (*B*) Image at arrival of contrast agent to the aorta (*arrow*). (*C*) Image at arrival of contrast agent to the renal cortex (*arrows*). (*D*) Washout of contrast from the aorta (*arrow*).

require a separate timing bolus include automated contrast agent detection (e.g., SmartPrep) and fluoroscopic triggering. These methods are more time-efficient than the use of a timing bolus sequence, as no additional injection of contrast agent is needed.

As with the timing bolus sequence, automated and fluoroscopic triggering involve observing for increased signal in the target vessel of interest. However, unlike the use of a timing bolus sequence, automated and fluoroscopic triggering involve determining when to begin image acquisition based on noting the initial arrival of the main bolus.

A rapid set of scout images of the target vessel are generated for both automated and fluoroscopic triggering. For the automated method, the signal intensity of the vessel is measured continually; and when it is noted, the image acquisition is automatically triggered. In most cases, the scout images that depict the signal intensity changes are not reconstructed.

For the fluoroscopy-triggering method, images are generated in real time; and when the operator observes enhancement of the target vessel (Fig. 23-7), MRA acquisition is triggered manually. Although there is no automated calculation of signal intensity, the requirement of real-time image generation places greater demand on the host computer, and operator vigilance and training are essential. However, by being in control the operator is less dependent on automated methods, and the likelihood of failure when the vessel signal does not reach a given threshold is probably lower.

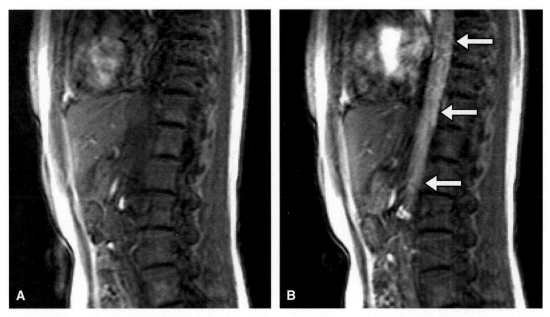

Figure 23-6
Sagittal T1-weighted single-slice gradient echo images without saturation pulses, used as a timing bolus sequence. (A) Unenhanced image. (B) Image at arrival of contrast agent to the aorta (arrows).

Time-Resolved MRA

The most robust technique for MRA is to obtain images rapidly enough to depict multiple slightly different phases of enhancement. This technique, referred to as time-resolved MRA, reduces the need to time image acquisition precisely relative to contrast agent administration. If images are continually obtained before, during, and after the first pass of the contrast agent, the most desirable sets of images can be chosen retrospectively. In clinical practice, this is analogous to conventional invasive angiography in that serial image acquisition begins before contrast agent arrival is anticipated and continues until after the vessels of interest have been depicted.

To reduce acquisition time sufficiently that time-resolved MRA can be accomplished, several strategies of fast imaging are usually combined, as detailed in Chapter 17. They may include minimizing the TR, partial Fourier imaging, asymmetrical sampling and zero-filling of k-space, view-sharing, and parallel imaging.

Multistation MRA

The principles and techniques described thus far in this chapter are concerned with acquiring a single volume of data, covering only a subset of a given patient's arterial system. To extend the examination, it is necessary to move the table and acquire more data. There are two basic methods for doing this.

The simplest, although less efficient, method is to give two injections of contrast material at different times. The advantage of this method is that once a reliable technique for conducting a three-dimensional enhanced MRA examination is established, it can simply be repeated in two locations. The disadvantage is that the total dose of contrast material must be approximately doubled without increasing the serum concentration of gadolinium chelate. Additionally, the

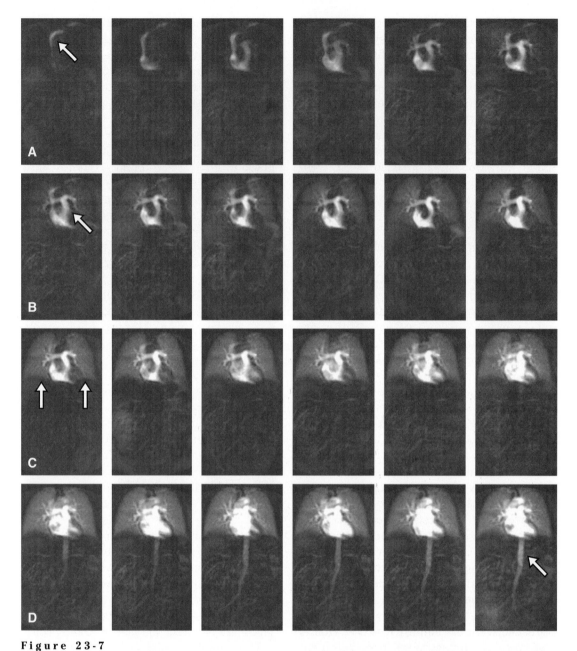

Figure 23-7
Thick slab rapid contrast-enhanced images reconstructed at real time to determine the timing for acquisition of abdominal MRA images. An unenhanced image has been subtracted from each, so only the contrast agent is shown. In the first image in row A, contrast agent enters the superior vena cava (*arrow*). In the first image in row B, contrast is in the pulmonary arteries (*arrow*). In the first image in row C, the lungs are enhanced (*arrows*). In the last image in row D, contrast has reached the abdominal aorta (*arrow*); at this point, the timing sequence is terminated, the patient is given breath-holding instructions, and MRA image acquisition begins.

second MRA examination is degraded by contrast remaining in the venous system and tissue interstitium from the first injection. Finally, this technique is not practical for accomplishing a three-station examination.

Although somewhat more challenging technically, the preferred method for extending a gadolinium-enhanced MRA examination is to use a *bolus chase* technique, analogous to that used for conventional catheter angiography. A single large injection of gadolinium chelate is given, and one set of images of the first station are acquired. Immediately following completion of this first acquisition, the table is moved, and a second image acquisition is begun, imaging the downstream arterial system. Following this step, a third set of images even more distal is often acquired.

To prolong the contrast agent injection, the injection rate may be lowered, such as to less than 1 cc/sec, rather than 2 cc/sec. Although this method reduces the contrast between background tissue and enhanced vessels, results are usually satisfactory. Using this technique it is possible to image well over a meter of a person's arterial system, typically extending from the upper abdominal aorta to the calves.

Recent developments in contrast-enhanced MRA have involved refining the methods used to image three contiguous portions of an individual's arterial anatomy sequentially. One important issue is the choice of an appropriate coil for multistation MRA. The simplest choice is to use the built-in body coil, as it involves the simplest setup. A high serum concentration of gadolinium chelate can be achieved with a high dose of contrast agent, resulting in an adequate SNR for many applications. However, a higher SNR, particularly useful for acquiring high-resolution images, can be achieved using a phased-array coil. Adapting phased-array technology to multistation MRA has been challenging.

One approach has been to use a single phased-array coil, typically one created to fit a torso, and to maintain this coil's position within a magnet bore as a patient slides through it. Commercial devices have been created that facilitate sliding a patient through a stationary coil to accomplish this. Another approach is to fit the patient inside a complex coil that extends along the entire length of the region of interest. As the table moves for each station, the portion of coil that is active is switched electronically.

If the exact same pulse sequence is executed for each station of a multistation examination, patient positioning is particularly important to ensure that the vasculature of interest lies within the acquired volume at each station. This usually involves elevating the legs. The closer the lower extremity arteries lie toward a plane parallel to the examination table, the smaller is the volume necessary to include them.

Advanced software for bolus chase MRA allows separately configuring each station to fit the anatomy and timing. For example, a thicker three-dimensional slab is needed for the iliac vessels than for the thighs or calves. The sequential view order may be used for the first station; because the gross contrast is not acquired until the middle of the acquisition, data acquisition may begin earlier. Subsequent acquisitions may use centric, or elliptical centric, view order. Another approach to multistation magnetic resonance imaging (MRI) involves segmenting the acquisition, so the central views of k-space are acquired from each station as the contrast bolus arrives; it is the central views that determine image contrast. After sampling the central views at each station, the scanner table returns to each station to complete acquisition of the peripheral views so that spatial resolution is sufficient.

Choice of Contrast Agent

Most experience with contrast-enhanced MRA involves obtaining images during or immediately after rapid bolus administration of extracellular-space gadolinium chelates. However, there are two additional types of contrast agent that show promise for contrast-enhanced MRA.

Tissue-directed gadolinium chelates, although developed primarily for hepatocellular enhancement, have some properties that are potentially desirable for MRA. Once injected, these compounds bind to plasma proteins, which facilitates their interaction with nearby water molecules. These agents have higher relaxivity than standard extracellular-space gadolinium chelates. Thus, a given dose of tissue-directed gadolinium chelate may reduce the T1 of blood twice as much as a comparable dose of extracellular-space gadolinium chelate.

The dual excretion of tissue-directed gadolinium chelates by the biliary and urinary systems decreases the blood half-time of these agents. Therefore, if more than one bolus is given, such as for repeat imaging or for MRA at multiple locations, background enhancement is reduced.

Blood-pool contrast agents are also potentially useful for MRA. If a contrast agent stays in the blood pool for a prolonged period, rapid imaging is no longer essential. High spatial resolution techniques, potentially using cardiac gating, can therefore be used; and images from multiple locations can be acquired following a single bolus. However, on delayed images, venous enhancement is comparable to that of arteries. Arteries and veins can be resolved anatomically by paging through contiguous images. Alternatively, strategies for distinguishing arteries and veins can be implemented, which can be based on differences in flow direction or pulsatility. Saturation techniques are difficult to implement owing to the short T1 of enhanced blood; recovery following saturation pulses is rapid. Alternatively, arteries and veins can be segmented from each other on postprocessed images based on continuity with manually selected vessels on a source image.

▼
Essential Points to Remember

1. Contrast-enhanced MRA usually utilizes 3D-FT gradient echo pulse sequences obtained so contrast enhancement of blood is maximal while the central views of k-space are being obtained.

2. 3D-FT gradient echo techniques for contrast-enhanced MRA should have minimized TE and TR and a relatively high flip angle (about 40°) so the background tissue is suppressed.

3. Higher doses of contrast agent generally improve image quality and decrease precise dependence on timing. However, with an optimized technique, satisfactory results can often be obtained at lower cost with a reduced dose.

4. MRA data acquisition must be timed so the center of k-space is acquired during optimum enhancement.

5. Timing of data acquisition with respect to the bolus of contrast agent can be ensured by using a timing bolus, by automated triggering, or by fluoroscopic triggering.

6. Time-resolved MRA involves obtaining sets of images rapidly at multiple phases relative to the bolus injection of contrast material. The most desirable image sets can then be determined retrospectively.

7. Multistation MRA can be accomplished by giving two separate boluses of contrast agent or by rapidly imaging different vascular anatomy as it becomes enhanced by the bolus traveling through the arterial system.

8. Tissue-directed gadolinium chelates are bound to plasma proteins, which increases their in vivo relaxivity and therefore allows the use of lower doses with comparable enhancement effects.

9. Blood-pool agents allow delayed or longer image acquisitions (or both). However, arteries and veins are both enhanced, so strategies must be applied to distinguish them.

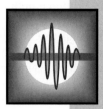

Chapter 24

Cardiovascular Techniques

If blood were not moving, its magnetic resonance (MR) signal intensity would result directly from its proton density, T1 and T2. Blood has more free water than almost any tissue in the body; its free water content is only somewhat less than cerebrospinal fluid and urine. Therefore, its proton density is higher than that of most other tissues.

Circulating blood has a relatively long T1 and a long T2. Therefore, if it were not moving it would have low signal intensity on T1-weighted images and high signal intensity on T2-weighted images.

The high iron content of blood has the potential to affect its signal intensity. Deoxyhemoglobin in deoxygenated red blood cells is weakly paramagnetic, which can lead to reduced T2 if it is unevenly distributed, as in subacute hemorrhage. The effect on the signal intensity of deoxyhemoglobin is weaker in circulating blood. Heavily T2*-weighted images are needed to distinguish oxygenated from deoxygenated flowing blood. This phenomenon is used to evaluate brain perfusion via blood oxygen level-dependent (BOLD) techniques (see Chapter 25).

The signal intensity of blood can be altered by many techniques, allowing many strategies for magnetic resonance angiography (MRA). Vessels can be depicted effectively by magnetic resonance imaging (MRI) using either "dark blood" or "bright blood" techniques.

First, we consider mechanisms that can produce low signal intensity of blood. Such mechanisms can be used to create images that depict vessel and myocardial walls, intraluminal thrombus, or tissue. We then consider three basic methods for producing bright blood images, all of which include strategies for avoiding dark blood mechanisms. Finally, we discuss methods for demonstrating perfusion and diffusion that do not involve depicting blood vessels.

315

Dark Blood Mechanisms

Because of the long T2 of blood, dark blood images are difficult to produce with T2-weighted techniques. The long T1 of blood, however, provides a strategy for reducing its signal intensity. In the absence of mechanisms that increase its signal intensity, blood is dark on T1-weighted images. The T1 of blood can also be used to null its signal throughout an image by applying an inversion recovery preparation pulse with an inversion time (TI) long enough to null the blood signal.

With single-slice acquisitions, blood flowing into an image slice between excitation pulses often has high signal intensity because it has not been affected by previous excitation pulses. With multislice acquisitions, blood is often bright on *entry slices*, that is, on slices at the edge of the imaged volume that flowing blood encounters first. The signal intensity of flowing blood is progressively lower on slices farther from the entry slice owing to increased saturation as the blood flows through more slices. One strategy for producing dark blood, therefore, is to use a multislice technique, so each excitation pulse saturates blood as it moves into adjacent image slices. Intravascular signal intensity can be reduced further by applying spatial saturation pulses, so flowing blood is saturated before it enters an image slice. This point is discussed in greater detail in Chapters 13 and 15.

Conventional spin echo and fast spin echo images are usually more effective than gradient echo images for depicting blood vessels as having low-signal-intensity lumens. For blood to generate signal intensity on spin echo images it must be exposed to both the excitation and refocusing pulses. If blood is excited but flows out of the image slice before the refocusing pulse, the rephasing lobe of the frequency-encoding gradient (Gf) causes further dephasing, rather than rephasing. Therefore, blood that leaves an image slice before the refocusing pulse generates no signal on spin echo images.

On conventional spin echo images, increasing the echo time (TE) is a mechanism for reducing the signal intensity of blood (Fig. 24-1). At some centers, for example, gated spin echo images of the heart are obtained with a TE of 20 to 30 msec,

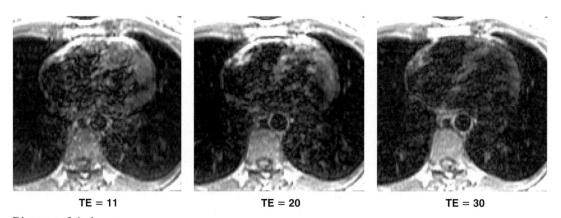

| TE = 11 | TE = 20 | TE = 30 |

Figure 24-1

Effect of echo time (TE) on intravascular signal intensity on cardiac gated axial SE images with a repetition time (TR) of 861 msec. With a TE of 11 msec (*left*), the intravascular signal and artifact are prominent, although they decrease with progressive increases in TE to 20 (*center*) and 30 (*right*) msec. However, myocardial signal intensity also decreases with increasing TE.

rather than the minimum TE, to decrease intraluminal signal intensity. This is only partially effective, however, because an increased TE also reduces the signal intensity of background tissue, which usually has a shorter T2 than blood and allows increased motion artifacts.

Loss of coherent phase in a voxel is probably the most important mechanism for signal intensity reduction of flowing blood. As discussed in Chapter 13, motion during the application of imaging gradients causes dephasing, which is not corrected by the rephasing gradient unless gradient moment nulling is used. If dark blood imaging is desired, gradient moment nulling is not used, and additional gradients may even be applied to dephase moving spins further. Even in the absence of gradient moment nulling, intravascular dephasing is minimal if the TE is very short (e.g., less than 3 msec).

A highly effective method for reducing the signal intensity of blood utilizes both the movement of blood into and out of an image slice and the T1 of blood. This method, nulling of blood signal by double inversion recovery, was discussed in Chapter 15. To review briefly, tissue throughout an image volume is inverted by use of a 180° inversion pulse. Then a second 180° inversion pulse is targeted to the slice of interest by use of a slice-encoding gradient. This second inversion pulse returns longitudinal magnetization to its equilibrium value because the spins in this slice have been rotated a full 360°. However, spins outside the slice remain inverted. Following an inversion time (TI) that allows the magnetization of blood outside the slice of interest to recover to zero (its null point), an excitation pulse creates transverse magnetization from the slice of interest. During the TI the double-inverted blood in the slice of interest has been replaced by inverted blood from outside the slice, so it has no signal.

Strategies for reducing the signal intensity of blood and their underlying mechanisms are summarized in Table 24-1.

Table 24-1 ■ STRATEGIES AND MECHANISMS FOR REDUCING THE SIGNAL INTENSITY OF BLOOD

Dark Blood Strategy	Mechanism
Short TR	Blood is saturated owing to long T1
Moderate TE	Allows motion-induced intravoxel dephasing
Inversion recovery	Nulls blood signal based on its T1
Spatial saturation	Saturates blood prior to entering region of interest
90°/180° washout	Blood leaves image section between 90° and 180° pulses
Gradient dephasing	Increases motion-induced intravoxel dephasing
Double inversion	Nulls signal of blood that flows into a slice

Bright Blood Techniques

One method for rendering blood bright on MR images is to administer intravascular paramagnetic contrast agents, as discussed in Chapter 23. Other bright blood techniques rely, at least in part, on time-of-flight (TOF) principles. All TOF techniques are based on the same basic principle: Blood flowing into an image slice has higher magnetization than the partially saturated stationary tissue in the slice. The *time* it takes for the *flight* of the blood into an image slice is the mechanism for vascular enhancement. This is a simple principle that does not require contrast agents, dedicated hardware, signal processing, or sophisticated software beyond that needed for a simple gradient echo pulse sequence. In fact, current two-dimensional TOF (2D-TOF) techniques are merely refinements of gradient echo pulse sequences that had been introduced and used clinically more than a decade ago.

High-quality bright blood imaging can be achieved using balanced steady state-free precession (B-SSFP) techniques, as discussed in Chapter 14. These techniques allow rapid acquisition of relatively motion-insensitive images, where blood has high signal intensity regardless of flow velocity. It must be remembered that B-SSFP images are anatomical images of blood based on its long T1 and long T2, rather than images of blood flow. In contrast, the high signal intensity of blood on TOF images is a direct result of the actual movement of the blood through an image. TOF imaging can therefore be thought of as a technique for imaging flow directly, whereas B-SSFP is a method for imaging fluid, including but not limited to blood.

Two-Dimensional Time of Flight

The basis of a 2D-TOF pulse sequence is slice-by-slice generation of individual images

on which blood is white and other tissues are dark or intermediate shades of gray. Stationary tissue in each image slice is exposed to repeated excitation pulses, causing it to be partially saturated. Between each excitation pulse, fresh unexcited blood flows into the image slice, replacing blood that had been exposed to the previous excitation pulse. Because it is less saturated than background tissue, flowing blood has higher signal intensity. The signal intensity of background tissue can be reduced further by the use of magnetization transfer (MT) saturation, which reduces the signal intensity of tissue without affecting blood. Projection MRA images can be created by combining the data from multiple 2D-TOF slices (Fig. 24-2). TOF techniques are sensitive only to flow perpendicular to the image plane, although sufficiently thin slices usually depict this component of

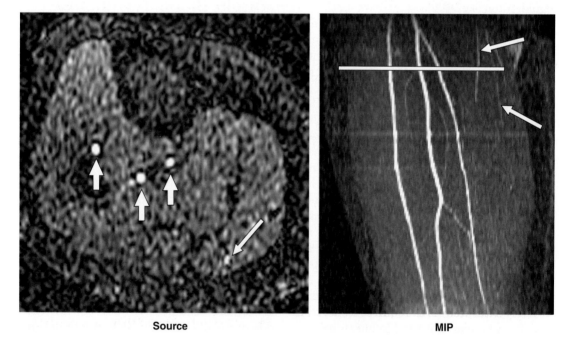

Source **MIP**

Figure 24-2

Axial source two-dimensional time of flight (2D-TOF) 37/7/60° image of the calf (*left*) shows anterior tibial, peroneal, and posterior tibial arteries (*thick arrows*) as high signal intensity relative to the partially saturated background tissue. *Thin arrow* indicates a small muscular branch vessel. The venous signal was suppressed by using inferior spatial saturation pulses. Coronal maximal intensity projection (MIP) image (*right*) depicts the patent arteries. *Arrows* indicate small muscular branches. The *horizontal white line* indicates the plane of the source image.

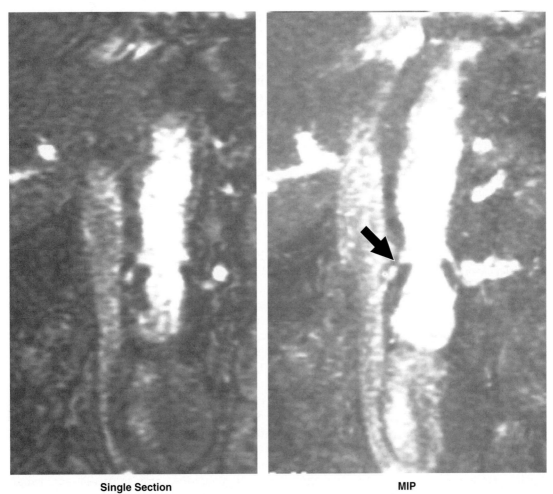

Single Section   **MIP**

Figure 24-3
Coronal 2D-TOF image (*left*) and MIP projection (*right*) show left renal artery stenosis (*arrow*). Even though the aorta and renal arteries are parallel to the imaging plane, the image slices are thin enough that the through-plane flow is adequate for their depiction.

flow even in vessels nearly parallel to the image (Fig. 24-3).

There are three basic requirements for successful 2D-TOF imaging.

1. Background tissue must be kept relatively saturated. This requires a short TR and an intermediate or high flip angle.
2. Enough blood must flow into the imaging slice or volume between excitations to increase signal intensity beyond that of nearby stationary tissue. This requires a sufficiently long TR and thin slices.

3. The phase of blood signals must remain coherent. This is accomplished by using the shortest possible TE, gradient moment nulling, or cardiac compensation or gating.

With these three basic principles in mind, the parameters are addressed individually. The effects of many of them are illustrated in Chapter 13.

REPETITION TIME

The TR should be long enough to allow sufficient inflow of unsaturated spins between repetitions and short enough to maintain saturation of stationary tissue. An additional benefit of short TR is less variation in the signal intensity of blood between successive echoes, which reduces artifacts from pulsatile flow. Most successful implementations of 2D-TOF techniques use TRs between 20 and 50 msec.

FLIP ANGLE

As the flip angle is increased, more transverse magnetization is created. Therefore, the transverse magnetization of unsaturated blood flowing into an image slice increases. An increased flip angle also results in greater saturation of stationary tissue in the image slice, decreasing the resultant transverse magnetization. Thus, the increased flip angle increases the signal intensity of flowing blood and decreases that of stationary tissue, increasing the contrast between flowing blood and background tissue.

The use of a high flip angle, however, reduces the signal intensity of slowly flowing blood, which is not completely replaced during the time between repetitions. During diastole there is little forward flow in many vessels; so high flip angles reduce the signal intensity of blood during diastole. Because the systolic signal intensity increases (more transverse magnetization created) and the diastolic signal intensity decreases (more saturation) with the high flip angle, view-to-view intensity changes, and the resulting phase artifacts due to pulsation, are exacerbated. In most instances, a flip angle between 30° and 60° yields satisfactory images, with the lower angle being reserved for minimizing artifacts from highly pulsatile flow.

SLICE THICKNESS

Slices should be thin enough to allow sufficient replacement of blood protons from inflow between repetitions but thick enough to ensure an adequate signal-to-noise ratio (SNR) and anatomical coverage. A slice thickness of 5 to 8 mm can provide a rapid "road map" of major vessels. Thin slices are especially important for imaging slow flow and flow in small in-plane vessels and for depicting details of vascular anatomy such as stenoses (Fig. 24-4). The use of 2D-TOF for detecting arterial stenosis requires a slice thickness of 2 mm or less for most applications. The use of thin slices also improves the quality of three-dimensional (3D) maximum intensity projection (MIP) reconstructed images.

ECHO TIME

Generally, the TE should be as short as possible within the limitations of the system hardware. Several user-selected parameters affect the TE, and the choice of these parameters involves a series of trade-offs. Desirable features of 2D-TOF implementations include thin slices to increase the sensitivity to slow flow, gradient moment nulling to decrease the loss of vascular signal intensity from phase differences in each voxel, and sufficiently low sampling bandwidth to ensure an adequate SNR. All of these measures increase the TE somewhat, but the trade-offs are usually acceptable or unavoidable.

MOTION COMPENSATION TECHNIQUES

Most current implementations of 2D-TOF use gradient moment nulling to compensate for the phase incoherence resulting from the first order of motion, constant velocity. During the short interval of echo sampling (usually less than 10 msec), constant velocity is a close enough approximation to compensate for phase errors resulting from even pulsatile flow. Higher orders of motion (e.g., acceleration and jerk) have little effect on the phase coherence of individual echoes. In fact, higher orders of gradient moment nulling are counterproductive because the

4.5 mm

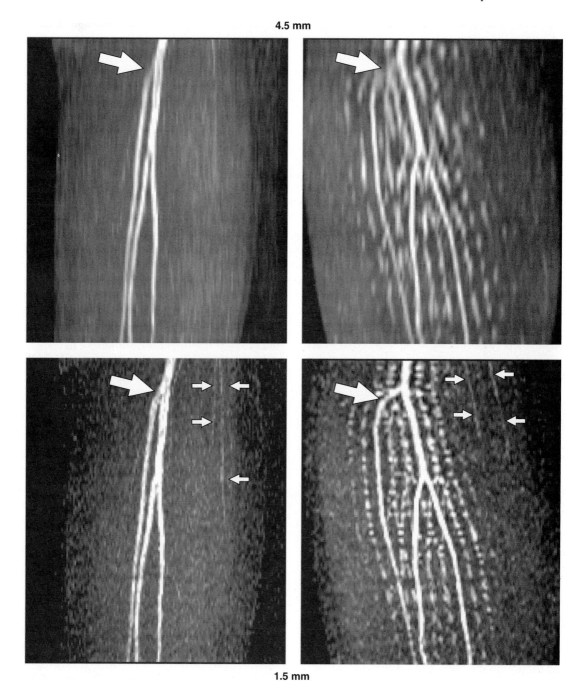

1.5 mm

Figure 24-4

Effect of slice thickness on 2D-TOF images of the calf acquired using axial 33/5/45° source images. The phase axis of the source images was left to right; the ghost artifacts from pulsatile flow are therefore depicted on the coronal projections (*right*) but not on the sagittal projections (*left*). Although the signal-to-noise ratio (SNR) is higher with 4.5 mm slice thickness (*top*), partially in-plane flow at the origin of the anterior tibial artery (*large arrows*) is depicted with greater clarity when using a 1.5 mm slice thickness (*bottom*), as are small peripheral vessels (*small arrows*).

resulting increase in TE leads to additional degradation of vascular signal intensity.

Artifacts due to pulsatile flow result primarily from variations in vascular magnetization between echoes, rather than from phase differences within each echo. Therefore, artifacts due to pulsatile flow are best reduced by decreasing magnetization differences between systole and diastole. These differences can be reduced by decreasing the TR, the flip angle (see above), or both or by using cardiac gating or triggering.

SIGNAL AVERAGING

Pulsation artifacts often *increase* with signal averaging, unlike spin echo images, where increased signal averaging reduces the conspicuousness of motion artifact. Motion artifacts on breath-holding images decrease when the central views of k-space, which determine tissue contrast, are acquired during a single cardiac cycle. Signal averaging requires sampling each point of k-space more than once, thereby increasing the time needed for sampling k-space. This usually splits the central views into two or more cardiac cycles, increasing the distance between ghost artifacts and the conspicuousness of ghosts and decreasing edge sharpness.

Decreasing the time required for sampling the center of k-space decreases pulsation artifacts. This can be accomplished by using one or fewer signal averages, decreasing the TR, or minimizing the field of view (FOV) in the phase-encoding axis by using a rectangular FOV.

SATURATION PULSES

Pulsation artifacts and the signal from overlapping arteries or veins can be reduced by judicious use of saturation bands, as discussed in Chapter 15. For example, axial images of carotid artery flow can be clarified by saturation bands placed immediately cephalad to each image slice to reduce the signal intensity of blood in caudad-flowing veins.

Similarly, jugular veins can be imaged without overlying arteries by inferiorly placed saturation bands.

For longitudinally oriented vessels such as those in the neck and extremities, the location of the saturation band can be changed for each image slice to saturate blood optimally immediately before it enters the image slice. Saturation bands that change their location with each image slice are sometimes referred to as *floating saturation pulses*. For some applications, such as imaging peripheral arteries, these saturation bands should not be immediately adjacent to the image slice but should be separated by at least a few millimeters. This ensures that reversed blood flow during diastole is not inadvertently saturated by a pulse too close to the image slice; inadvertent saturation of reversed diastolic flow would decrease arterial signal intensity.

It must be remembered that 2D-TOF "MR arteriograms" and "MR venograms" do not necessarily depict only arteries or only veins. Rather, they depict inferiorly flowing or superiorly flowing blood. For example, retrograde arterial flow in collateral vessels is not depicted on a typical TOF MR arteriogram.

Floating saturation pulses can cause inadvertent saturation of desired blood vessels in body parts with complex vascular anatomy, such as the abdomen. For example, renal arteries commonly curve so their distal portions are angled cephalad. Images obtained with floating inferior saturation pulses therefore show the aorta and proximal (inferiorly oriented) renal arteries but fail to depict any portion of the artery with upward angulation. Similarly, saturating blood immediately above each image slice eliminates the signal intensity from a patent splenic vein (Fig. 24-5), which usually courses inferiorly toward the confluence with the superior mesenteric vein. Portal vein flow voids may result. If used at all in body parts such as these, saturation pulses should have a fixed location that does not overlap any portion of the vessel of interest and that does not vary as the location of a

Floating Superior Saturation

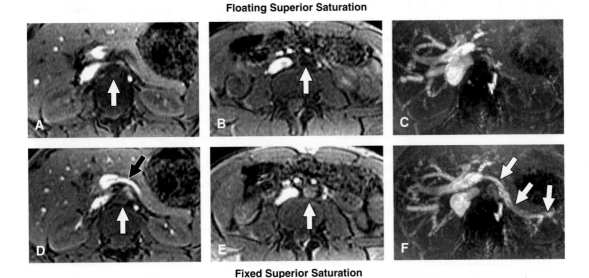

Fixed Superior Saturation

Figure 24-5

Effects of floating (*A–C*) versus fixed (*D–F*) superior saturation pulses on axial 2D-TOF images of the abdomen. (*A*) and (*D*) are at the level of the splenic vein (*black arrow in D*). (*B*) and (*E*) are at an inferior level. (*C*) and (*F*) are axial MIP images covering the splenic vein (*arrows in F*). With floating saturation pulses, the signal intensity of inferiorly flowing blood in the aorta (*arrows in A, B, D, E*) is suppressed more completely. However, the splenic vein is seen only if the superior saturation pulse has a fixed location superior to that of this vein (*arrows in D, F*).

slice changes. Because of the complexity of the vascular anatomy in the abdomen, application of 2D-TOF techniques is limited. They can be used with floating superior saturation pulses to determine the patency of the inferior vena cava and superior mesenteric vein, but other veins may be saturated as well. Similarly, the gross anatomy of the aorta can be seen using 2D-TOF with inferior floating saturation pulses, but many aortic branches become partially saturated. Alternatively, 2D-TOF techniques can be used without any saturation pulses to depict all vessels with a component of through-plane flow as bright, regardless of direction; vessels that flow primarily within the image slice, such as renal vessels in an axial image, are partly saturated. To depict vessels with flow in all directions as bright, B-SSFP techniques may be preferable to 2D-TOF.

If a 2D-TOF technique is optimized, the administration of gadolinium chelates does not improve depiction of vessels. The high signal intensity of unsaturated blood flowing into an image slice does not depend on its T1 relaxation time; because unsaturated blood has not experienced an excitation pulse, the time for recovery of longitudinal magnetization is not necessary. Therefore, shortening the relaxation time of blood via contrast agents is not beneficial for optimized 2D-TOF techniques. The signal intensity of background tissue, however, increases after administration of contrast agents, potentially obscuring vessels. If, in fact, administration of current gadolinium chelates improves 2D-TOF images, the 2D-TOF technique itself is not optimized for depicting slow or in-plane flow. However, if thick image slices are used to increase the SNR and reduce the acquisition time, gadolinium chelates increase the intravascular signal from slow or in-plane flow.

Paradoxically, the severity of ghost artifacts may actually decrease after administration of gadolinium chelates because the intensity of flowing blood becomes more uniform throughout the cardiac cycle. During systole, blood magnetization is high because blood entering an image slice has not been exposed to an excitation pulse. Reducing its T1 therefore does not affect its signal intensity; however, blood may remain within an image slice during diastole, so it *is* affected by the prior excitation pulse. Its magnetization recovers faster from the resulting saturation when a contrast agent has been administered. The resulting signal intensity of blood during diastole is thus closer to that during systole after contrast agent administration, reducing artifacts from view-to-view intensity changes.

Time-of-flight images can be highly sensitive to slow flow but sometimes do not completely depict complex flow in aneurysms or distal to stenoses. Contrast-enhanced MRA techniques generally depict vascular lumens with greater accuracy in these situations (Fig. 24-6).

Three-Dimensional Time of Flight

Three-dimensional TOF techniques consist of gradient echo acquisition of a volume into which blood is flowing. The advantage of 3D-TOF over 2D-TOF is generally higher spatial resolution in the slice direction and a greater SNR. The 3D-TOF techniques have been most useful for imaging rapid flow such as that in the carotid arteries and circle of Willis (Fig. 24-7); however, 3D-TOF techniques are usually suboptimal for imaging slow flow, such as that in the abdominal vessels. It is also more difficult to adapt the 3D-TOF technique to allow suspended respiration.

Unlike optimized 2D-TOF techniques, 3D-TOF techniques can benefit from the administration of contrast agents to shorten the T1 relaxation time of blood. This is because blood within the imaged volume is partially saturated when using

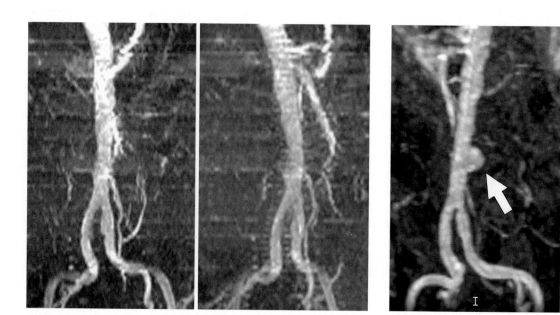

Time-of-Flight **Gadolinium**

Figure 24-6
Coronal and oblique 2D-TOF MIP images acquired from 2 mm thick axial source 37/6.5/50° images (*left* and *center*) show aortic and iliac ectasia but no aneurysm. The gadolinium-enhanced 3D 11.2/2.3/60° MIP image (*right*) clearly depicts a saccular aneurysm (*arrow*).

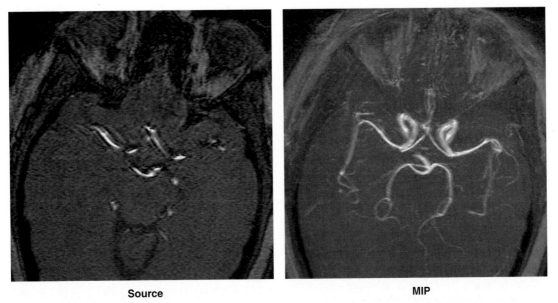

Source   MIP

Figure 24-7
Three-dimensional TOF axial source (*left*) and MIP (*right*) images using TR/TE/flip angle of 59/6.9/30°. Background signal has been partially suppressed using magnetization transfer saturation. The 3D-FT acquisition has resulted in a high SNR.

3D-TOF techniques; longitudinal magnetization recovers more rapidly after contrast agent administration, thereby increasing vascular signal intensity. In fact, some so-called contrast-enhanced 3D-TOF techniques are not really TOF techniques at all, as they depict blood vessels based on the short T1 of enhanced blood rather than the actual TOF principle.

One method for increasing the sensitivity of 3D-TOF techniques to moderate velocity flow is to use multiple overlapping thin-slab acquisitions (MOTSA). MOTSA can be thought of as a compromise between 2D-TOF and 3D-TOF. By decreasing the slab thickness, sensitivity to slow and moderate flow velocities is increased. Anatomical coverage is maintained by using multiple acquisitions. Smooth transitions between slabs is ensured by overlapping the slabs. Compared to 2D-TOF, MOTSA has a higher SNR but less sensitivity to slow flow (Fig. 24-8). Compared to 3D-TOF, MOTSA has a lower SNR but greater sensitivity to slow flow.

Phase-Contrast Technique

One disadvantage of all pulse sequences discussed thus far for depicting flowing blood is the possibility of ambiguous signal. On dark blood images (e.g., those with spatial saturation pulses), air, bone, and other substances also have low signal intensity. On bright blood images based on TOF or contrast enhancement, other tissues may have high signal intensity. On phase-contrast (PC) pulse sequences, the phase changes due to motion itself are used to depict flowing blood. The principal advantages of PC sequences are better suppression of background tissue and greater potential for measuring blood flow.

In Chapter 13 we discussed how phase changes that result from motion can create artifacts during phase-encoding. We also described how these effects can be reduced by altering the gradient waveforms through gradient moment nulling. The same

2D-TOF

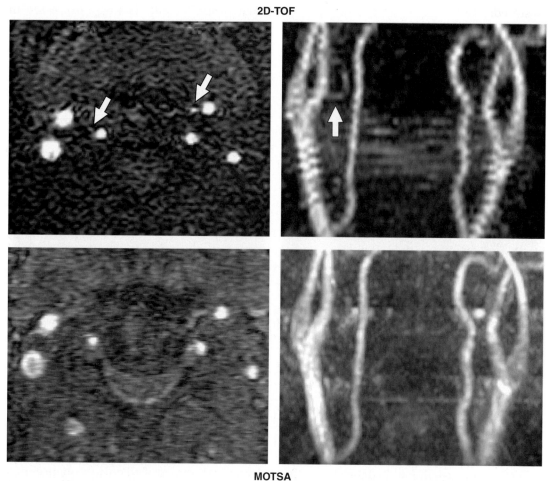

MOTSA

Figure 24-8
Two-dimensional-TOF 38/8.6/60° (*top*) and multiple overlapping thin slab acquisitions (MOTSA) 57/6.9/30° (*bottom*) images of the neck. Axial source images are at left and coronal MIP images at right. Patient motion and vascular pulsations during acquisition has resulted in a stair-step pattern in the 2D-TOF MIP. The MOTSA images have higher SNRs but greater background signal. *Arrows* indicate small vessels that are better depicted by 2D-TOF owing to its greater sensitivity to slow flow.

principles provide the basis for using phase changes to depict and measure blood flow.

Phase contrast images are reconstructed from two or more data sets, usually acquired simultaneously in an interleaved manner. These two data sets are identical except for the phase changes due to motion along a particular axis. For example, two data sets may differ because gradient moment nulling is applied in the frequency-encoding axis in one set but not in the other. The difference between these two data sets is the phase shifts along the frequency-encoding axis. Subtraction of these data sets produces an image of motion along this axis. Images of flow along the phase-encoding and slice-select axes can be similarly created (Fig. 24-9).

The phase difference between the flow-compensated and flow-encoded sequences is proportional to g (the gyromagnetic ratio, as discussed in Chapter 2), Dm (the difference between the two series in the first gradient moment), and v (velocity):

$$\text{Phase difference} = g \times Dm \times v$$

Restated:

$$\text{Velocity} = \text{phase difference}/(g \times Dm)$$

The amount of phase change that arises from motion of a given velocity can be varied by altering the gradient waveform. This flow-sensitive gradient adjustment is often referred to as the *velocity-encoding variable* (v_{enc}), which is the value that produces a phase shift of 180°. The v_{enc}, expressed in centimeters per second, determines the highest and lowest velocities measurable by a phase contrast technique. The v_{enc} is inversely related to the area (the product of the strength and duration) of a gradient. Stronger gradient amplitudes are required to encode smaller velocities. The v_{enc} represents the practical upper limit of velocities that can be depicted unambiguously. Flow velocity

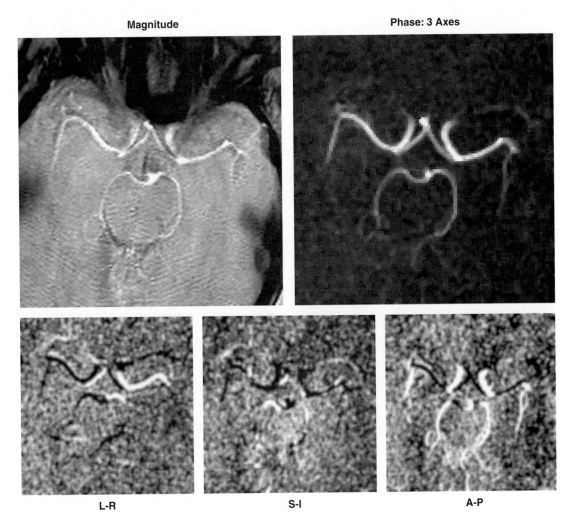

Figure 24-9
Two-dimensional phase contrast (2D-PC) 28/7.4/20° acquisition of a single 1.5 cm thick slice at the circle of Willis (same patient as in Fig. 24-7). The received magnitude (amplitude) of the MR signals is used to construct the image at top left. Separate phase images are depicted at bottom, sensitive to flow directions of left to right (*left*), superior to inferior (*center*), and anterior to posterior (*right*). Flow in one direction is *white* and flow in the other *black*, and static tissue is represented as *neutral gray* noise. The reconstructed phase image, sensitive to flow in all three axes, is depicted at top right without directional sensitivity, showing flow in any direction as *white* and nonmoving tissue as *black*.

higher than the v_{enc} may be misrepresented owing to velocity aliasing, depicted as if it were flow in the opposite direction (Fig. 24-10). In other words, if the v_{enc} is set too low, aliasing results; hence, small and large velocities are associated with similar phase shifts. Slow flow is depicted more sensitively with a lower v_{enc}. If the v_{enc} is set too high, slow velocity flow may not be detected. Also, with high v_{enc}, the influence of noise increases, which reduces the accuracy of the flow measurement.

The signal intensity on PC images is proportional to the velocity of motion in the encoded axis. The accuracy of the data, however, depends on the strength of the signal (i.e., on the SNR). Therefore, gradient echo techniques are usually used for PC because flowing blood has higher signal intensity on these images. Paramagnetic contrast agents can also increase the signal intensity of flowing blood, thereby increasing the sensitivity and accuracy of PC images. The measurement is most accurate if the image is perpendicular to the direction of the flow.

One disadvantage of PC images, compared to other pulse sequences, is their generally longer acquisition time. To encode motion or flow along one axis, two data sets must be compared. To encode flow in three orthogonal directions, four data sets must be acquired, consisting of one motion-compensated set and three sets with flow-encoding in each of the three axes.

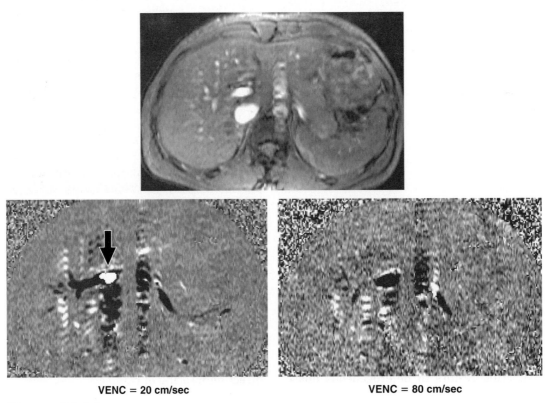

VENC = 20 cm/sec   **VENC = 80 cm/sec**

Figure 24-10
Effect of different velocity-encoding values (v_{enc}) on 2D-PC 18/9/20° images sensitive to flow in the superoinferior axis. Magnitude image is at top. With a low v_{enc} of 20 cm/sec (*bottom left*), the velocity of flow in the portal vein is above the limit for unambiguous encoding of direction, causing aliasing in the portal vein (*arrow*). With a higher v_{enc} of 80 cm/sec (*bottom right*), flow in the portal vein is encoded unambiguously. Fewer small intrahepatic vessels are depicted, however, owing to less sensitivity to slow flow.

Two-Dimensional Phase Contrast

Two-dimensional phase contrast (2D-PC) is useful for obtaining images during suspended respiration or different phases of the cardiac cycle. On these images, background stationary tissue is usually gray; flow in one direction is light, and flow in the other direction is dark. The shade of gray depends on the velocity of flow; rapid flow is depicted as white or black. These images are analogous to the color portion of color Doppler ultrasound images. In fact, PC images can be encoded in color and superimposed on gray-scale magnitude images, as with color Doppler imaging.

Two-dimensional PC images are useful for measuring the velocity and volume of blood flow. Velocity is directly proportional to the phase shift, whereas the volume of flow depends in addition on the cross-sectional area of the blood vessel.

Imaging and measurement of pulsatile flow is usually most accurate if cardiac gating techniques are used to produce 2D-PC images at different phases of the cardiac cycle. These techniques are often referred to as *cine phase contrast*.

Three-Dimensional Phase Contrast

Three-dimensional phase contrast (3D-PC) images are useful for depicting flow with a high SNR, high spatial resolution, and high background suppression. The major disadvantage of 3D-PC is the long acquisition time required for encoding motion along three orthogonal axes. Additionally, complex flow often results in heterogeneous phase changes in a voxel, reducing the vascular flow signal. Although it can exaggerate the severity of vascular abnormalities or give false-positive results, this property of 3D-PC can be useful for confirming disturbed flow distal to a stenosis, implying hemodynamic

significance (Fig. 24-11). If a vessel is not depicted on 3D-PC images distal to a stenosis, hemodynamic significance is likely.

Cardiac MRI Techniques

Despite its tremendous potential, cardiac MRI has been perhaps the most difficult application to implement in clinical practice for several reasons. One is that radiologists, the group of physicians most involved in advancing clinical MRI applications, are less involved in imaging the heart; most clinical cardiac imaging is performed or supervised by cardiologists. As with many musculoskeletal imaging applications, cardiac MRI involves acquiring multiple oblique planes relative to the heart. These imaging planes are not referred to as coronal, axial, and sagittal but, rather, by less familiar terms such as short axis, long axis, inflow, and ouflow, among others. Most of the techniques used for cardiac MRI are not designed primarily to achieve T1- or T2-weighted contrast but, rather, to render blood bright or dark and to depict various aspects of motion. Finally, cardiac and respiratory motions must both be taken into consideration and their effects minimized.

Although artifacts due to cardiac motion can sometimes be adequately reduced by pulse oximetry monitoring, the variable delay between cardiac events and pulsations at the fingertips prevents accurately assigning the cardiac phase of a given image or data acquisition. Therefore, any technique that depends on determining the phase within the cardiac cycle depends on direct monitoring of cardiac events, usually through electrocardiographic (ECG) gating or triggering. This has been a challenge because the radiofrequency (RF) pulses used to excite tissue can increase the ECG lead impedance and thereby interfere with cardiac gating.

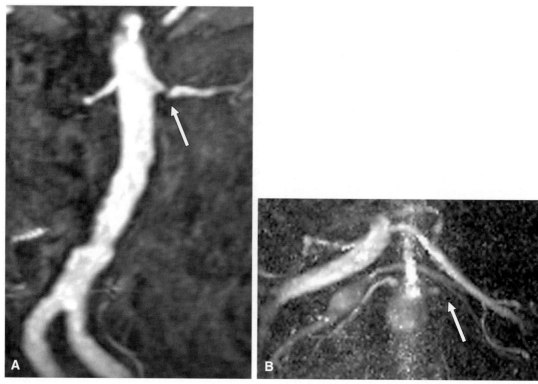

Figure 24-11
High-grade stenosis (*arrow*) depicted by a gadolinium-enhanced 3D-gradient echo (GRE) 7.5/2.2/50° MIP (*A*) and exaggerated by a 3D-PC 33/7.7/20° technique (*B*) owing to dephasing of complex flow distal to the stenosis (*arrow*).

Cardiac Gating

Although discussed in Chapter 13, we review here some principles of cardiac gating. The earliest techniques of cardiac gating involved sampling one echo and filling one line of k-space for a given image following each R wave. A different slice was then excited, generating an image of a different location at a different phase of the cardiac cycle. The TR was therefore set as the R-to-R interval (time between R waves).

Alternatively, a short TR can be used to excite a given slice repetitively, with each echo sampled to fill a line of k-space of a different image. When image acquisition for such a series is complete, images at numerous phases of the cardiac cycle are reconstructed at one or more slice locations. This set of images is usually displayed as a cine loop, resembling real-time images.

In either case, the acquisition time of a cardiac gated sequence was defined as the product of the R-R interval, the phase axis resolution, and the number of signals averaged (NSA).

$$\text{Acquisition time} = \text{R-R} \times \text{phase resolution} \times \text{NSA}$$

The acquisition time can be decreased greatly by segmented filling of k-space. This involves filling more than one line of k-space for a given image within a cardiac cycle. As the TR becomes increasingly shorter, the amount of cardiac motion between two successive MR signals becomes negligible. Therefore, with very short TR techniques, several consecutive MR signals can be used to fill several lines of k-space for a given image, representing a single cardiac phase. The number of consecutive signals contributing to one cardiac phase is referred to as the number of *views per segment*.

As the number of views per segment increases, fewer segments are needed to fill k-space, so the acquisition time decreases. However, a large number of views per segment increases the amount of time represented by each cardiac phase, which decreases the temporal resolution and increases motion-induced blurring. The number of cardiac phases represented in a final cine series can be increased by using the principle of view sharing, discussed in Chapter 17 and illustrated in Figure 24-12.

Cardiac gating can be applied prospectively or retrospectively. For prospective gating, the R wave triggers data acquisition, which continues for a predetermined interval each cardiac cycle. At the end of this data acquisition period, no data are collected until the next R wave. However, repetitive RF excitation usually continues,

so the amount of recovery prior to each excitation pulse is not altered; that is, a consistent TR throughout the series is maintained. The time between the end of data collection and the next R wave may vary and functions to decrease the influence of variations in cardiac rate throughout image acquisition.

Retrospective cardiac gating involves continuous data collection throughout the cardiac cycle. Data are then assigned retrospectively to images that represent different phases in the cardiac cycle based on the time of data collection relative to the appearance of the R wave. The main advantage of retrospective gating is that it allows measurement of blood flow throughout the cardiac cycle, whereas prospective gating does not record blood flow immediately prior to each R wave.

We now discuss the standard image planes that are acquired for imaging cardiac anatomy and function. Techniques for dark blood and bright blood, as well as other unique techniques employed specifically for cardiac imaging, are evaluated.

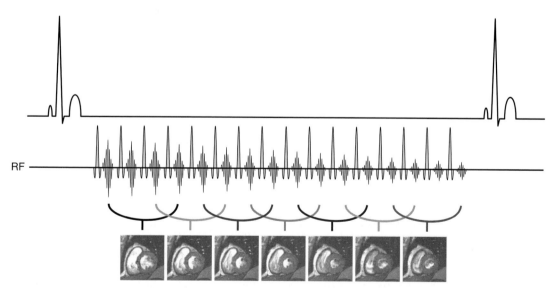

Figure 24-12
Segmented cine cardiac imaging using view-sharing to increase the number of cardiac phases shown. In this example, there are four echoes (views) per segment, providing four lines of k-space. The second image shares two of the views from the first image and two of the views from the third image. Therefore, the 16 echoes in this R-R interval provide data for seven cardiac phases, rather than only four.

Oblique Planes

One of the most important planes for cardiac imaging is the short axis plane through the left ventricle. This image is best obtained by double oblique projection, which can begin from either coronal or axial scout images (Fig. 24-13). A long axis scout image is obtained from either of the original scout images. If this process is begun with a coronal image, the plane should be prescribed along the axis from the cardiac apex to either the aortic root (left ventricular outflow) or the left atrium (left ventricular inflow). Alternatively, with a standard axial image, a two-chamber scout image can be obtained through the left ventricle and left atrium along a plane parallel to the ventricular septum. A short axis plane is then defined that is perpendicular to both the standard and oblique scout images.

The short axis view should then be used to prescribe a horizontal long axis plane, which is referred to as the four-chamber view. This plane bisects both the left and right ventricles in the short axis. Long axis scout imaging should also be used to make sure that the new image plane is oriented along the long axis of the left ventricle. Finally, the short axis and four-chamber views should be used to prescribe a vertical long axis view, which is the left ventricular two-chamber inflow view. An additional plane, the left ventricular outflow view, can be prescribed from the original axial images along the axis of the aortic root.

Dark Blood

Traditionally, cardiac anatomy has been depicted on images where myocardium has moderate signal intensity, contrasted against the signal void of flowing blood. Mechanisms of signal loss secondary to motion, as discussed in Chapter 13, combine to depict contrast between myocardium and flowing blood. Initially, the standard gated spin echo technique was used, but the long

acquisition time and incomplete suppression of blood signal were disadvantages.

More recently, the double inversion recovery technique has been implemented to null more completely the signal intensity of flowing blood, described earlier in this chapter and in Chapter 15. To allow acquisition during suspended respiration of dark blood images of the heart, the single-shot fast spin echo (FSE) or long echo train multishot FSE technique is usually used for double inversion recovery dark blood image acquisition. The echo train obtained with these techniques can be reduced using parallel imaging techniques (see Chapter 17).

Most protocols for cardiac imaging involve obtaining at least one set of dark blood images. These images are particularly valuable for depicting cardiac masses as well as the thickness and morphology of myocardium (Fig. 24-13).

Bright Blood Imaging of Cardiac Motion

Bright blood imaging is usually obtained using a short TR, so several signals are acquired during each cardiac cycle. Depending on the TR and the temporal resolution of the resulting series, one or more consecutive signals contribute to an image at a particular phase of the cardiac cycle.

Bright blood during cardiac imaging is usually achieved using one of two basic methods. The older of the two methods relies on TOF principles, discussed earlier in the chapter. The quality of blood–myocardial contrast using these techniques is inconsistent, however, owing to the complex geometry of intracardiac flow and the limited replacement of blood that can occur during the increasingly short TRs that are used to acquire breath-holding cine images.

A more consistent quality of bright blood images results when using B-SSFP (see Chapter 14). Another advantage of B-SSFP is that an MRI system's minimum possible TR can be used; this is not possible for TOF techniques, as a minimized TR does not allow sufficient time for saturated blood in a slice to be replaced by unsaturated blood entering the slice between excitation pulses. The extremely short TR used to obtain B-SSFP images results in a short acquisition time, and the inherent characteristics of B-SSFP lead to a high SNR, high contrast between balanced steady-state blood and myocardium, and low sensitivity to motion-induced artifacts. Therefore, this technique is becoming the preferred method for obtaining bright blood cardiac images.

When multiple strategies of fast imaging are combined, such as short TR, parallel imaging, and alternate k-space filling (see Chapter 17), the acquisition time of an ungated image can be sufficiently short to allow "snapshot" imaging of cardiac activity. This generates a series of real-time images rather than a gated cine loop.

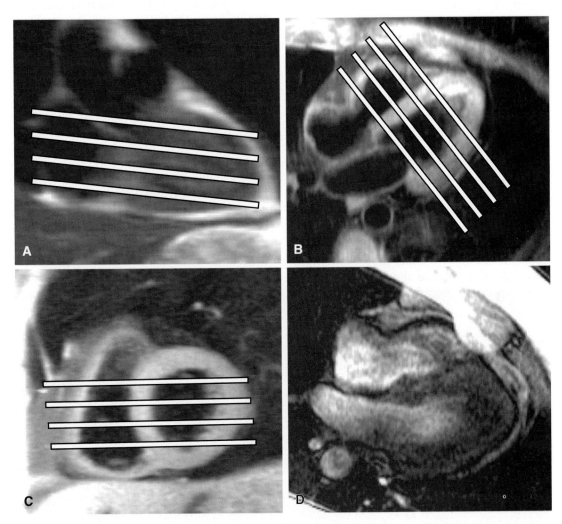

F i g u r e 2 4 - 1 3
Graphic prescription of oblique and double-oblique projections. A coronal single-shot FSE image (*A*) is used to prescribe a left ventricular inflow plane through the left atrium and left ventricle. One such image, obtained using double inversion recovery for blood nulling, is shown in (*B*); this image is then used to prescribe a left ventricular short axis plane, one of which is shown in (*C*). This image is then used to prescribe a four-chamber cardiac plane; one frame from a segmented cine acquisition is shown in (*D*).

Myocardial Tagging

A series of RF prepulses can be applied to generate an array or grid of thin saturation stripes on the first image of a cine series corresponding to the time point immediately following the R wave of the ECG trigger. On each successive image, the stripes are distorted by myocardial motion. This allows a precise view of local as well as global myocardial motion. One method for generating a series of equally spaced stripes is to generate two RF pulses separated by a gradient pulse. This produces a periodic *spatial modulation of the magnetization* (SPAMM). The result is a grid of finely spaced saturation bands (Fig. 24-14).

The saturation band voids are seen most clearly on the first cine image immediately following the saturation. The mixing of blood leads to rapid dissipation of the saturation, so contrast between blood and tissue is accentuated. As the myocardium contracts, the grid lines become deformed. This facilitates visual appreciation of myocardial wall motion and provides the basis for detailed calculation of focal wall motion physiology as well as alterations with disease.

Flow Measurement

Phase contrast imaging, as described earlier in the chapter, can be used to measure blood flow by detecting phase changes due to motion. The signal intensity of a given pixel is proportional to the velocity of blood flow along its axis of encoding. The volume of blood flow in a vessel is the sum of the velocities of each pixel. As with Doppler applications, pressure gradients can be calculated from the peak velocity measurement at a site of stenosis; the pressure gradient is four times the square of the peak velocity ($P = 4 \times V_{max}^2$).

Myocardial Contrast Enhancement

Suspected myocardial ischemia can be evaluated using either of two contrast enhancement techniques. One depends on rapid multiphasic acquisition during and immediately following a bolus of contrast material to depict myocardial perfusion. An area of decreased perfusion is depicted as an area of decreased myocardial enhancement on these early postcontrast images.

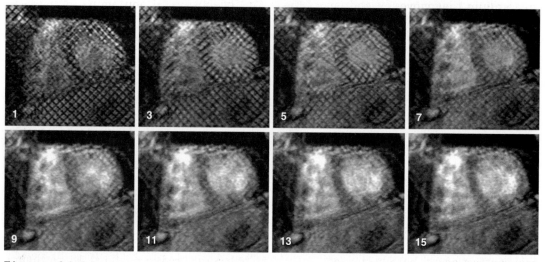

Figure 24-14
Two-dimensional myocardial tagging using *spatial modulation of the magnetization* (SPAMM), on a ventricular short axis 15/8.7/30° segmented cine left image. Every other image is shown. The grid lines are clearest in image 1 and become deformed and less distinct during later cardiac phases. End-systole corresponds to image 5.

Alternatively, T1-weighted images can be obtained several minutes after injecting gadolinium chelate, by which time the agent has diffused throughout the extracellular space (see Chapter 21), including the interstitium of tissues such as fibrous scar. Healthy myocardium is composed primarily of intact myocardial cells, which do not accumulate the contrast agent. In contrast, infarcted myocardium consists primarily of fibrous scar, which contains a paucity of intact cells and therefore a relatively larger volume of extracellular (primarily interstitial) space. On delayed images, therefore, infarcted myocardium is depicted as *increased* enhancement relative to healthy myocardium, even though it has less blood flow.

Numerous techniques have been used to show delayed enhancement of infarcted myocardium, including gated spin echo and cine spoiled gradient echo methods. The most effective results have been achieved with gated segmented inversion recovery gradient echo techniques, which were discussed in Chapter 15. For demonstrating delayed enhancement, a nonselective (no slice-select gradient) inversion pulse occurs at a set delay following the R wave. There is no slice-select gradient to ensure that myocardium that moves in and out of the slice is uniformly inverted. A TI of about 300 msec is generally appropriate to null normally enhanced myocardium; hyperenhanced fibrosis has a shorter T1 and therefore recovers beyond zero. Hence it appears as high signal intensity.

Coronary MR Angiography

A variety of approaches to MRA, discussed earlier in the chapter, have been applied to nonenhanced coronary imaging. Additionally, first-pass gadolinium-enhancing techniques, as well as imaging after injection of a blood pool contrast agent, have been used.

Coronary MRA is one of the most challenging areas of MR imaging. At the time of this writing a consensus regarding the preferred technique has not emerged, and coronary MRA remains in development, not ready for routine clinical use. With the advent of multidetector row computed tomography (CT), it appears likely that CT angiographic techniques may become clinically useful for coronary imaging earlier than will MRA. However, the promise of coronary MRA is that it can become part of a single comprehensive examination that provides more additional information (e.g., cardiac function, coronary flow, status of the ischemic myocardium) than is possible using CT techniques.

Stress Imaging

The use of cardiac stress to induce myocardial ischemia is well established for other modalities of cardiac imaging, including scintigraphy and echocardiography, and these principles have been extended to MRI. Stress can be induced by exercise, but this is difficult to accomplish during MR imaging without disturbing the process of image acquisition. Therefore, stress is usually induced pharmacologically by agents such as dobutamine, dipyridamole, or adenosine. Dobutamine stimulates cardiac contractility at low doses; increasing the dose increases oxygen consumption and thereby induces ischemia in vulnerable myocardial segments. This manifests as a focal reduction in cardiac contractility. It is extremely important that the patient be adequately monitored for complications of induced ischemia, especially during high-dose dobutamine studies.

Dipyridamole and adenosine are sometimes used for vasodilation. They have no effect on ischemic segments of myocardium, however, because the arterioles in these segments are already maximally dilated. Therefore, reduced flow to ischemic myocardial segments is recognized more readily following administration of a pharmacological vasodilator.

▼

Essential Points to Remember

1. Stationary oxygenated blood has low signal intensity on T1-weighted images and high signal intensity on T2-weighted images.

2. Saturation pulses can be applied to reduce the signal intensity of blood before it flows into an image slice.

3. The flow of blood out of an image slice between the excitation and refocusing pulses causes decreased intravascular signal.

4. Loss of phase coherence secondary to different flow velocities in a voxel causes decreased intravascular signal intensity.

5. Administration of a gadolinium chelate reduces the T1 of blood, increasing its signal intensity.

6. Gadolinium-enhanced bright blood arteriographic images are best obtained using 3D-FT techniques, timed so the weak phase-encoded views are acquired during the first pass of contrast agent through the vessels of interest.

7. TOF techniques depend on saturating background tissue with rapidly repeated excitations. Blood flowing into the image slice has higher signal intensity because it has not been saturated.

8. Two-dimensional TOF techniques are highly sensitive to slow flow owing to the short distance the blood must flow to leave the image slice between excitations.

9. Three-dimensional TOF techniques have a higher SNR and lower sensitivity to slow flow than do 2D-TOF techniques.

10. MOTSA is one method of increasing the sensitivity to the slow flow of 3D-TOF techniques at the expense of a lower SNR.

11. Phase contrast techniques use phase changes due to motion to encode flow. They allow measurement of flow velocity and usually have high background suppression, although the acquisition time is longer than for most other vascular imaging techniques.

12. For cardiac MRI, multiple orthogonal planes relative to the heart should be obtained.

13. The blood signal can be suppressed by the double inversion recovery technique, which consists of a nonselective inversion pulse followed immediately by a selective reinversion pulse and an inversion time (TI) prior to excitation so the blood signal relaxes to zero.

14. Bright blood cine images utilize short TRs. Preferably, they are based on a balanced steady-state free precession technique. With sufficiently short image acquisition time, imaging can be done in real time.

15. A series of saturation lines can be applied at the beginning of the cardiac cycle, tagging myocardium so its motion can be observed in detail.

16. Myocardial viability can be assessed on delayed postcontrast images; fibrous scar has a larger extracellular space than does viable myocardium, and therefore scar is hyperintense on delayed postcontrast images.

C h a p t e r **25**

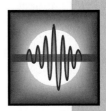

Perfusion and Diffusion Techniques

T he previous chapter focused on anatomical depiction of blood vessels. Vascular pathology and physiology can also be investigated with methods that rely on depiction of perfusion or diffusion rather than vascular anatomy. Many of these methods follow directly from principles introduced earlier in this book, including contrast agents, signal loss due to motion or susceptibility, and the use of magnetization preparation pulses. Techniques for studying perfusion and diffusion are discussed in this chapter.

Perfusion

Perfusion is a measure of blood flow though a volume of tissue. It is conventionally quantified in milliliters per milligram of tissue. However, because the densities of body tissue and blood are similar (both about 1 mg/ml), perfusion is often expressed as a dimensionless number.

Volume conservation requires that the blood flowing into a region is compensated by an identical volume of blood flowing out. Perfusion differs from bulk flow, however, in that it refers to the amount of blood (and by extension nutrient) that actually reaches the tissue. The blood *flow* through the aorta, for example, is enormous, but it does not *perfuse* the aortic tissue itself. Similarly, cerebral arteriovenous malformations bypass the brain and may result in perfusion deficits even though they support substantial blood flow. In many cases it is practical to assess perfusion as the flow of blood through the capillary bed: So long as the capillaries themselves are healthy and support normal exchange of nutrients, tissue perfusion is essentially proportional to capillary blood flow. Perfusion is a more direct indicator of tissue vascular health than is bulk blood flow.

337

Perfusion is an area of highly active research interest because of its substantial potential impact. Clinical applications include the acute management of stroke, the characterization and classification of tumors, and the field of functional magnetic resonance imaging (MRI) (i.e., localization of brain function via MRI). Emerging applications include evaluation of tumor perfusion prior to and following antiangiogenesis therapy and assessment of tissue ischemia. Extracerebral applications are likely to expand in the near future.

The currently available approaches to perfusion vary significantly. Generally, the trade-offs must include quantitative accuracy, invasiveness, volume coverage, and resolution. Therefore, the choice of technique must be matched carefully to the clinical question.

Bolus Methods

When contrast agent is injected as a tight bolus, it is possible to track its passage through the vasculature or tissue using proper imaging technique. Such dynamic imaging requires rapid scanning, as the interval from the venous injection of the agent and its transit through the heart and lungs and into the arterial circulation and end-organ, is typically less than 20 seconds.

Depending on the specific choice of contrast agent, the optimal contrast behavior of the imaging sequence may differ. In particular, gadolinium chelates affect both T1 and T2 relaxation rates. As discussed in Chapters 2 and 4, paramagnetic materials in a magnetic field increase the field strength in their immediate vicinity, causing local magnetic field heterogeneity. This decreases the T2* relaxation time, thereby decreasing the signal intensity, particularly on gradient echo images with moderate to long TEs.

In low concentrations the T2 effects are relatively modest and the T1 shortening dominates the signal changes, increasing the signal intensity on T1-weighted images with a sufficiently short TE. At high concentrations, however, the T2 effects are substantial. Even with a short to moderate TE (about 20 msec), the signal intensity is greatly reduced, particularly using techniques that do not have spin echo refocusing radiofrequency (RF) pulses. Following a bolus injection, therefore, T2- or T2*-weighted methods show the passage of gadolinium through the vasculature as an overall *loss* of the magnetic resonance (MR) signal.

Pulse sequences that are sensitive to susceptibility-induced signal loss are referred to as T2*-weighted. Sensitivity to T2* contrast can be minimized by refocusing transverse magnetization via a 180° refocusing pulse transmitted at one half the TE or effective TE (TE_{ef}). Conversely, T2* contrast can be *increased* by omitting 180° refocusing pulses and by using a long TE or TE_{ef}. Particularly fast and efficient T2*-weighted images can be obtained using echo planar techniques, as introduced in Chapter 16.

The susceptibility effect of uneven distribution of contrast agent extends farther than the more local paramagnetic effect of T1 reduction. Heterogeneous susceptibility causes signal loss extending beyond the boundaries of the vessels into the surrounding tissue, whereas increased signal intensity due to paramagnetic substances affects only water protons in the blood vessels themselves (Fig. 25-1).

Although small doses of superparamagnetic contrast agent (e.g., iron oxide particles or dysprosium chelates) can shorten T2* substantially, they are not currently approved for rapid bolus administration in clinical practice. Fortunately, currently available gadolinium chelates produce sufficient T2* shortening when unevenly distributed in tissue, as when present only within capillaries during initial arrival in a tissue. Echo planar techniques are ideal for perfusion imaging because of their rapidity and sensitivity to T2* enhancement (Fig. 25-2).

Dilution of the contrast agent during the passage from peripheral vein to the tissue of interest produces unavoidable broadening of the effective bolus. A tighter bolus, for more

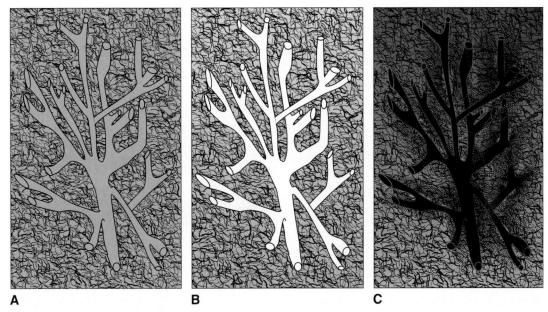

Figure 25-1
Effects of gadolinium chelates on brain parenchymal signal intensity using T1-weighted and T2*-weighted pulse sequences. (*A*) Baseline. (*B*) On T1-weighted images, signal intensity increases markedly within vessels, but the effect on parenchyma is minimal. (*C*) Susceptibility effects of gadolinium chelate extend beyond the vessel walls, decreasing parenchymal signal intensity on T2*-weighted images.

precise depiction of tissue perfusion, could be obtained by direct intraarterial injection just proximal to the tissue of interest; however, unacceptably invasive techniques are generally necessary for this approach.

The source images that show the contrast agent passage are difficult to interpret on their own, even when viewed as a movie or cine loop. Therefore, most practitioners use some sort of processing strategy to analyze the series. Usually this amounts to numerical integration of the signal change, although the more sophisticated methods *model* the time course of the bolus and perform statistical fits that can be used to give a quantitative estimate of perfusion. These methods must rely on assumptions about the relationship between contrast agent concentration and signal change and, in some cases, on reperfusion by the second or later passage of the contrast bolus. The mean transit time (MTT) describes the average time for a contrast bolus to reach a specific location and is a useful measure for describing

circulation deficits. The MTT also must be calculated by integrating the signal change and then finding the time point at which half of the signal change occurred.

For practical clinical examinations, power injector systems give a well-controlled, continuous dose of contrast intravenously over a short period—typically 6 seconds or less. For quantization, the timing of the injection relative to the image acquisition must be known precisely. For practices that perform these examinations only occasionally, it may be acceptable to inject the bolus manually and simply accept the resulting loss of accuracy. Many commercial MR systems now include the software for quantitative analyses of perfusion under such conditions.

Magnetic Labeling

An alternative approach for evaluating perfusion is to tag the blood magnetically. This can be accomplished with a spatial

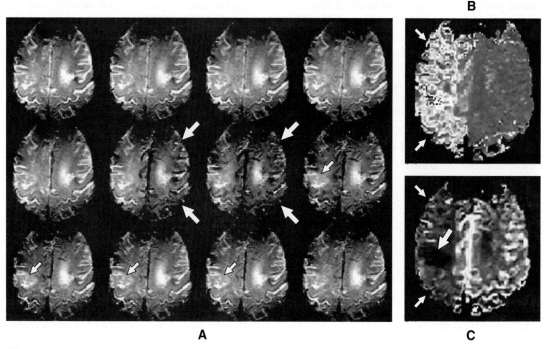

A   **C**

Figure 25-2

Acute cerebral infarction depicted by echo planar perfusion imaging following a bolus of gadolinium chelate (0.1 mmol/kg). (*A*) Twelve T2*-weighted images at the same location, each of which was acquired as part of a multiplanar whole-brain set of images at 40 phases after contrast agent injection. These 12 images were acquired during an interval of 42 seconds. Upon arrival of the contrast agent, the signal intensity of the normally perfused left hemisphere decreases (*large arrows*); perfusion to the right hemisphere is delayed. In the right hemisphere, the infarct is not perfused (*small arrows*). (*B*) Mean transit time map depicts slow transit through the right hemisphere secondary to ischemia (*arrows*). (*C*) Regional cerebral blood volume (rCBV) map depicts decreased blood volume of the ischemic region (*small arrows*) and nonperfusion of the infarct (*large arrow*). (Courtesy of M. Moseley, M. Marks, D. Tong, and G. Albert, Department of Radiology and Stanford Stroke Center.)

saturation pulse, so that arterial blood flowing into an image slice or volume is more saturated. The effects of saturation pulses are most apparent on large vessels, but there are more subtle effects on signal intensity. These are somewhat greater if 180° selective inversion pulses are used. Even so, the change in parenchymal signal intensity produced by such inversion pulses can be as little as 2%; and depiction of these small changes requires postprocessing techniques such as image subtraction. The methods that magnetically encode inflowing blood are generally known collectively as arterial spin labeling (ASL). Because the spins are labeled when they are outside the imaging slice and must flow into it, there is

a significant transit time involved that depends on distance. Unfortunately, substantial T1 relaxation can occur during transit times of only seconds, so the label becomes diminished. Because neither the transit time nor the T1 of blood are completely known, there is always residual error in the ASL-based perfusion maps. Furthermore, the transit times into any given slice of tissue may be quite variable by region; the vascular paths may differ, and the flow in a single blood vessel is not at constant velocity.

If two images of the same site, one acquired with a preceding inversion pulse and one without, are subtracted from each other, the difference image reflects the tissue perfusion. This is the basis of the *echo planar imaging signal targeting with alternating radiofrequency* (EPISTAR) method. There are many practical problems, however, with simple applications of EPISTAR, and investigators have come up with alternatives. As there is still no broad consensus on the relative merits of these many competing methods, their details are not covered here. The reader should be aware, however, of some of the values and limitations of such spin labeling. Unlike any of the other perfusion methods presently available, ASL offers, at least potentially, the valuable combination of noninvasiveness and quantitation.

Blood Oxygen Level-Dependent (BOLD) Techniques

In the preceding section we discussed the use of T2*-weighted gradient echo or echo planar images obtained following a bolus of paramagnetic contrast agent for depicting perfusion. Disadvantages to the use of contrast agents include the added time, effort, and invasiveness of injections and the direct cost of the contrast agent. Additionally, it may be necessary to wait several minutes or hours before repeating the observation. However, intravascular deoxyhemoglobin may be used as an endogenous contrast agent for obtaining images that show changes in perfusion after a variety of physiological provocations.

Deoxyhemoglobin has four unpaired electrons, rendering it paramagnetic, whereas oxyhemoglobin is diamagnetic and has little effect on MR images. On heavily T2*-weighted pulse sequences, the signal intensity is related inversely to the deoxyhemoglobin concentration. Pulse sequences that are sensitive to the concentration of deoxyhemoglobin are commonly referred to as blood oxygenation level-dependent (BOLD) techniques. Shortly after their introduction investigators realized that the blood oxygen signal may be

a useful marker for cellular activity, as the oxygen needs of tissue change with other metabolic processes (Fig. 25-3).

The BOLD technique has been used to evaluate renal function (Fig. 25-4). The most significant application of BOLD imaging, however, has been to interrogate the function of neurons in the brain, whose oxygen consumption increases with the electrical firing rate.

The effect of neural activity on the BOLD signal is somewhat paradoxical, however, as the vascular system responds to the increased demand by increasing blood flow to maintain a large oxygen gradient across the capillary vessel wall. The combination of increased flow and high intravascular oxygen levels results in an increased concentration of intravenous oxygen. Therefore, increases in neural activity lead quickly to increases in the MR signal. The BOLD signal response to a short neural event is a gradual rise over about 5 seconds followed by a return to baseline in about 15 seconds.

Because there is a short period between the time at which oxygen consumption increases and when the vasculature can respond with increased blood flow, there is a short period of signal *decrease* that peaks less than a second after the neural events. This "fast response" may be important for understanding the dynamics of neural processes, but it is so small that available imaging methods do not show it reliably.

Functional MR imaging (fMRI) of the brain using BOLD is performed using rapid T2*-weighted imaging, usually echo planar imaging (EPI), while the subject performs behavioral or mental tasks. During presurgical planning fMRI can demonstrate which brain regions are needed for important functions. Such areas of "eloquent" cortex can be marked for potential sparing during brain surgery or ablation. Finding the brain locus for hand motion, for example, is extremely important during management of tumors near the parieto-occipital junction. More complex, higher level functions, such as human language and memory, require greater sophistication to identify, as

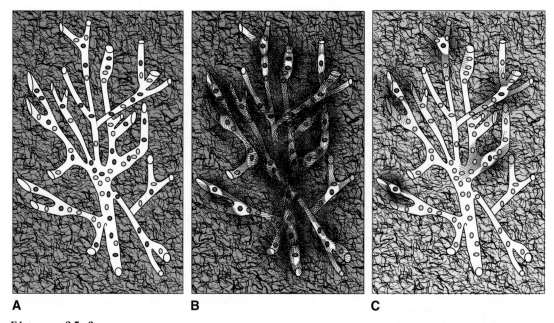

Figure 25-3
Principles of the blood oxygen level-dependent (BOLD) technique. (*A*) *Light and dark ovals* represent, respectively, oxygenated and deoxygenated red blood cells in the microvasculature. (*B*) The paramagnetism of deoxyhemoglobin in deoxygenated red blood cells induces a higher local magnetic field, creating local field heterogeneities that extend beyond the blood vessels and decreasing the parenchymal signal intensity on T2*-weighted images. (*C*) With increased flow, more oxygenated blood cells are delivered to the tissue, decreasing the concentration of deoxyhemoglobin and thus increasing signal intensity.

the required stimuli may be subtle. As the field of clinical fMRI evolves, it is likely to require close integration of radiologists, neurologists, neuropsychologists, and neurosurgeons. Higher field strength appears particularly beneficial for fMRI, as sensitivity to magnetic field heterogeneity increases with the square of the magnetic field and signal intensity increases directly with the magnetic field (see Chapter 12). Like most bolus injection methods, BOLD fMRI images are not useful on their own. They must first be processed to show the relationships between signal changes and the ongoing mental or behavioral tasks. For this, investigators usually rely on statistical analyses that relate ("correlate") the signal change with the timing of the subject's behavior. For reasonable accuracy, these methods must also include modeling of the time course of the BOLD signal change. In most cases the resulting images are presented as maps of a statistical parameter that indicate

the likelihood that a particular brain region is involved in processing the particular task or behavior (Fig. 25-5). Importantly, these regional activation maps are thresholded, so brain areas with a small likelihood of task involvement are not colorized. If the voxel is not colored or labeled, however, one should not assume that the region is not involved in the task. In statistical jargon, the methods currently used do not control for "type II" errors. Therefore, if used in applications such as surgical planning, one cannot be certain that removal of any specific brain region will result in spared function.

Diffusion

In Chapter 10 we discussed the loss of signal intensity caused by uncompensated motion during the interval between excitation and

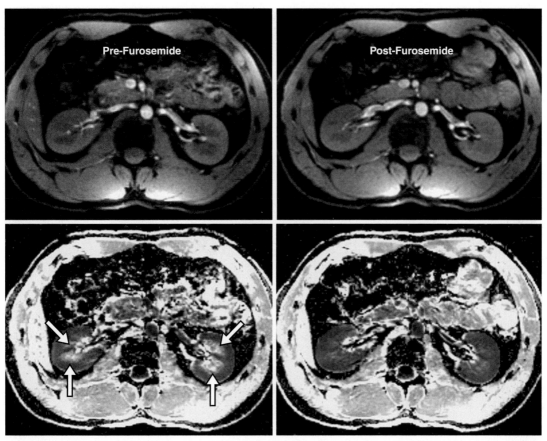

Figure 25-4
BOLD imaging of the kidneys at 3.0 T at rest and following diuresis accomplished by intravenous administration of 20 mg of furosemide, which increases renal blood flow and activity [Prasad et al. Circulation 1996;94:3271–5]. Multiecho gradient echo images were obtained using TR 65 msec, flip angle 30°, and TE 7–40 msec; these were used to create R2* maps by depicting the signal intensity change with increasing TE. Images at the top are gradient echo images prior to (*left*) and following (*right*) furosemide administration. At the bottom, an R2* map at rest (*left*) shows high signal intensity of the renal medulla (*arrows*) owing to its low concentration of deoxyhemoglobin. Following furosemide injection (*right*), the renal medulla has lower signal intensity, indicating oxygenation approaches that of cortex. (Courtesy of Luping Li and Pottumarthi Prasad, Evanston Northwestern Healthcare, Evanston, IL.)

signal measurement; this motion can reduce the amplitude of the resultant echo through intravoxel phase dispersion. This principle can be applied to generate images in which gross loss of signal intensity results from random microscopic motion of water in relatively unstructured tissues such as fluid collections. When this random motion results in displacement of molecules, it is referred to as *diffusion*.

Water diffuses freely across capillaries and within the cellular interstitium. Water also diffuses readily across cell membranes and among tissue compartments. Pure water at 37°C diffuses at a rate of approximately 0.003 mm²/sec; this value is called the *diffusion coefficient* (D) of water. The diffusion of water in tissue is restricted and less random, so an apparent diffusion coefficient (ADC, or D*) is used. The ADC is smaller than the unrestricted value of D, and it continues to decrease as the time of its measurement (the diffusion time, T_d) increases because free water molecules have an

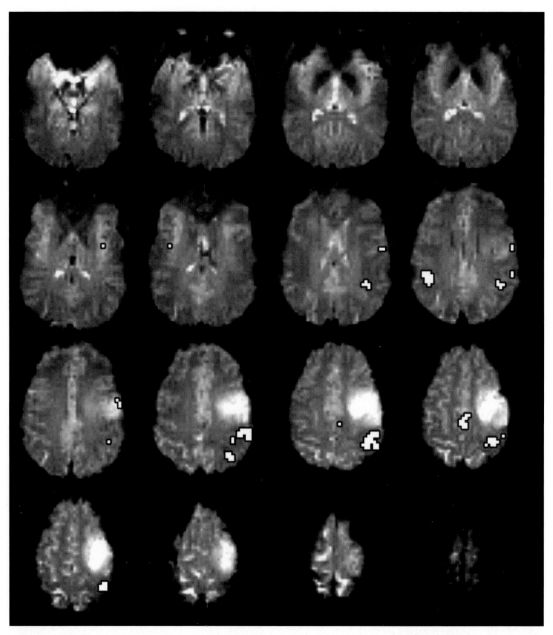

Figure 25-5
BOLD activation map for hand motion. Outlined white areas showed a statistically reliable increase in MR signal during periods in which the patient moved the fingers of her right hand. Typically, such maps are presented as colored overlays showing active brain regions. Note that the highlighted regions suggest that removal of the obvious parietal lesion will result in spared motor function, a prediction validated post-surgically. (Courtesy of Keith R. Thulborn, M.D., Ph.D., University of Pittsburgh.)

increasing probability of encountering physical restrictions. T_d can be increased to reduce the contribution from restricted diffusion, rendering the pulse sequence more specific for unrestricted diffusion.

One of the most intriguing structural features of water diffusion in tissue is its directionality. In cells such as muscle fibers and neuronal axons, water within and outside the cell membrane diffuses more readily along the membrane's long axis and less freely across the cell membranes. This results in diffusion "anisotropy," indicating that the diffusion rates are not the same in all directions. Anisotropic diffusion is apparent within the white matter of the brain and in muscle tissue. Several quantities can be used to describe the anisotropy, including the directional diffusion rate (a set of vectors), the difference in diffusion with direction (a quantity called simply diffusion anisotropy) and the total ADC. Each has been used to evaluate tissue health. In particular, measurements of both ADC and anisotropy can change rapidly, falling after ischemic insult to the brain and some other tissues. Because intervention for stroke with thrombolysis [e.g., using tissue plasminogen activator (TPA)] is indicated only within hours after acute events, there is a need for tools that can be used to guide the interventional team on the possibility of

tissue sparing. Currently, there is good indication that diffusion imaging may provide just such a tool.

Diffusion anisotropy is the basis for *diffusion tensor* imaging. A tensor is a mathematical construct that describes the three-dimensional properties of an ellipsoid. Diffusion anisotropy can thus be described in three dimensions, using the spatial coordinates *x, y, and z*, relative to the main magnetic field. The combination of these vectors can be simplified mathematically as the eigen values l_1, l_2, and l_3. Further discussion of the mathematics of diffusion tensor imaging is beyond the scope of this book.

Diffusion imaging is accomplished by incorporating into a pulse sequence pulsed gradients that increase sensitivity to diffusion. These diffusion-sensitizing dephasing gradients are analogous to the flow-sensitizing dephasing gradients used for phase contrast magnetic resonance

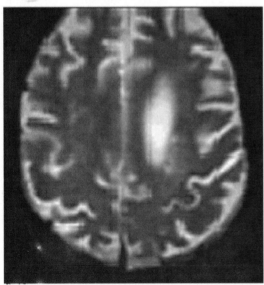

T2WI **DWI**

Figure 25-6
Depiction of an acute cerebral infarction by diffusion-weighted images (same patient as in Fig. 25-2). The T2-weighted echo planar image (*left*) shows no abnormality owing to the relative lack of edema in this acute infarct. On the diffusion-weighted image with $b = 1000$ sec/mm^2 (*right*) there is markedly decreased signal intensity in the left lateral ventricle (*small arrows*) owing to the high apparent diffusion in the free fluid. There is moderate apparent diffusion in brain parenchyma but little in the infarct (*large arrow*). (Courtesy of M. Moseley, M. Marks, D. Tong, and G. Albert, Department of Radiology and Stanford Stroke Center.)

angiography (MRA) techniques but are usually applied at higher amplitudes and for longer durations. The sensitivity of these pulse sequences can be altered by adjusting the strength and timing of the diffusion-sensitive gradients, expressed by the diffusion sensitization parameter b. Generally, b values of 500 to 1500 sec/mm^2 are used. As the b value increases, the TE (typically about 100 to 200 msec) must increase as well. Notably, the b values increase with the square of the gradient amplitude and the cube of its duration.

Diffusion-weighted images tend to resemble the inverse of T2-weighted images because both are generally sensitive to free water, which is depicted as low signal intensity on diffusion-weighted images and as high signal intensity on T2-weighted images. However, diffusion-weighted images depict certain abnormalities better than do T2-weighted images. In particular, acute cerebral infarction involves decreased axonal cytoplasmic streaming owing to interruption of the sodium-potassium-ATPase pump, which results in decreased diffusion. Additionally, the resulting cell swelling causes decreased interstitial and intravascular volume. These changes are depicted as markedly reduced diffusion in the slice-select direction on axial diffusion-weighted images. At this early stage, T2-weighted images are often normal owing to the absence of edema (Fig. 25-6).

▼

Essential Points to Remember

1. Perfusion can be determined by analyzing a series of images acquired immediately after rapid bolus injection of contrast agent.

2. For depicting perfusion following contrast agent injection, T2*-weighted images are useful because the intravascular contrast agent causes heterogeneous susceptibility and a heterogeneous magnetic field that extends across vessel walls into the parenchyma.

3. For perfusion imaging, T2*-weighted images can be obtained after a bolus of either a particulate agent (e.g., iron oxide) or a gadolinium chelate.

4. Perfusion imaging can be accomplished via arterial spin labeling by magnetically tagging blood using a saturation or inversion preparatory pulse before its entry into a region of interest.

5. Deoxyhemoglobin is paramagnetic and is normally present only in blood vessels. It therefore creates magnetic field inhomogeneity within tissue and decreased signal intensity on T2*-weighted images.

6. Stimulated by neural activity, cerebral blood flow increases (and therefore so does the delivery of fully oxygenated blood). This decreases the concentration of venous deoxyhemoglobin, increasing brain parenchymal signal intensity.

7. Activation-related effects of perfusion and BOLD on images may be subtle. Thus, with fMRI the BOLD images are formed into statistical maps that show the likelihood of a given brain region's involvement in tasks.

8. Diffusion of water molecules in blood vessels or interstitial fluid causes intravoxel phase dispersion, which decreases signal intensity on sensitive images. Sensitivity to diffusion can be increased by applying additional pulsed gradients.

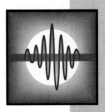

Chapter 26

Artifacts

During the course of our discussion of magnetic resonance imaging (MRI) principles we have explained the basis of several artifacts. Now, we review several common artifacts and methods by which they can be avoided.

Wraparound

Two-Dimensional Wraparound

As discussed in Chapters 7 and 9, spatial resolution of an image can be improved by decreasing its field of view (FOV). Often the FOV is smaller than the body part being imaged. These situations can lead to wraparound artifacts in which image data outside the FOV are "wrapped around" and represented on the opposite side of the image.

Wraparound artifacts can occur in both axes of an image slice and in the slice-encoding axis of a three-dimensional Fourier transform (3D-FT) acquisition. This artifact, also referred to as *aliasing*, occurs with ultrasound imaging and Doppler as well.

In the frequency-encoded axis, image data are represented according to the frequency of received magnetic resonance (MR) signals. The range of frequencies sampled is defined by the sampling bandwidth. The highest frequency that can be sampled unambiguously, also referred to as the *Nyquist frequency*, is half of the sampling bandwidth. Signals above the Nyquist frequency may appear at half their actual frequency, which results in those portions of the data appearing in the wrong portion of the image, specifically displaced by one half the size of the image. Figure 26-1 illustrates how a wave with a frequency higher than that of the sampling rate might be sampled such that its frequency appears to be lower.

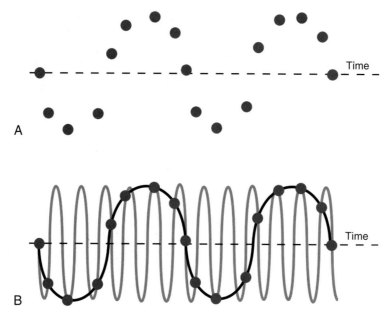

Figure 26-1
Frequency ambiguity results because waves of high and low frequency can both fit a given set of data samples. (*A*) A finite set of data samples is shown as points that fit the low-frequency waveform shown as a *dark line* in (*B*). To determine the high frequency shown with the *light line* unambiguously, a faster sampling rate would have been needed.

In older imaging systems, frequencies just above the sampled range would be encoded as if they were at the low end of the range, producing wraparound in the frequency-encoded axis. On these imaging systems, wraparound in the frequency-encoded axis could be avoided by using a sufficiently large FOV or by obtaining more frequency samples than are needed. For example, 512 samples could be obtained, even though the frequency-encoded resolution was only 256. The drawback of this technique is that it lengthens the sampling time. On modern equipment, wrap-around in the frequency axis is avoided by digital filtering, which eliminates signals with frequencies outside the desired range.

Wraparound in the phase-encoded axis is more difficult to prevent. Typically, an image is encoded for 360° of phase. A phase change of slightly more than 360° is identical to a small phase change. For example, a phase of 405° is the same as a phase of 45° (Fig. 26-2). In addition to overlapping structures on opposite sides of a body part,

a wraparound artifact can produce a distinctive "zebra stripe" moireá fringe artifact on gradient echo images of large body parts (Fig. 26-3). Magnetic field heterogeneities outside the FOV produce artifacts that overlap the primary image. Stripes are caused by the resulting phase interference.

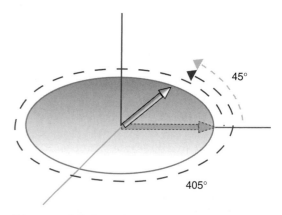

Figure 26-2
Phase ambiguity. Rotations of 45° and 405° produce the same phase, resulting in ambiguous phase-encoding, which is depicted as aliasing.

Wraparound artifact is another example of the fundamental similarity between frequency- and phase-encoding. Unfortunately, sampling at a higher frequency along the phase-encoding axis can be performed only by acquiring more raw data lines (equivalent to sampling at a faster rate). In general, then, eliminating the wraparound artifact along the phase-encoding axis necessitates an increase in the minimum total sampling time. This is effectively identical to increasing the FOV but discarding the data outside the region of interest. Although the pixel data from the unwanted region are discarded, acquisition of the views (echoes) that allowed the creation of these pixel data was not a wasted effort. It must be remembered that for 2D-FT techniques *every view contains information and thus contributes to the signal-to-noise ratio (SNR) for every pixel in the image slice.* For 3D-FT techniques, every view contains information for every pixel in the image volume. This principle allows some vendors to eliminate phase wrap in a way that is nearly transparent to clinical users; choosing a "no phase wrap" option eliminates the phase wraparound artifact without any apparent effect on the image or slowing of the acquisition time.

Consider an image with a 256 × 256 matrix, a 20 cm² FOV, and the number of signals averaged (NSA) being 2. The number of views obtained is therefore 256 × 2 = 512. Phase wrap can be eliminated by doubling the FOV in the phase-encoded axis from 20 cm to 40 cm. If the pixel size is not changed, it is necessary to double the number of phase-encoding views from 256 to 512. The matrix is now 256 × 512, and the FOV is 20 × 40 cm. If the NSA is decreased from 2 to 1, the total number of views obtained remains the same: 512. Spatial resolution is determined by the pixel size. Because the pixel size and the number of views have not changed, the spatial resolution and SNR do not change (Fig. 26-4). Vendors may choose to label this image as having an increased FOV and matrix and decreased NSA, or they may choose simply

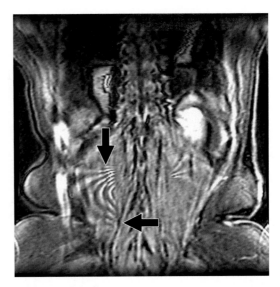

Figure 26-3
Zebra stripe artifact (*arrows*) at the periphery of a gradient echo 11/2.2/30° image results from phase interference between tissue in the image and aliased artifact due to magnetic field heterogeneity outside the field of view.

to display image annotation as if nothing had changed because, indeed, the spatial resolution, SNR, and apparent FOV have not changed.

The principal disadvantage of phase axis oversampling is an increased acquisition time for pulse sequences without signal averaging. If the number of signal averages is already the minimum, phase axis oversampling cannot be accomplished without increasing the total number of views obtained. For applications such as high-resolution dynamic imaging after a bolus of contrast material, other approaches are needed. Phase axis wraparound can often be avoided by a judicious choice of the FOV and the phase-encoding axis, so the shortest body dimension is chosen as the phase-encoding axis. When wraparound occurs, careful viewing of images is essential so the wraparound artifact is not mistaken for disease (Fig. 26-5). It is possible also to use additional 90° radiofrequency (RF) "suppression" pulses targeted at the regions outside the FOV. Immediately after the RF pulse, a dephasing gradient is applied so

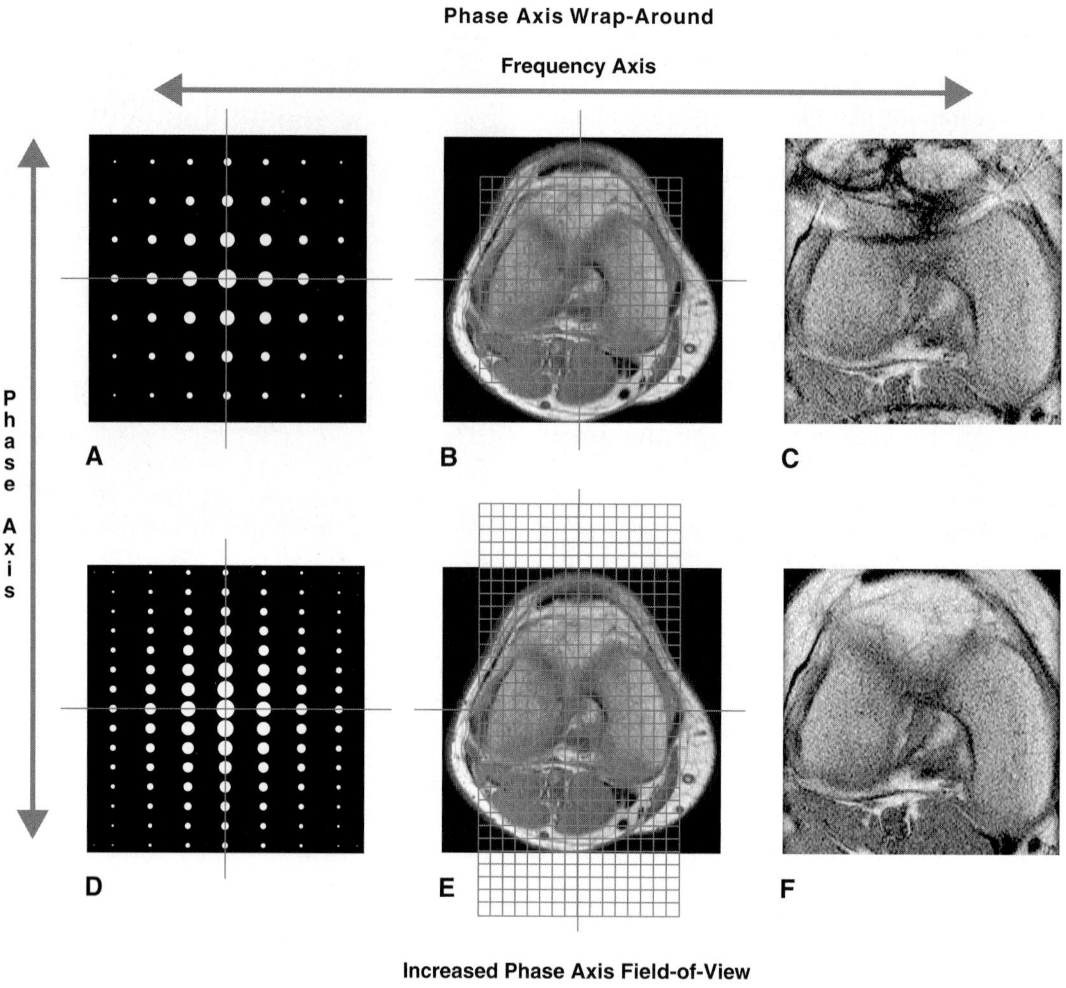

Phase Axis Wrap-Around

Frequency Axis

Increased Phase Axis Field-of-View

Figure 26-4

Phase axis wraparound results from a body part extending beyond the field of view (FOV) in the phase axis (*top*). (*A*) The map of k-space for the small FOV is depicted by the grid in (*B*). The part of the knee that extends outside the acquired FOV is depicted ambiguously as wraparound artifact in (*C*). This artifact is eliminated if the acquisition FOV in the phase axis is increased, even if the reconstructed FOV is not changed (*bottom*). (*D*) Map of k-space for the increased FOV depicted by the grid in (*E*). There are twice as many points in k-space. Two signal averages of the top scenario and one signal average of the bottom scenario have the same total number of views, so the signal-to-noise ratio (SNR) is unchanged. Pixel size is unchanged, so (*F*) has the same spatial resolution as (*C*) but without wraparound artifact. Wraparound in the frequency axis is eliminated by digital filters.

the transverse magnetization from those tissues does not contribute to the signal.

A process similar to phase axis oversampling can be implemented to allow simultaneous excitation of two image slices in a two-dimensional (2D) multislice technique. A complex excitation pulse is transmitted that consists of the multiplex of individual pulses needed to excite each of the two slices. Each image is then phase-encoded for only 180° so their phase encodings can

be separated. The resulting image is doubled in the phase axis, so both image slices fit within it, without overlapping. For the final image display, the composite image is split so the images are displayed in an anatomically correct order in the series. This technique has been called a phase axis multiplanar (POMP) or dual-slice technique. Unfortunately, the RF power required for POMP can be quite high, so there may be limitations in the total number

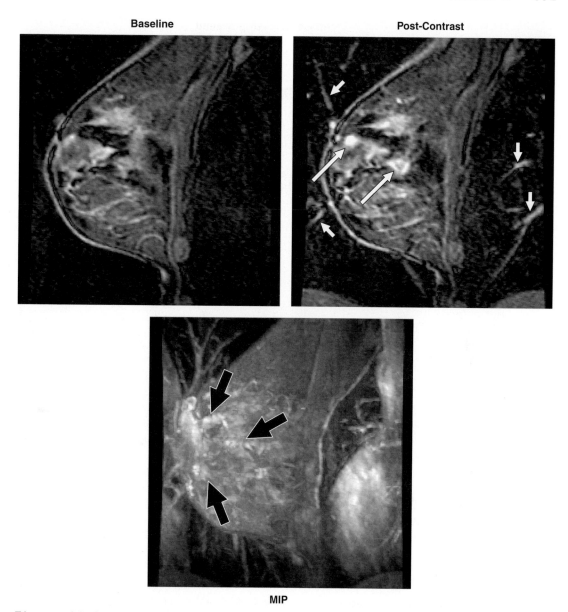

Baseline   **Post-Contrast**

MIP

Figure 26-5

Pseudonodules on sagittal images of the breast result from aliased pulmonary and hilar vessels. The phase axis is anteroposterior. Baseline image (*top left*) shows no breast lesions. On the postcontrast image, two round, enhancing structures (*large arrows*) project over the breast. *Small arrows* indicate pulmonary vessels. *Bottom.* Maximum-intensity projection (MIP) image shows the hilar structures (*arrows*) overlying the breast, accounting for the enhancing pseudonodules.

of slices that can be collected, particularly at high magnetic fields.

Recently, methods have been implemented that use the signal intensity profile of a phased-array coil to provide information about the location of spins. These *parallel imaging* techniques are discussed in Chapter 17. One of these techniques,

sensitivity encoding (SENSE) involves obtaining a reduced number of k-space lines in the phase-encoding direction, so a severely aliased image would result if conventional reconstruction were used. SENSE involves calculating the missing lines of k-space, so the image is unwrapped. If the number of calculated lines is not sufficient,

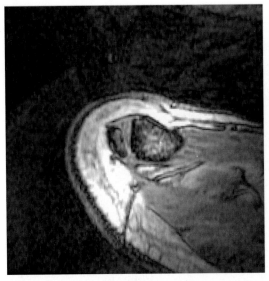 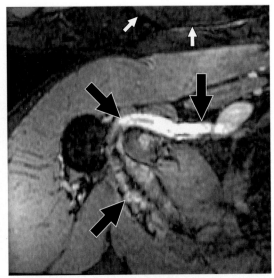

Top Section   **Bottom Section**

Figure 26-6
Wraparound artifact in the slice-encoded direction in axial three-dimensional Fourier transform (3D-FT) images of the shoulder. At right, a ghost of the top of the shoulder *(black arrows)* is projected onto the bottom slice. *White arrows* indicate wraparound artifact in the phase axis.

some wraparound artifact persists. However, unlike the wraparound artifact in conventionally reconstructed images, the wraparound artifact in SENSE images is visible in the center of the image, rather than at the edges. If the map of the coil sensitivity profile is not completely accurate, noise artifact may be present in the mid-portion of the image.

Three-Dimensional Wraparound

Because they use phase-encoding to separate slices, 3D-FT techniques are prone to wraparound artifacts in the slice-encoding axis as well as in the phase-encoding axis. This is unlike 2D-FT techniques, which use phase-encoding in only one axis.

To review briefly: For 2D-FT techniques, slice thickness is determined by selectively exciting, along the slice-select gradient, protons of a desired range of frequencies. Protons with frequencies outside this range are not excited, so wraparound artifact does not occur in the slice-select axis. With 3D-FT techniques, however, slices are phase-encoded, so phase wrap can occur in the slice-encoded direction (Fig. 26-6).

Wraparound in the slice-encoded direction can be avoided by encoding additional slices beyond the region of interest. Acquisition of the data for these slices contributes to the SNR of all other slices, regardless of whether these slices are reconstructed; each echo measured contributes information to all voxels throughout the volume of a 3D-FT acquisition. Slice-encoding wraparound can also be reduced by increasing the precision of the slab-selective excitation pulse, although this increases power deposition and is therefore practical only when using small excitation flip angles.

Edge Artifacts

Detail of an image can be reduced by a variety of edge artifacts, even if the voxel

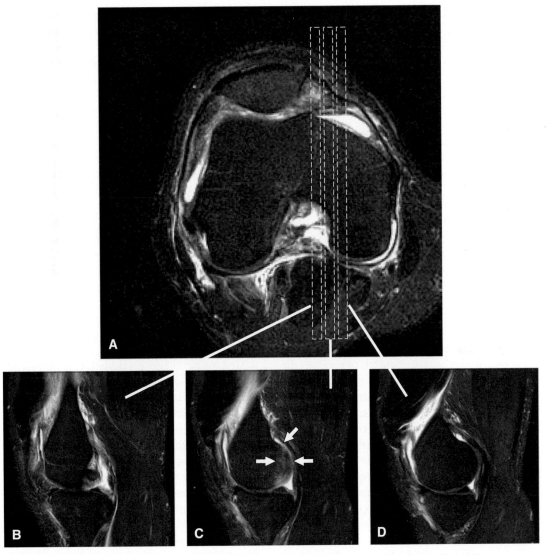

Figure 26-7
Partial volume artifact on fat-suppressed T2-weighted sagittal fast spin echo (FSE) images of the knee. The image slices for (*B–D*) are indicated by *white-dotted rectangles* on the axial fat-suppressed T2-weighted FSE image in (*A*). (*C*) *Arrows* indicate moderately high signal intensity mimicking bone marrow edema caused by a partial volume artifact between the high signal intensity of synovial fluid in (*B*) and the low signal intensity of bone and marrow in (*D*).

size is small and ghost artifacts are avoided. Many edge artifacts occur as a result of the FT processing of the image data.

Partial-Volume Artifacts

Partial-volume artifacts are intrinsic to essentially all volume imaging methods owing to finite limits of image resolution. With MRI and other digital techniques, image resolution is limited by the size of the image voxels. The signals of different tissues or structures in a voxel are averaged so they are not resolved. Thus, the interface between two objects with different signal intensities may be depicted as intermediate signal intensity (Fig. 26-7).

Chemical Shift Edge Artifacts

The difference between the precessional frequencies of water, lipid, and silicone protons produces chemical shift artifacts. Chemical shift *misregistration* artifact is erroneous mapping of protons with different chemical shifts (see Chapter 5). High-signal bands result when protons with different chemical shifts are mapped as if they were in the same pixel, causing summation of their signals. Signal voids result when protons with different chemical shifts are mapped more distant from each other than their true separation. Chemical shift misregistration artifact is most visible on MR images when the magnetizations of different chemical shifts are *in phase* with respect to each other so summation bands may be observed.

The amount of lipid displacement relative to water depends on the magnetic field strength and the bandwidth per pixel. In an image with a frequency-encoding axis resolution of 256 and a sampling bandwidth of 32 kHz, the bandwidth per pixel is 125 Hz (32,000 ÷ 256 = 125). The chemical shift between lipid and water protons, about 3.5 parts/million, increases with magnetic field strength. With this bandwidth, at 1.5 T the shift is about 220 Hz, slightly less than the bandwidth of two pixels. Thus, the displacement of lipid relative to water is slightly less than two pixels.

The frequency shift between lipid and water depends on the magnetic field and thus cannot be changed by the MR operator. The physical distance that corresponds to this chemical shift, however, can be decreased by increasing the frequency-encoding resolution, so a given number of pixels corresponds to a smaller displacement. In practice, this is performed by increasing the sampling bandwidth, so the chemical shift corresponds to a smaller number of pixels. For the example above, if the bandwidth is doubled to 250 Hz per pixel, the chemical shift displacement would be reduced to less than one pixel.

Chemical shift misregistration can also produce image aberrations when water and fat are not immediately adjacent, as when they are separated by a thin, low-signal-intensity structure. Examples include cortical bone, such as vertebral end-plates separating vertebral fat from water in intervertebral discs. Water in the intervertebral disc is misregistered toward the high end of the frequency-encoding axis relative to fat on the other side of the vertebral end-plate, decreasing its apparent thickness on the MR image. The water in the disc is misregistered away from the opposite end-plate, increasing its apparent thickness on the MR image (Fig. 26-8). Similarly, fat in the medullary cavity of a long bone is misregistered along the frequency axis relative to surrounding muscle (Fig. 26-9) or articular cartilage (Fig. 26-10), producing errors regarding the apparent thickness of cortical bone in these sites.

Silicone (Si) is an elongated molecule consisting of a siloxane (Si–O–Si–O) backbone with two or three methyl (CH_3) molecules attached to each Si atom. The chemical shift between silicone and water protons is even larger than the shift between fat and water (Fig. 26-11).

Chemical shift *cancellation* artifact occurs when the magnetizations of different chemical shifts are *out of phase* with respect to each other. For example, opposed phases of lipid and water proton magnetizations reduce signal intensity because the effect is signal cancellation rather than signal summation. Edge artifacts result from chemical shift differences when water and lipid protons occupy the same voxel owing to partial volume artifact. Phase cancellation results from destructive interference between these signals and their discrepant phases. Chemical shift cancellation artifacts can be minimized by obtaining standard spin echo or fast spin echo images, in which the refocusing pulses correct for chemical shift differences.

On gradient echo images, chemical shift cancellation artifacts are eliminated by choosing the echo time (TE) so magnetizations of lipid and water protons are in phase. The conspicuity of both chemical shift artifacts can be minimized by suppressing

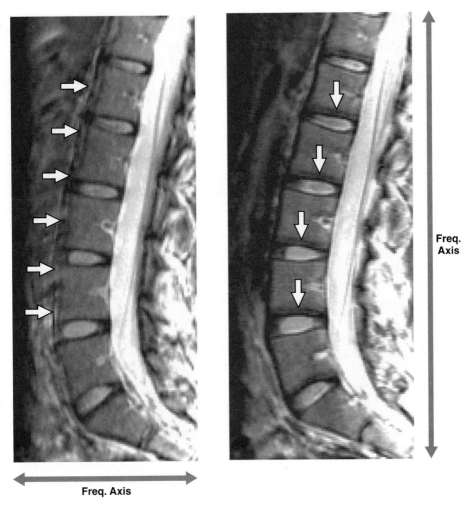

Figure 26-8
Chemical shift misregistration artifact affecting vertebral bodies. With the frequency axis anteroposterior (*left*), the anterior and posterior vertebral cortices (*arrows*) appear indistinct owing to misregistration of fat in vertebral marrow relative to water. With the frequency axis superoinferior (*right*), misregistration of water in intervertebral discs relative to vertebral fat has produced indistinct images of the vertebral end-plates (*arrows*).

the signal of lipid using chemical shift fat suppression, chemically selective water excitation, or inversion recovery fat-nulling techniques.

Some earlier scanner products were set up such that the relative displacement of fat and water along the slice-selection axis differed for the 90° and 180° pulses in a spin echo sequence. This resulted in relative suppression of the signal from fat on such images. At least one vendor has enabled a special "classic" mode of operation that maintains this behavior of the contrast, which is attractive to some radiologists.

Inversion Recovery Bounce Point Artifact

Inversion recovery bounce point artifact, discussed in Chapter 15, has an appearance similar to that of chemical shift cancellation artifact. To review: There are times when an inversion time is long enough that

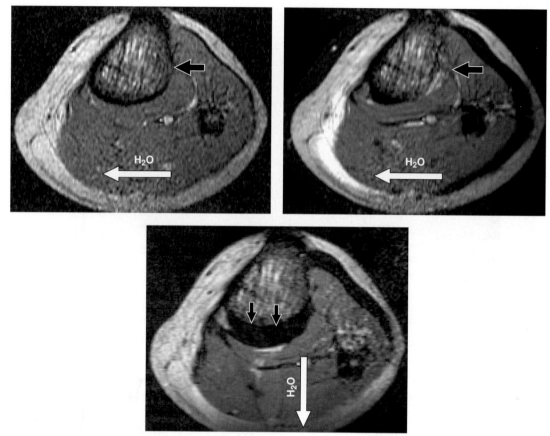

Figure 26-9

Erroneous depiction of cortical bone thickness results from chemical shift misregistration between muscle and fatty marrow on axial gradient echo 100/40/45° images. Water in muscle is shifted toward the right relative to lipid (*white arrows*). With a sampling bandwidth of 32 kHz (*top left*), the shift is about one pixel, resulting in thinning and indistinctness of the left side of the cortex (*black arrow*). With a sampling bandwidth of 4 kHz (*top right*), the chemical shift misregistration is several pixels. When the axis of frequency-encoding is switched to anteroposterior (*bottom*), muscle is misregistered several pixels posteriorly relative to fatty marrow, producing a large signal void and exaggerating the thickness of the posterior cortex (*small black arrows*).

magnetization of a tissue with a short T1 has recovered past zero, so it is positive. Other tissues, however, with a longer T1 may still have negative longitudinal magnetization at the same inversion time. These two tissues, with very different T1s, may have similar signal intensity on standard-magnitude reconstructed images, as negative magnetization is not distinguishable from positive magnetization on these images. Two such adjacent tissues, however, can be distingished because there is a bounce point cancellation signal void between them.

Truncation Artifacts

Magnetic resonance signals are electromagnetic waves that are mapped spatially according to their frequency and phase. To form a perfect representation of these waveforms it would be necessary to sample them for an infinite time, which is obviously not possible. Instead, the typical readout periods for MR scanners comprise a few milliseconds, so the waveforms must be truncated. After Fourier-transforming the data, this truncation results in a characteristic

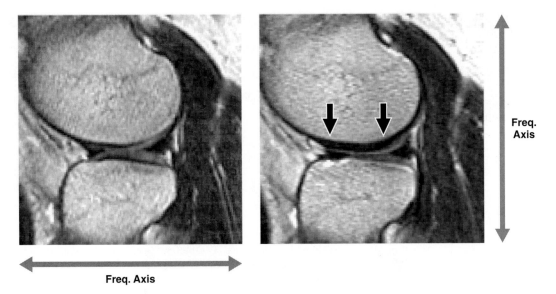

Figure 26-10
Chemical shift misregistration artifact in a sagittal image of the knee. In the image on the right, with a superoinferior frequency-encoding axis, lipid signals of bone marrow are misregistered superiorly relative to the water signal of hyaline cartilage (*arrows*), exaggerating the thickness of the femoral articular cortex and decreasing the apparent thickness of tibial articular cortex.

edge ringing (sometimes called Gibbs ringing), which appears as alternating light and dark bands (Fig. 26-12). This artifact can be quite serious, and there are now documented cases of such edge ringing being misinterpreted clinically as disease (e.g., syringomyelia).

The conspicuousness of truncation artifacts can be reduced by increasing the spatial resolution of the image or by decreasing the contrast of the interface. For example, truncation artifact adjacent to adipose tissue on a T1-weighted image can be reduced by suppressing the signal from fat.

Relaxation Artifacts

Edge artifacts result from any process that changes the signal amplitude during image acquisition. For example, fast spin echo techniques rely on obtaining echoes with several TEs. Signal decay increases with a longer TE owing to T2 relaxation. Thus, the signals from echoes with long TE are weaker than the signals from echoes with a

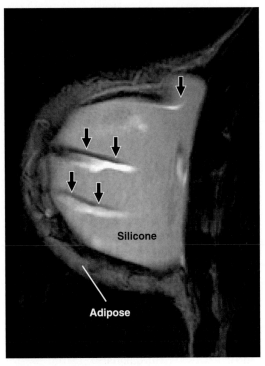

Figure 26-11
Chemical shift misregistration between water and silicone in a breast implant. Water in the folds of the silicone capsule (*arrows*) is misregistered inferiorly relative to the silicone.

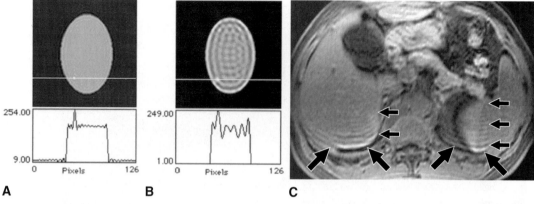

Figure 26-12

Truncation artifacts. (*A*) With a matrix of 64 × 64, the ovoid phantom is degraded by concentric lines. (*B*) They are more severe with a 32 × 32 matrix. The graphs below each of these images plot the signal intensity along the *white line* in the images. Note that there is a single bright pixel along that line, which is obscured almost completely by the edge ringing in (*B*). (*C*) Truncation artifact degrades an axial three-dimensional gradient echo 7/2.2/20° image of the abdomen with a (*left to right*) 256 × 128 (anteroposterior) matrix, and 5 mm slice thickness. The low slice-encoding and anteroposterior spatial resolution has resulted in a truncation artifact in the anteroposterior and through-plane axes that manifest as a ring-down artifact (*small arrows*) originating from the high-contrast borders posteriorly (*large arrows*).

short TE. These edge artifacts are minimized in modern implementations of the fast spin echo technique by carefully designing the order of phase-encoding gradient strengths and by minimizing the time between echoes so signal intensity changes between successive echoes are small. Even so, the change in MR signal strength during the readout process results in some blurring.

Ghost Artifacts

Patient motion is a major cause of ghost artifacts. These artifacts and ways to prevent them are discussed in Chapter 13. Such measures include spatial presaturation, gradient moment nulling, averaging, cardiac or respiratory monitoring, and decreased repetition time (TR) (Fig. 26-13). Ghost artifacts can also result from severe changes in signal intensity during image acquisition, such as with the fast spin echo technique with incorrect phase-encoding order or with long echo spacing.

Stripes

Zipper Artifacts

Zipper artifacts consist of a stripe, often at the center of the frequency-encoding or phase-encoding axes. Alternating black and white spots produce a zipper appearance. At zero phase, a zipper parallel to the frequency-encoding axis can be caused by unwanted residual transverse magnetization before a radio pulse. This unwanted transverse magnetization can come from nondecayed free induction decay (FID) or from stimulated echoes.

If the side lobes of 180° refocusing pulses overlap the FID signal before it decays, a zipper artifact along the frequency-encoding axis at zero phase can result. The FID is the signal emitted immediately after creation of transverse magnetization by the excitation pulse. Normally, this signal decays rapidly, and later an echo is formed by the rephasing lobe of the frequency-encoding gradient. If the TE of a spin echo pulse sequence is

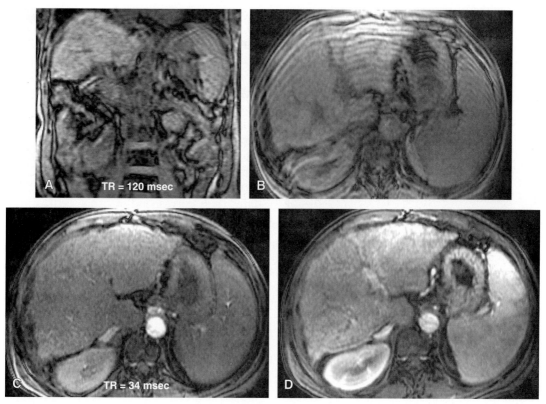

Figure 26-13
Reduction of respiration-induced ghost artifacts achieved by reducing the repetition time (TR) in a patient who could not suspend respiration during imaging. Within-view errors are minimal owing to the short echo time (TE) of 2.2 msec for all images. Coronal (*A*) and axial (*B*) images with TRs of 120 msec show pronounced artifact. When the TR was reduced to 34 msec, unenhanced (*C*) and gadolinium-enhanced (*D*) images showed less artifact. With a shorter TR, there is less variability between views, so the artifact is generally less pronounced.

short enough, the refocusing pulse may occur before the FID has fully decayed. A zipper results at the midpoint of the phase-encoding axis. This can be corrected by increasing the TE, which allows complete decay of the FID before the 180° refocusing pulse.

Zipper artifact at zero phase can also result if stimulated echoes are not adequately spoiled. Stimulated echoes are additional signal echoes that occur with virtually any combination of three RF pulses (with the notable exception of a series consisting of an exact 90° pulse followed by two 180° pulses). It is not possible, in general, to form perfectly shaped pulses with exact flip angles, and such stimulated

echoes are an unwelcome addition to all MR pulse sequences. The magnetization for stimulated echoes can be stored along the longitudinal axis, where it cannot be removed by gradient spoiling; therefore, it is necessary to suppress the stimulated echoes during the time that the magnetization is in the transverse plane. This is done by adding gradient pulses during periods of the pulse sequence where the desired signal is not present or where the gradient pulses can become self-canceling for the wanted MR signal. Depending on the details of the imaging sequence, stimulated echo artifacts may appear as lines in the image, complete images that are offset spatially from the planned study, or signal cancellations.

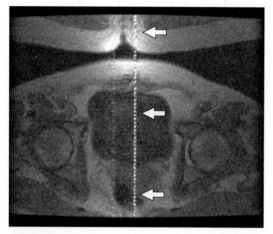

Figure 26-14
Radiofrequency feedthrough artifact *(arrows)* along the phase axis at the point of zero frequency-encoding. Note also the phase axis wraparound artifact, projecting the posterior tissues anteriorly.

A similar zipper artifact along the *phase-encoding* axis, at the point of zero frequency-encoding, can be caused by RF feedthrough, which occurs when the excitation RF pulse is detected directly by the receiver coil. It is located in the center of the frequency-encoding axis because it matches the frequency of the excitation pulse, which corresponds to the central frequency of the sampled bandwidth (Fig. 26-14). An RF feedthrough artifact can be eliminated by alternating the polarity of the excitation pulses if more than one excitation is averaged. The positive and negative feedthroughs are averaged, producing zero artifact. If there is no signal-averaging, RF feedthrough zipper artifacts can be eliminated by omitting the data that correspond to this central frequency and replacing them with data interpolated from adjacent points.

Zipper artifacts along the phase-encoding axis, away from the point of zero frequency-encoding, can result from extraneous radio noise, which is collected along with the sampled MR signals (Fig. 26-15). There are numerous sources of electronic noise, such as radio and television signals, fluorescent lighting, and electrical monitoring equipment such as pulse oximeters. The unwanted signals are mapped at the specific locations along the frequency-encoding axis that correspond to their frequencies.

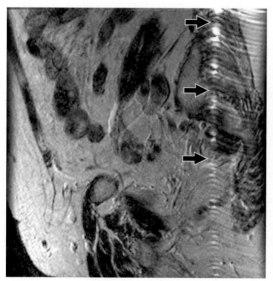 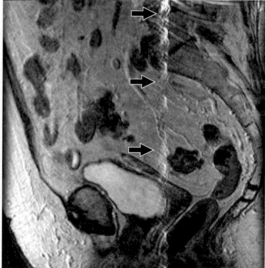

Figure 26-15
Zipper artifact *(arrows)* from extraneous radio noise on two image slices from the same acquisition.

Data Errors

Occasionally, mistakes in the filling of k-space lead to bad data points, which may result from static electricity in the magnetic bore caused by blankets or the patient's clothing. The data errors are visible in maps of k-space as points of increased amplitude, and they produce a corduroy-type pattern on the resulting image. Fast imaging techniques that rely on interpolation based on the symmetry of k-space, such as partial echo sampling or partial Fourier techniques, are particularly prone to these artifacts, as the data errors are duplicated in the other half of k-space. The artifacts are less common and less severe when all of k-space is sampled at least once. The artifact can be reduced or eliminated if the causative data point is eliminated or if the image acquisition is repeated. Usually, only one image, or a few, in a multislice acquisition are affected (Fig. 26-16).

Altered Signal Intensity

Susceptibility Artifacts

Magnetic susceptibility is discussed in Chapter 4. As with chemical shift artifact, image distortion results from incorrect frequency-encoding. Heterogeneous susceptibility causes magnetic field heterogeneity, which in turn alters the frequency of protons. Protons exposed to a higher magnetic field spin with increased frequency. These protons are thus mapped at a location that corresponds to a higher position along the frequency-encoding gradient, and they produce a signal void in the image where they should have been represented. A white band is commonly noted at the edge of this void that reflects overlapping signals of the mismapped protons.

When the field distortions become very large or when the image bandwidth is very low, susceptibility inhomogeneities can result in complete loss of signal. Such signal voids are a serious problem in echo planar images of the inferior frontal lobes of the brain, for example.

Susceptibility artifact can be minimized by using the spin echo technique with the shortest possible TE or the fast spin echo technique with the shortest possible echo spacing. Susceptibility artifact is generally more pronounced with gradient echo techniques, although it can be reduced by using the shortest possible TE (Fig. 26-17). The sampling bandwidth should be as high as possible, and image gradients should have maximum strength; gradient strength can usually be maximized by using a small FOV and thin image slices. The susceptibility artifact is greatest on gradient echo techniques, as the transverse magnetization is not refocused. On gradient echo images, the susceptibility artifact increases dramatically with even small increases in TE.

To restate: Susceptibility artifacts can be reduced by refocusing the transverse magnetization (using a spin echo technique), reducing the time for dephasing to occur (short TE and short echo spacing for fast spin echo), and reducing the distance over which it spreads (by increasing the sampling bandwidth per pixel). Total signal voids can sometimes be eliminated with echo planar imaging collections simply by reducing the voxel volume (smaller pixels or thinner slices).

Cross-Talk

Radio pulses targeted to one slice of a multislice acquisition may affect adjacent slices (see Chapter 7). This produces more saturation effects than would be expected from a given TR because some saturation occurs during the TR. The result is equivalent to a decrease in the "effective" TR. Thus, a given pulse sequence may have a lower SNR and may appear more T1-weighted and less T2-weighted.

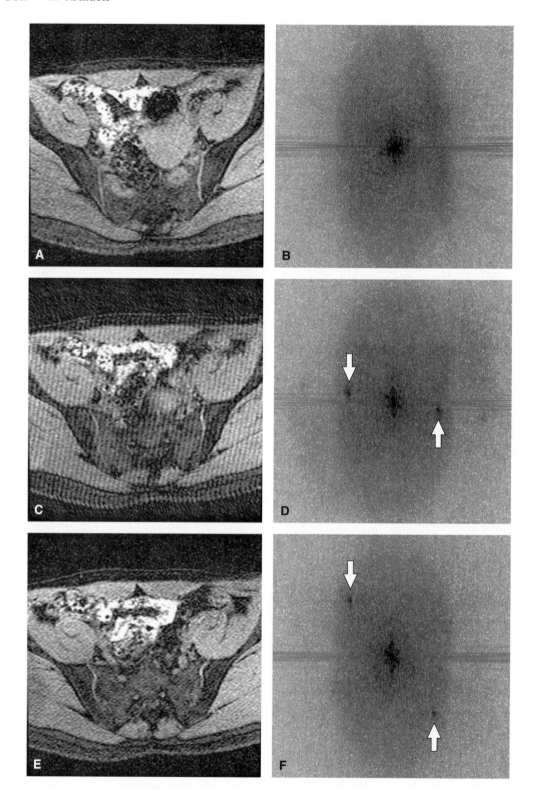

Heterogeneous Fat Suppression

Fat suppression via chemical shift saturation techniques involves exciting lipid protons by a radio pulse that matches their resonant frequency. If all lipid protons in the region of interest are precessing at the same frequency, they can be excited by a single radio pulse; however, if the main magnetic field is heterogeneous or if the radio pulse is not transmitted uniformly throughout this region, excitation of lipid protons is not uniform. Heterogeneous fat suppression is one of the most common artifacts because the chemical shift between water and lipid protons is only about 3.5 parts per million. Slight variation of the main magnetic field causes lipid protons to precess at a different frequency from that of the narrowly focused chemical shift saturation pulse.

The homogeneity of even a perfect main magnetic field is disturbed once a patient lies in it. The most common causes of patient-induced magnetic field heterogeneity are the air–tissue interfaces, whether in the patient or at the skin surface. Air and water have different magnetic susceptibilities, which results in different local magnetic fields. Bone and water also have different susceptibilities, but the disturbance of magnetic field homogeneity for these tissues is less pronounced.

With severe magnetic field heterogeneity, as in the presence of metal objects, most fat-suppression techniques should be avoided (Fig. 26-18). Generally, fat nulling by short inversion time recovery (STIR) is less affected than are fat-suppression techniques (Fig. 26-19). In some instances, magnetic field heterogeneity causes the frequency of water protons in some portions of the image to correspond to the frequency of a fat-suppression pulse, resulting in unintended water saturation (Fig. 26-20).

Magic-Angle Effects

The decay of transverse magnetization is facilitated by nonrandom structure, particularly by a structure that includes oriented parallel components. Examples are tendons and ligaments, which contain parallel fibrous bands. The T2 is thus particularly short for these tissues, leading to low signal intensity on most MR images. However, if these parallel bands are oriented at 55° relative to the main magnetic field, the T2 facilitation is decreased, leading to increased signal intensity. For this reason, focal areas of increased signal intensity in tendons and ligaments are common on images with a short or moderate TE (i.e., <25 msec). The location of the increased signal varies with the position and angle of the fibers relative to the main magnetic field (Fig. 26-21).

Eddy Currents

Eddy currents are small electrical currents caused by rapidly switching the gradients on and off. These currents produce persistent undesirable magnetic gradients that result in faster dephasing of transverse magnetization. Affected images show areas of reduced signal intensity that is most conspicuous at the periphery, where gradient profiles are often less adequate.

Figure 26-16
Artifact on fat-suppressed two-dimensional gradient echo (2D-GRE) 120/2.6/90° images from bad data points in k-space. The image in (*A*), corresponding to the k-space map in (*B*), shows no significant artifact. A prominent striped pattern overlies the adjacent image in (*C*). This is caused by bad data points (*arrows*) in the k-space map in (*D*). The striped artifact in (*E*) is more subtle because the bad data points (*F, arrows*) are farther from the center of k-space.

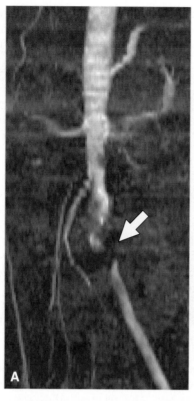

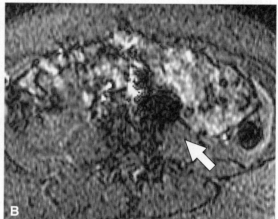

Time-of-Flight

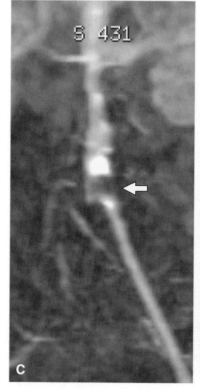

Gadolinium

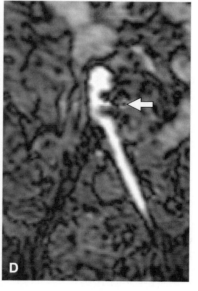

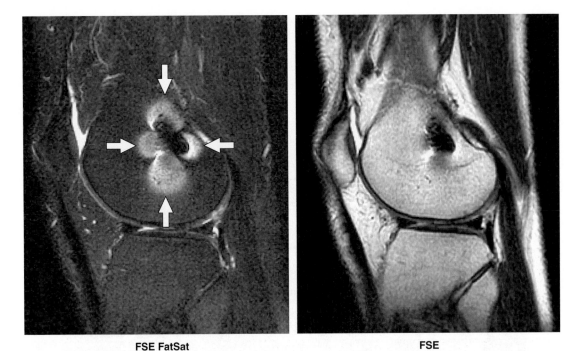

FSE FatSat   **FSE**

Figure 26-18
Left. Pronounced artifact *(arrows)* on fat-suppressed fast spin echo (FSE) 4500/100 image from uneven fat suppression due to a metal implant. *Right.* Distortion is less on a comparable fast spin echo image without fat suppression.

Figure 26-17
Signal void *(arrows)* due to metallic surgical clips: effect of echo time (TE) on severity. (*A*) There is a large void in the coronal MIP, constructed from axial 37/6.5/60° two-dimensional time of flight (2D-TOF) source images (*B*). (*C*) The signal void is much smaller in the coronal MIP image constructed from coronal gadolinium-enhanced three-dimensional gradient echo (3D-GRE) 11/2.2/60° source images (*D*) owing to the shorter TE.

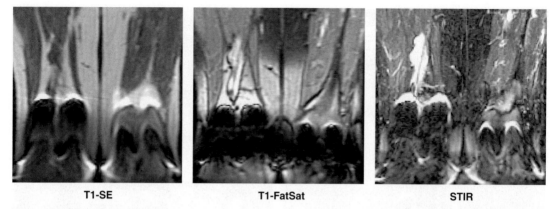

T1-SE   **T1-FatSat**   **STIR**

Figure 26-19

Susceptibility artifact from a metallic prosthesis is exacerbated by uneven fat suppression. The local distortion and signal voids are comparable for the T1-weighted spin echo (T1-SE) 417/8 image (*left*), T1-weighted fat-suppressed (T1-FatSat) gradient echo 250/1.6/90° image (*center*), and fast spin echo-short inversion time inversion recovery (STIR) 6250/60/150 image (*right*). Image degradation is exacerbated on the T1-weighted fat saturation image (*center*) due to heterogeneous fat suppression. Fat nulling is more homogeneous on the STIR image (*right*).

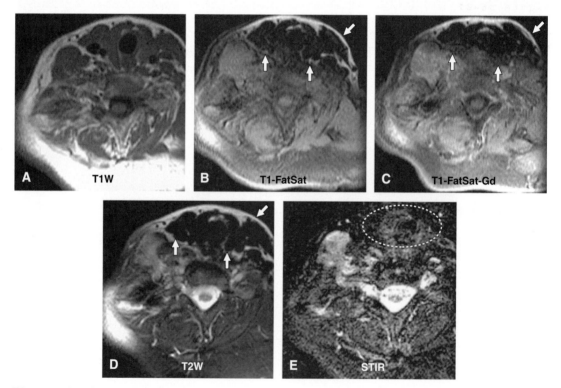

A **T1W**   **B** **T1-FatSat**   **C** **T1-FatSat-Gd**

D **T2W**   **E** **STIR**

Figure 26-20

Artifactual water suppression (*arrows*) on fat-suppressed images (from magnetic field heterogeneity). (*A*) The T1-weighted spin echo 467/8 image shows increased signal intensity posteriorly owing to a nonuniform profile of the local receiver coil. (*B*) The T1-weighted, fat-suppressed gradient echo 250/1.6 image shows water suppression of the anterior tissues of the neck. (*C*) Following administration of gadolinium chelate (Gd) it is not possible to determine whether any tissue in this region is enhanced, as water signal is suppressed. (*D*) Anterior water signal is also suppressed on the T2-weighted fat-suppressed fast spin echo (FSE) 6100/98 image. (*E*) These tissues are depicted (*dotted circle*) on the FSE-STIR 8571/75/150 image.

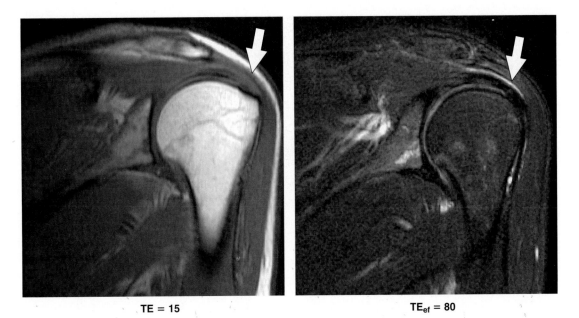

TE = 15 TE_{ef} = 80

Figure 26-21
Left. Magic angle effect produces an area of increased signal intensity (*arrow*) of the supraspinatus tendon on a spin echo 600/15 image. *Right.* On the FSE 3000/80 image the tendon has uniformly low signal intensity owing to the longer effective echo time (TE_{ef}).

Table 26-1 ■ CAUSE, APPEARANCE, AND CORRECTION OF VARIOUS ARTIFACTS

Artifact	Cause	Appearance	Correction
Wraparound	Field of view too small for body part	Body part extends beyond one edge of image and is projected at the opposite side	Sample data sufficient for a larger field of view Use local coil to reduce sensitivity of tissue outside image
Partial volume	More than one tissue is included within a voxel, usually because of thick slices	Edges of a structure contain tissues from two adjacent slices	Increase spatial resolution, particularly in the slice direction
Chemical shift misregistration	Water and fat are misregistered relative to each other	Bright band on one slice and a dark band on the other side of a water structure surrounded by fat along the frequency-encoding axis	Increase sampling bandwidth per pixel
Chemical shift edge cancellation	Water and lipid signals in a voxel at fat–water interfaces interfere destructively	Black line at fat–water interfaces	Use spin echo or in-phase gradient echo technique Suppress lipid signal intensity
Truncation	Abrupt, high contrast, boundaries cannot be accurately represented by Fourier transform	Ring-down artifact at high-contrast interfaces	Increase spatial resolution
Motion-induced ghost	Motion causes phase changes during signal sampling or intensity changes between signals. Both result in phase-encoding errors	Repetitive patterned noise that resembles the source structure, repeated at regular intervals along the phase-encoding axis	Average multiple signals Complete image acquisition rapidly Trigger acquisitions so the anatomy is constant from view to view Balance gradients to eliminate gradient moment Reduce signal of moving tissue

Zipper	Nondecayed transverse magnetization, RF feedthrough, or extraneous noise	Band of alternating white and black dots	Improve spoiling of transverse magnetization Alternate polarity of excitation pulses Eliminate source of noise
Corduroy appearance	Bad data points	Corduroy appearance across some images	Increase sampling of k-space
Susceptibility	Magnetic field altered by heterogeneous magnetic properties in body part	Signal loss and distortion	Eliminate source of heterogeneous susceptibility Maximize sampling bandwidth Minimize TE Refocus echoes
Cross-excitation	RF pulse targeted to one slice partially excites an adjacent slice	Reduced signal intensity	Use gaps between slices in 2D multislice acquisitions Allow sufficient time for recovery between radial overlapping slice acquisitions
Suboptimal fat saturation	Magnetic field heterogeneity causes the lipid resonance to vary within the field of view, so the fat-suppression RF pulse does not correspond to all lipid	Increased signal intensity of lipid, possibly with suppression of water signal	Improve magnetic field shimming Improve tuning of the fat-suppression pulse
Magic angle	T2 of oriented fibers depends on angle relative to magnetic field	Variable signal intensity of tendons and other structures	Use sufficiently long TE for structure to have low signal intensity regardless of angle
Eddy current	Electrical currents caused by rapidly switching gradients	Reduced peripheral signal intensity	Improve precision of gradient pulses Use eddy current compensation

RF, radiofrequency.

Ghost artifacts in the phase axis, indistinguishable from motion artifact, can also occur.

The artifacts discussed in this chapter are listed in Table 26-1 along with their causes, appearances, and methods for correction.

▼
Essential Points to Remember

1. Wraparound artifact, or aliasing, involves representation of a body part on the opposite side of an image when it extends beyond the acquired FOV.

2. Wraparound artifact can be prevented by acquiring data for a larger FOV. If the pixel size and the total number of echoes sampled do not change, the SNR and spatial resolution are not affected.

3. With 3D-FT techniques, image slices are phase-encoded, so wraparound can occur in the slice-encoding axis.

4. Partial volume artifact results when two structures are included in the same voxel.

5. Chemical shift misregistration artifact is most conspicuous on images in which fat and water magnetizations are in phase and both have moderate or high signal intensity.

6. Chemical shift misregistration artifact can be reduced by increasing the sampling bandwidth but at the cost of a loss in the SNR.

7. Chemical shift cancellation artifact occurs when fat and water magnetizations have opposed phases.

8. Truncation artifacts, which appear as alternating series of bright and dark bands, occur because the FT reconstruction cannot accurately depict abrupt high-contrast borders.

9. The conspicuousness of truncation artifact can be reduced by increasing the spatial resolution or decreasing the contrast of the border, as by fat suppression.

10. Any change in the echo amplitude during acquisition, for whatever reason (e.g., variable TEs in an echo train), can cause ghost artifacts.

11. Zipper artifacts can be caused by a variety of pulse sequence deficiencies or by extraneous radio signals that are detected by the MRI receiving coil.

12. A corduroy-like banding pattern can result from a single bad data point in k-space, which may be due to from static electricity as from a patient's clothing or blankets.

13. Heterogeneous susceptibility can be caused by air or metal, producing areas of signal loss and image distortion. Spin echo images with a short TE and fast spin echo images with short echo spacing are least affected.

14. A nonhomogeneous magnetic field results in nonhomogeneous fat suppression because the resulting various lipid frequencies cannot be matched by the single frequency of the fat-suppression pulse.

15. The T2 of tissues with oriented fibers is highest when these fibers are aligned at 55° (the magic angle) relative to the main magnetic field. Homogeneous low signal intensity of these tissues can be achieved by using a sufficiently long TE.

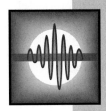

Chapter 27

Clinical MRI Techniques

In this final chapter, we discuss the magnetic resonance imaging (MRI) techniques used for common clinical neurological, musculoskeletal, and body applications. It is expected that the comments in this chapter will differ from actual practice at many centers, and it is not our purpose to insist that the suggestions included here are necessarily superior to those of other individuals. Rather, our purpose is to provide examples of how these techniques might be implemented in practice; we invite readers to obtain other opinions and to form their own.

At the risk of oversimplification, we include a table of typical pulse sequences for neurological, musculoskeletal, and body applications. It is not expected that all pulse sequences listed here will be part of a routine examination, although individual sequences may be combined to suit the clinical information needed from the examination. The tables included are not meant to be completely inclusive or absolute, but readers may find them useful.

Neurological MRI Techniques

Various considerations predominate when imaging the head and spine. For both applications, clear delineation of cerebrospinal fluid (CSF) is needed, as is the depiction of an altered T2 due to brain or spinal parenchymal abnormalities. For imaging the brain and head, the volume of interest is roughly cubic, so a standard quadrature volume coil fitted to the head is often adequate, although phased-array technology can improve the signal-to-noise ratio (SNR). For imaging the neck, an inferior extension or component is needed.

For brain imaging, the only adipose tissue is in the scalp or bones or below the

371

skull base, so chemical shift techniques are not needed for routine imaging. The relative absence of fat in the brain also allows use of a low sampling bandwidth to increase the SNR. Fat suppression may be desirable, however, for imaging the skull base and orbits so any adipose tissue present is clearly distinguished from fluid or enhancing tissue.

For the spine, the region of interest is elongated, so a posterior-predominant phased-array architecture is clearly preferable. There is abundant adipose tissue in vertebral bodies and soft tissues, so fat suppression is commonly employed.

Standard T1-weighted spin echo and T2-weighted fast spin echo (FSE) images are generally used in multiple planes, supplemented by postcontrast T1-weighted images. Recently, additional techniques, such as fluid-attenuated inversion recovery, diffusion and perfusion techniques, magnetic resonance angiography (MRA), and proton spectroscopy, have become routine at many centers.

T1-Weighted Images

Most T1-weighted imaging of the brain, neck and spine utilizes the conventional spin echo technique, with the field of view (FOV) fitted to the body part. A matrix size of 256×256 pixels is standard, although a larger matrix is preferable for spinal imaging if large FOVs are used to image long regions. Although three-dimensional (3D) gradient echo techniques may be used to reduce the acquisition time, decrease the slice thickness, or both, image degradation at the skull base due to air–tissue interfaces is a potential problem; such degradation can be reduced using the shortest possible TE.

Another alternative technique for obtaining T1-weighted contrast with minimal artifact at the skull base is FSE imaging with a short TR, short effective TE (TE_{ef}), and short echo train. These images are slightly blurred relative to standard spin echo images, but they can be obtained more rapidly, which allows dynamic contrast-enhanced imaging, such as for the pituitary gland. For most applications, however, the gradient echo technique is more efficient than the FSE method.

T2-Weighted Images

The conventional dual spin echo (SE) technique has been a standard component of protocols for imaging the brain and spine, but at most centers it has been replaced by the far more efficient FSE techniques. FSE imaging yields images with a high SNR, improved spatial resolution, and superior depiction of CSF spaces with shorter acquisitions. The rapid repetition of multiple refocusing radiofrequency (RF) pulses reduces motion artifacts due to CSF motion. The dual FSE technique can be used to generate intermediate-weighted images with a long TR and a short TE, such as for the spine, but these images are often omitted. The improved efficiency of FSE allows the use of higher spatial resolution (e.g., 512×512 matrix) for imaging the brainstem.

The abandonment of standard SE T2-weighted images is not universal, however. Advantages of standard SE include increased sensitivity to the susceptibility effects of hemorrhage and an improved dynamic range resulting from lower signal intensity from CSF compared with most T2-weighted FSE images. The images often have less blurring, and small subtle white matter lesions may be depicted with greater clarity. One option is to obtain two planes of T2-weighted imaging: one with FSE and one with SE.

If no standard SE T2-weighted images are obtained, alternative sequences should be obtained that are more sensitive to magnetic field heterogeneity from iron in hemorrhage. Typically, a supplementary T2*-weighted gradient echo pulse sequence is obtained.

For routine brain imaging, there is no need to suppress the signal from adipose tissue. Fat saturation techniques are desirable, however, for imaging the head and neck as well as the spine.

For high-resolution imaging in the internal auditory canal, the 3D steady-state free precession technique can yield thin slices with a high SNR and high contrast between fluid and tissue.

T2*-Weighted Gradient Echo Images

T2*-weighted gradient echo images can be obtained using either two-dimensional (2D) multislice or 3D acquisition. For either, the TE should be about 25 to 30 msec. At this TE, there is substantial signal loss in regions of magnetic field heterogeneity, leading to sensitive depiction of hemosiderin or deoxyhemoglobin from a prior hemorrhage. The long TE allows the use of a low sampling bandwidth to increase the SNR; the longer sampling time resulting from use of a low bandwidth does not allow a short TE. The use of a low bandwidth and the associated weak imaging magnetic gradients further increases the sensitivity to magnetic field heterogeneity (see Chapter 9).

The use of a long TE without a refocusing RF pulse leads to substantial unwanted signal loss from other causes of magnetic field heterogeneity, such as air–tissue and bone–tissue interfaces at the skull base. The use of long TE also leads to an overall increase in the acquisition time and a decreased SNR. Slightly lower TEs reduce some of these artifacts and increase the SNR/acquisition time ratio but at the expense of lower sensitivity to blood. The most popular balance of these considerations has been to use a TE of about 25 msec.

If diffusion-weighted images are obtained, the $b = 0$ image can be used as an alternative susceptibility-sensitive technique.

Fluid Attenuated Inversion Recovery (FLAIR)

The use of standard T2-weighted spin echo or FSE images for evaluating periventricular white matter or superficial cortical gray matter has been challenging owing to the extremely high signal intensity of CSF. A clever solution to this problem is to use a long TR and TE to generate T2-weighted contrast but to null fluid using an inversion pulse with an appropriately long inversion time (TI); at 1.5 T this is about 2200 msec. With this TI, simple fluid is nulled; all other tissues, with shorter T1s, have relaxed past their null points and therefore have positive longitudinal magnetization at the time of the excitation pulse. Because the TI is so long, imaging efficiency is maintained by interleaving inversion and excitation of other image sections during each TI.

Contrast-Enhanced Images

The most common use of contrast agents for imaging the brain is to detect blood-brain or blood-cord barrier disruption due to ischemia, neoplasm, or other disease. For this purpose rapid scanning is not necessary. The most commonly used technique for depicting contrast enhancement remains the spin echo technique, although the 3D gradient echo technique with minimum TE is also useful if a series of thin sections or dynamic scanning is desired. For dynamic scanning of the pituitary, the FSE technique with a short echo train (e.g., three) and a short TE_{ef} (< 20 msec) can yield rapid imaging with little artifact from the air–tissue interfaces at the skull base.

For imaging the cranial nerves, orbits, soft tissues of the neck, and the spine, fat suppression improves the clarity of enhancing tissue by increasing its contrast relative to adipose tissue.

At lower field strengths, such as those below 0.5 T, the shorter T1 of brain parenchyma reduces the effect of gadolinium contrast agents. To achieve contrast comparable to that at 1.5 T or higher, the contrast agent dose may be doubled. Alternatively, magnetization transfer saturation may be used; this reduces the signal intensity of brain parenchyma with an intact blood-brain barrier more than that of damaged brain or enhancing lesions. These two options—doubling the dose or using magnetization transfer saturation (or both)—can also be used at 1.5 T to increase the sensitivity for detecting small metastatic lesions for specific clinical indications, such as when minimally invasive ablation of a lesion is contemplated.

Magnetic Resonance Angiography

Numerous alternative techniques, discussed in Chapters 23 and 24, are used for magnetic resonance angiography (MRA) of the extracranial and intracranial circulations. They include two-dimensional time-of-flight (2D-TOF) techniques for maximum sensitivity to slow flow and for covering large areas (e.g., neck), 3D-TOF techniques for improved SNR but decreased sensitivity to slow flow, multiple overlapping thick slab acquisitions (MOTSA) for a balance of sensitivity and SNR and for extending coverage, and the gadolinium-enhanced 3D technique for high SNR and fast acquisition. Phase-contrast techniques can be used to determine direction of flow or to measure velocity or volume of flow, which is useful for detecting hyperdynamic CSF flow in patients with shunt-responsive normal-pressure hydrocephalus.

Diffusion

Diffusion-weighted techniques, described in Chapter 25, are used most commonly for evaluating patients with acute ischemia. Edema caused by brain infarction and failure of sodium-potassium exchange increases tissue pressure, thereby reducing diffusion of water. The diffusion-induced loss of signal on diffusion-weighted images is reduced or absent in infarcted brain. These findings are visible prior to abnormalities seen on T2-weighted images. Diffusion-weighted techniques also help distinguish between solid tissue and fluid and between an abscess and a tumor.

Diffusion-weighted images of the brain are typically obtained using the single-shot echo planar technique, with a b value of about 1000. These images are compared to similar images with a b value of 0. To maintain the SNR and speed, spatial resolution is generally low, such as a 96×128 matrix.

Perfusion

Perfusion techniques, described in Chapter 25, are used to measure cerebral blood volume and flow and the mean transit time. These parameters can be helpful for evaluating some patients, especially those with acute ischemia or brain tumors. In patients with acute ischemia, reduced perfusion in areas that are normal on diffusion-weighted images is thought by some to indicate reversible ischemia, with the patient at risk for extended infarction. (This concept is still under investigation.)

Most often dynamic T2*-weighted gradient echo or echo planar images are obtained after bolus injection of a gadolinium chelate contrast agent. Perfusion is depicted as reduced signal intensity secondary to a heterogeneous magnetic field, as the magnetic field is slightly higher in blood vessels than in brain parenchyma.

Blood Oxygen Level-Dependent Techniques

At the present time, functional MRI (fMRI) using a blood oxygen level-dependent (BOLD) technique is rarely included in a routine imaging protocol. However, these images may be useful for helping to map important areas of cerebral function prior to surgery or tumor ablation. BOLD fMRI is currently one of the most active areas of MRI research, so clinical applications for this technique may expand in the near future.

Table 27-1 ■ PULSE SEQUENCES USED FOR NEUROLOGICAL IMAGING

Pulse Sequence	Purpose	Typical Technique
T1-weighted	General anatomy	SE
T2-weighted	CSF spaces, pathology	Fast SE
T2*-weighted	Calcification, blood	GRE with TE 25–30 msec
FLAIR	Periventricular white matter	Inversion recovery prepared FSE
Contrast-enhanced	Disrupted blood-brain barrier	SE or 3D GRE
MRA	Vascular anatomy	TOF or Gad-enhanced
Diffusion	Ischemia; mass characterization	Echo planar
Perfusion	Ischemia, tumor evaluation	Echo planar
BOLD	Cerebral function	Echo planar
Spectroscopy	Characterize metabolites	PRESS

SE, spin echo; GRE, gradient echo; FLAIR, fluid attenuated inversion recovery; MRA, magnetic resonance angiography; BOLD, blood oxygen level-dependent; CSF, cerebrospinal fluid; PRESS, point resolved spectroscopy; Gad, gadolinium; TOF, time of flight.

Spectroscopy

Spectroscopy, described briefly in Chapter 5, involves analyzing the resonant frequencies of a tissue, thereby obtaining some potentially useful chemical information about that tissue. Clinical use of spectroscopy has been implemented most commonly for brain evaluation. Proton spectroscopy is used most often, utilizing the same transmit and receive hardware as that used for standard MRI. In the brain, proton signals from adipose tissue are less problematic; the SNR is high because of the use of appropriate local coils, and the body part remains stationary. A 2D or 3D point resolved spectroscopic (PRESS) technique is usually used.

There are a few proton spectroscopic peaks that provide relevant insight into brain chemistry and may affect the clinical evaluation. *N*-Acetyl aspartate (NAA) is a marker of normal neurons, creatine is a marker of energy utilization, choline is a marker of membrane turnover, and *myo*-inositol is a sugar that is involved in osmotic homeostasis.

A potential clinical application of proton spectroscopy involves the observation of decreased NAA (indicating loss of neurons) and perhaps increased choline and creatine in areas of neurodegeneration. Brain tumors generally contain increased choline and decreased NAA, allowing viable tumor to be distinguished from radiation changes. Central necrosis in tumors shows the by-products of membrane breakdown, consisting of altered lipid peaks as well as lactate.

There is some controversy as to whether proton spectroscopy should be performed before or after gadolinium chelate administration. If spectroscopy follows contrast agent administration, the shorter T1 of enhanced tissues should be considered; among other effects, it reduces the relative height of the choline peak by about 15%. One reason to consider injecting a contrast agent prior to spectroscopy is so necrotic tissue can be avoided when performing image-guided localized spectroscopy.

Pulse sequences commonly used for musculoskeletal imaging are summarized in Table 27-1.

Musculoskeletal MRI Techniques

For musculoskeletal imaging, high spatial resolution and the SNR are of paramount importance. Tissues that must be distinguished from each other include fluid, adipose tissue, hyaline cartilage, collagenous tissues, muscle, inflammation, tumor, and cortical bone. Commonly used pulse sequences include T1-weighted spin echo or gradient echo, intermediate-weighted, T2-weighted fast spin echo, short TI inversion recovery (STIR), and 3D gradient echo techniques. Some applications benefit from addition of fat-suppressed imaging after administration of gadolinium chelates.

T1-Weighted Images

Many musculoskeletal structures are delineated by surrounding adipose tissue. Therefore, at least one pulse sequence should depict adipose tissue clearly and unambiguously, with high spatial resolution and high SNR. Spin echo and in-phase gradient echo techniques can be used for this purpose.

Most applications do not depend on heavy T1-weighting, rather, just enough to show adipose tissue clearly. Therefore, precise choice of the TR and flip angle are not as important as they are for other applications, such as body imaging, where depiction of subtle T1 contrast depends heavily on these parameters. For musculoskeletal imaging, as the TR increases, the SNR of tissues such as muscle, hyaline cartilage, and ligamentous or meniscal tears increases. For example, at 1.5 T choosing a TR of more than 500 msec reduces T1 contrast, but TRs as high as 1000 msec or longer may provide a useful SNR and contrast for depicting normal structures and diagnosing abnormalities.

Intermediate-Weighted Images

At least one T1-weighted pulse sequence is recommended so adipose tissue is clearly distinguished from fluid, inflammation, or tumor. However, for many purposes, intermediate-weighted sequences provide superior depiction of normal anatomy or tears of ligaments, tendons, and fibrocartilage (e.g., menisci and labra). As mentioned above, increasing the TR improves the SNR of tissues with a long T1, such as muscle,

hyaline cartilage, fluid, inflammation, and tears. If the TR is about 2000 msec or more, most of these tissues have maximum signal (TRs of nearly 10,000 are often needed to maximize the SNR of simple fluid). To depict these tissues most clearly as having a higher SNR than intact ligaments, tendons, and fibrocartilage, the latter tissues must have nearly absent signal. This can be accomplished using a moderate TE (e.g., 25 to 30 msec). If the TE is shorter, normal ligaments, tendons, and fibrocartilage begin to show internal signal intensity that may resemble degeneration or injury. In fact, because of magic angle dependence (see Chapter 26), this internal signal varies depending on the angle of the structure relative to the main magnetic field. If the TE is long enough, these effects are less problematic.

Therefore, an optimum sequence for depicting common musculoskeletal abnormalities may have a long TR and a moderate TE. Although the conventional spin echo technique may be used with such parameters, a nonminimized TE reduces acquisition efficiency. Therefore, the fast spin echo technique is recommended, preferably with a short echo train. These intermediate-weighted images may be considered mildly T2-weighted because, in fact, the distinction between intact and injured structures is primarily based on T2 differences between intact collagenous tissues and inflammation or injury.

T2-Weighted Images

At least one T2-weighted set of images is recommended to define synovial and other fluid unambiguously. These images also help depict inflammatory tissues and tumors. They may depict ligamentous, tendinous, and meniscal injuries but usually not as sensitively as do pulse sequences with a moderate or short TE.

Fast spin echo techniques should be used for T2-weighting, as they are far more efficient than the conventional spin echo technique and they more clearly distinguish fluid from inflammatory and other high-intensity-signal tissues without requiring the use of an extremely long TE_{ef}. The TE_{ef} should generally be about 80 to 100 msec, although a higher TE may be used to suppress tissues other than fluid.

Fat suppression can be used to distinguish better fluid and other high signal tissues from adipose tissue. Depiction of high-signal-intensity tissues and fluid can generally be accomplished adequately with a shorter TE_{ef} if the lipid signal is suppressed. An alternative method for reducing the signal intensity of adipose tissue is to use short TI inversion recovery (STIR) sequences.

Short TI Inversion Recovery Imaging

STIR images commonly are used to create images of musculoskeletal body parts that show adipose tissue as low signal intensity and tumors and inflammation as high signal intensity. A "conventional" STIR sequence has a long TR, a short TE, and a TI chosen to null the triglyceride signal. Contrast on these images is primarily based on the inverse of T1-weighted images, so tissues with a long T1 are depicted as bright.

The main disadvantage with STIR is that it has a lower SNR than do comparable pulse sequences without an inversion pulse. Additionally, the TI is often "dead time," where no data acquisition occurs. The loss of acquisition efficiency of STIR can be reduced if a fast spin echo technique is used. For example, with an echo train of 8, there will only be 1/8 as many TIs and therefore only 1/8 as much dead time. Another advantage of the fast spin echo technique for STIR imaging is that a longer TE_{ef} can be used without increasing the acquisition time.

Although conventional STIR images may resemble fat-suppressed T2-weighted images, there is little T2-weighting because the TE is short. However, increasing the

TE on STIR sequences creates T2 contrast in addition to inverse T1 contrast. These images depict fluid more clearly because they have a longer T2 than other tissues. Additionally, marrow injury, inflammation, and tumor can be more clearly distinguished from hematopoietic marrow because the latter has a shorter T2. Muscle pathology such as edema and injury is also delineated because normal muscle has a short T2 and therefore has lower signal intensity on T2-weighted images, STIR or otherwise. However, the low signal of muscle on T2-weighted STIR images reduces the depiction of normal anatomy, as most normal tissues are dark.

In many respects, fat-suppressed fast spin echo and STIR images have similar uses. STIR images generally have more homogeneous fat signal reduction and depict synergistic T2 and inverse T1 contrast, whereas fat-suppressed fast spin echo images are faster, have a higher SNR, and can be more heavily T2-weighted. A common practice is to obtain fat-suppressed fast spin echo images in one plane and STIR images in another. STIR images are particularly appropriate for large FOV images, as fat saturation is often suboptimal at the edges of large FOVs. Fat-suppressed fast spin echo images have higher SNRs and are therefore better suited to small FOVs.

Gradient Echo Images

Although gradient echo images are not included in every routine protocol, they have numerous uses. On many systems, in-phase T1-weighted gradient echo images, whether two-dimensional Fourier transform (2D-FT) or 3D-FT, may be substituted for T1-weighted spin echo images if the edge detail is sufficient. Other applications include more sensitive depiction of calcium, thin section imaging of hyaline cartilage and other joint structures, and postgadolinium imaging.

As a replacement for spin echo T1-weighted images, gradient echo images should use the shortest possible TE at which fat and water magnetizations are in phase. Otherwise, edge artifacts obscure the fine detail necessary to optimize musculoskeletal images. For some applications, opposed-phase gradient echo images add complementary value; by comparing them with in-phase images, it is possible to distinguish hematopoietic marrow from tumor or hypercellular marrow. Tumor and hypercellular marrow contain virtually no lipid, so their signal intensities on in-phase and opposed-phase images are similar; normal cellular marrow contains both lipid and water and therefore is less intense on opposed-phase images.

A disadvantage of MRI for skeletal imaging is that it cannot depict calcium as sensitively as can computed tomography (CT), although acquisition of appropriate pulse sequences can improve this sensitivity. $T2^*$-weighted gradient echo images with a TE of 15 msec or greater depict signal voids at calcium–tissue interfaces due to differences in susceptibility between the two. These signal voids are sometimes referred to as "blooming." Whereas in-phase T1-weighted, fat-suppressed T2-weighted, and STIR images are useful for depicting marrow, $T2^*$-weighted images may be more useful for depicting bone.

The use of thin-section 3D imaging for musculoskeletal MRI has been advocated by some for nearly two decades, but it has not been universally adopted owing to disagreement regarding the usefulness of their soft tissue contrast. For menisci and labra, thin-section gradient echo images can depict tears and allow multiplanar reformatting. However, there is a tendency to depict increased signal intensity in normal structures, especially if the TE is too short. Unfortunately, the use of a TE long enough to reduce the unwanted signal in normal structures leads to increased acquisition time, increased susceptibility artifact, and reduced SNR. Some investigators have found specific implementations of fat-suppressed 3D-FT gradient echo techniques ideal for evaluating hyaline cartilage, but

high-resolution fast spin echo may also be useful.

Contrast-Enhanced Images

Although most musculoskeletal MRI examinations are performed without the use of contrast agents, gadolinium chelates are commonly administered. Benefits include improved depiction of inflammation, muscle injury, and some tumors, although these entities can usually be seen on STIR or fat-suppressed T2-weighted images. For most applications, a dynamic multiphasic injection is not needed, although it can be useful for evaluating the vascularity of tumors and for depicting vessels. When contrast agents are administered, fat-suppressed T1-weighted images are usually obtained to depict enhancement using either 2D-FT multislice or 3D-FT techniques.

Intravenously injected gadolinium chelate diffuses into synovial fluid, leading to an "indirect arthrographic" effect, which can be useful for evaluating joints. However, a direct injection of dilute (approximately 20:1) gadolinium chelate also distends the joint and allows determination of whether compartments communicate. Direct injection is particularly useful for evaluating labral tears in the hip or shoulder and ligament tears in the wrist.

Pulse sequences commonly used for musculoskeletal imaging are summarized in Table 27-2.

Body MRI Techniques

The three most important technical considerations for body MRI are contrast, motion artifact, and coverage. Pulse sequences generally include at least one of the following: T1-weighted, T2-weighted, chemical shift, and contrast-enhanced techniques. The specific techniques used to obtain these images have evolved considerably, especially on

Table 27-2 ■ PULSE SEQUENCES USED FOR MUSCULOSKELETAL IMAGING

Pulse Sequence	Purpose	Typical Technique
T1-weighted	General anatomy, marrow	SE
Intermediate-weighted	Anatomy, tendons, ligaments, fibrocartilage	SE or fast SE, with or without FS
T2-weighted	Synovial spaces, marrow, injury, cartilage	Fat-sat fast SE or STIR
3D GRE	Cartilage, menisci	Nonspoiled GRE, SSFP, or driven equilibrium
Contrast-enhanced	Tumor, vessels, inflammation, tissue viability	2D or 3D GRE

SE, spin echo; STIR, short TI (tau) inversion recovery; FS, fat suppression; GRE, gradient echo; SSFP, steady-state free precession.

modern MRI instruments at 1.5 T or higher. In particular, the approach to motion has evolved from averaging to motion compensation to suspended respiration or subsecond imaging (or both of the latter).

Abdominal Imaging and Breath Holding

Examinations of cooperative patients using modern MRI equipment consist primarily of acquisitions during breath holding. For a given pulse sequence, imaging the entire region of interest during a single breath hold simplifies the examination and avoids misregistration secondary to an inconsistent position of the body organs. In some circumstances, divided breath holds are used, but image misregistration between breath holds is a potential problem. This can be partially avoided by obtaining overlapping stacks of images, rather than interleaved acquisitions. For all multiple breath-holding techniques, interleaved slices should be avoided. A stack of images with a gap of 1 mm or less should be acquired, followed by another stack of images, with a 1-cm overlap.

In particular, the arterial phase of dynamic extracellular-space contrast agent imaging can only be acquired during a brief interval of about 20 seconds. Whenever possible, patients should be triaged to MRI units that have this capability. The abdomen ranks along with the heart and vascular system as body parts that benefit most from examination using the most up-to-date MRI hardware and software.

At the time of this writing, most modern body MRI sequences require the patient to be able to suspend respiration for approximately 25 seconds, although implementation of parallel imaging techniques can reduce this interval (see Chapter 17). If possible, administration of oxygen inhalation, such as by nasal cannula, improves the ability of patients to suspend respiration for longer periods.

Practices differ as to the use of end-inspiration or end-expiration for breath-holding imaging. Although patients can generally suspend respiration longer at full inspiration, it has been found that breath holding is more consistent and there is less motion during breath holding if respiration is suspended at relaxed end-expiration. Rather than blow all the air out, patients should simply exhale and hold.

If suspended respiration is not possible, longer pulse sequences may be acquired using the motion-compensation techniques described in Chapter 13, but dynamic multiphasic contrast-enhanced imaging is not possible.

On systems equipped with respiratory bellows or other methods of monitoring respiratory movements, these devices should be used on all patients, even if they are not used to trigger acquisitions or otherwise guide respiratory compensation techniques.

The MR technologist can view the resulting respiratory waveform, revealing whether a patient in fact is successfully suspending respiration. Alternatively, subsecond imaging can be initiated at the end of an exhalation, during the period of least motion in the respiratory cycle.

The first motion-sensitive breath-holding technique should be viewed carefully for artifact. Depending on the order of the pulse sequences, this may be a spoiled gradient echo (GRE) pulse sequence with a TR greater than 100 msec, a 3D acquisition, or a multishot T2-weighted technique. However, any image acquisitions that are completed in 2 seconds or less (e.g., GRE sequences with TR < 10 msec and single-shot sequences) are relatively insensitive to motion and therefore may have little artifact even if breath holding was not successful.

If significant motion artifact is visible on the initial GRE motion-sensitive sequence, the patient should be instructed to improve his or her efforts; alternatively, the acquisition time can be reduced by decreasing the coverage or spatial resolution, or the slice thickness can be increased. If the patient is unable to cooperate, less-motion-sensitive sequences should be substituted.

Pelvic Imaging

The technical issues involved in high-quality imaging of the pelvis differ from those involved for imaging the abdomen. Motion artifact can degrade images but not as severely as in the abdomen. Therefore, longer, breathing-averaged techniques remain an option. Contrast enhancement, although useful, is not required for many applications; and in many of these cases static delayed-phase images are more useful than are dynamic techniques. Although dynamic multiphasic contrast-enhanced images should generally be included whenever extracellular space agents are administered, precise timing of the arterial phase is less critical than it is for abdominal or thoracic imaging. Therefore, a timing bolus or other method for determining the precise timing for bolus administration and scanning is less critical than for abdominal imaging or MRA.

For imaging the pelvis, spatial resolution is highly important, as fine morphological detail is often important for the differential diagnosis or tumor staging. Therefore, the image FOV should be as small as possible and the matrix as large as possible.

To maintain the SNR with small FOVs, appropriate local coils should be used. In most instances, this is a pelvic or torso phased-array coil or an appropriate endo-coil. Use of an appropriate coil for imaging the pelvis is more important than having an advanced gradient subsystem, whereas the latter is most important for MRA; both are critical for abdominal imaging.

T2-Weighted Techniques

Although single-shot techniques may have limited contrast, SNR and spatial resolution, their consistent image quality and relative insensitivity to motion renders them particularly important for body imaging, particularly in the abdomen. An initial set of coronal single-shot FSE images can serve as localizer images for the subsequent axial sequences and provide a useful initial survey.

Single-shot FSE with a TE_{ef} of about 180 to 200 msec is useful for distinguishing solid tissue (e.g., hepatic metastases) from nonsolid lesions (e.g., cysts or hemangiomas) and for delineating fluid collections and ducts. An additional set of images with a shorter TE_{ef}, about 60 to 100 msec, is useful for depicting more subtle T2 contrast, such as between liver and solid tumor or between zones of the uterus. In most instances, multishot FSE depicts this type of contrast better than does single-shot FSE.

Single-shot FSE is also used for MR cholangiopancreatography (MRCP). One effective MRCP technique is the acquisition of thick-slab slices (3 to 4 cm thick) oriented radially about the biliary system.

These images should have effective TEs between 500 and 1000 msec, often chosen as the final echo in the echo train. These thick-slab MRCP images should be supplemented by a set of thinner slices, 5 mm or less. The latter set of images may have a lower TE_{ef} (e.g., about 200 msec) so surrounding soft tissue structures are visible for an anatomical perspective. Although thin-slice MRCP images may be used to generate maximum projection images, there may be misregistration between slices, and the resulting projection images are often inferior to those obtained directly by thick-slab techniques. A third technique for MRCP is 3D-FSE, with the images preferably acquired during suspended respiration. Fixed slab heavily T2-weighted images are used most commonly to evaluate the biliary and pancreatic ducts, but these images are also effective for imaging the unenhanced renal collecting system, which can be referred to as MR urography. Such T2-weighted MR urographic images must be obtained prior to intravenous administration of any water-soluble contrast agents such as gadolinium chelates because these agents reduce the T2 of urine and therefore its signal intensity on these images.

MRCP images may be obtained after administration of gadolinium contrast agents; this practice slightly lowers the signal intensity of blood, the renal collecting system, and the surrounding tissues on these heavily T2-weighted images, reducing the background signal. If MRCP images are obtained using a torso phased-array coil, fat suppression, and a TE_{ef} of 500 msec or greater, wraparound artifact is not a problem, even with a small FOV. This is because solid tissue at the periphery of the body has minimal signal on images such as these.

T1-Weighted and Chemical Shift Techniques

Because of the importance of identifying lipid in parenchymal organs and tumors, chemical shift techniques should be included in most body examinations. For abdominal imaging, comparable in-phase and opposed-phase images provide maximal sensitivity to small amounts of lipid, such as in fatty liver, hepatic and renal carcinomas, and adrenal or hepatic adenomas. If possible, in-phase and opposed-phase images should be obtained as a dual-echo sequence. The TEs of this sequence depend on field strength. If this is not available, separate in-phase and opposed-phase acquisitions should be obtained. In most instances, both sets should be acquired by a gradient echo technique. An alternative is to obtain opposed-phase gradient echo images and conventional spin echo images with the same TE; because of the refocusing pulse at the center of the TE, the spin echo images are in phase. The latter approach is particularly effective at low magnetic field strength, as the TE necessary for obtaining in-phase gradient echo images is particularly long.

In the pelvis, detecting minimal amounts of fat is usually less important than in the abdomen. Fatty tumors such as ovarian teratomas can be diagnosed by obtaining in-phase and fat-suppressed T1-weighted images. The latter images are useful for depicting subtle T1 contrast, methemoglobin in hemorrhage, and enhancement after administration of gadolinium chelates. At low field strength, where fat suppression is usually not possible, similar-appearing water images can be calculated using the raw data obtained from in-phase and opposed-phase acquisitions.

Dynamic Multiphasic Imaging

In the past, 2D multisection imaging was preferred for most dynamic body imaging. Improvements to the 3D technique, however, have made it the method of choice for contrast-enhanced MRA, as discussed in Chapter 23. A similar technique can be used for dynamic imaging throughout the body, with some slight modifications. As with MRA, zero-fill interpolation can be used to generate overlapping thin slices with a high SNR, and segmented methods of fat suppression can be used to produce effective fat suppression with a minimum time penalty.

As with MRA, the TR and TE should be as short as possible. However, the 3D-GRE techniques used for dynamic multiphasic contrast enhancement should have a lower flip angle than those used for MRA. For MRA, a high flip angle (usually 40° or more) is used to saturate background tissue so it produces little signal on the eventual images. In contrast, a low flip angle, about 15°, saturates soft tissue less, so soft tissue on the dynamic images has a better SNR. In addition, compared with MRA, thicker image slices are sometimes needed to provide adequate anatomical coverage.

Dynamic multiphasic contrast-enhanced imaging usually includes at least four sets of images that correspond to four physiological phases relative to the dynamic bolus administration of the contrast material.

1. *Baseline precontrast images* help determine whether the technical quality and anatomical coverage are adequate. These images also provide a basis of comparison to determine the presence or absence of perfusion, which in turn allows confident differentiation between fluid and tissue. If a timing bolus was used prior to acquiring the baseline images, there is visible contrast in the kidneys and collecting systems and minimal intravascular enhancement, but there is no significant effect on the liver or other tissues.

2. *Arterial (capillary, presinusoidal) phase images* are useful for detecting hypervascular tissues, such as the pancreas, renal cortex, uterus, and many malignancies and for depicting arteries. All the arteries are hyperintense on these images, as are hypervascular tissues such as those mentioned above. There may be some contrast enhancement of large, rapidly filling veins such as the portal and renal veins. However, because the hepatic sinusoids should not have filled on these images, there should be little enhancement of the liver and no enhancement of hepatic veins.

3. *Blood pool (venous) phase images* show enhancement of the entire vascular system, including arteries, veins, capillaries, and sinusoids. These images show maximal contrast between the liver and hypovascular lesions and are best for depicting the portal venous system. Because most administered contrast material is present throughout the vascular system at this time, these images are analogous to blood-pool phase images. Beyond the first minute, with increasing time after administration, a large proportion of contrast material has leaked across the capillary membranes of most tissues, so a larger amount of visible enhancement is of interstitial water, rather than intravascular water. This occurs because the currently used gadolinium chelates are extracellular space (not blood pool) contrast agents.

4. *Extracellular (delayed) phase images* are acquired 2 minutes or more after injection of contrast material, by which time the contrast material has diffused into the interstitium of non-central nervous system (CNS) tissues. Because for most tissues these are extracellular space contrast agents, the delayed phase, which is near equilibrium, reflects enhancement of the entire extracellular space, which is a combination of the vascular and interstitial spaces. For healthy CNS and testicular tissues, whose capillaries are not permeable to these contrast agents, delayed images still depict enhancement of the blood pool, although over time the contrast enhancement diminishes owing to renal excretion and diffusion into the interstitium of other tissues.

Delayed contrast enhancement is particularly prominent in edematous tissues such as in neoplasms, areas of inflammation, and fibrosis. If the lipid signal is suppressed via frequency-selective saturation, interstitial enhancement is particularly conspicuous.

To depict delayed extracellular enhancement most effectively, these images should be acquired at least 5 minutes after injecting the contrast material. To do this as part of an efficient imaging protocol, at least one set of required images should be obtained after acquiring the dynamic contrast-enhanced images but before the delayed images. Candidates for this early post-contrast sequence include a set of moderately T2-weighted images and MRCP images, both of which benefit slightly from prior injection of a gadolinium chelate.

Moderately T2-Weighted FSE with Fat Suppression

Moderately T2-weighted FSE fat-suppressed images can be obtained after, rather than before, gadolinium administration. Other than causing lower signal intensity of the kidneys and renal collecting structures, the previously administered gadolinium has little effect on the image, although there may be slightly improved conspicuity of solid liver lesions. Other advantages of performing this sequence after contrast agent administration include obtaining the important contrast-enhanced images earlier and allowing a longer interval before obtaining the delayed postcontrast images.

Single-Slice Gradient Echo with Fat Suppression

Although single-slice GRE images have a lower SNR than comparable multislice or 3D images, these images have some advantages, particularly as delayed postcontrast images for applications where high spatial resolution is not required; because of the inherently low SNR, voxel size cannot be minimized. On these images the TR should generally be between 10 and 30 msec. These images show delayed extracellular space contrast, and all vessels are white because of the combined effects of gadolinium

enhancement and TOF. Motion artifact is minimal because the relatively short TR allows completion of each image in less than 2 seconds.

Potential Problems

There are three common major potential problems encountered during body imaging examinations. Patients may not be able to suspend respiration, the timing of gadolinium administration may be incorrect, or an artifact from internal or external metal may degrade the images. Image degradation due to all three of these problems can be minimized by attention to technique.

Respiratory artifact can be addressed by reducing the acquisition time so the patient can suspend respiration successfully. If this is not possible, the breath-holding sequences may be eliminated, substituting motion-compensated techniques, as discussed in Chapter 13. Although these images generally have a longer acquisition time, this additional time often allows the use of a higher image matrix, and the SNR is often higher.

For dynamic contrast-enhanced imaging, long motion-compensated images are not applicable; imaging must be completed within about 30 seconds or less. One approach to reducing the motion artifact on 3D imaging is to use the shortest possible TR (so view-to-view changes are minimal) and one or more averages to reduce the conspicuity of motion-induced ghosts. Alternatively, gradient echo images can be obtained with short-TR (≤ 10 msec) single-section T1-weighted sequences with a flip angle of about 30°. These images are less sensitive to motion because their acquisition is completed within about 1 second, unlike 2D multislice or 3D images, which generally require about 20 seconds or more. However, 2D single-slice images may have lower contrast than longer acquisition images. Also, vessels generally have high signal intensity on these images, even without contrast agents, owing to replacement of some blood with unsaturated blood flowing into the

Table 27-3 ■ PULSE SEQUENCES USED FOR BODY IMAGING

Pulse Sequence	Purpose	Typical Technique
T1-weighted	General anatomy, fat-water	Dual GRE
T2-weighted	CSF spaces, pathology	Fast SE with FS, or T2-STIR
Heavily T2-weighted	Calcification, blood	Single-shot fast SE; TE ~ 200 msec
Dynamic contrast-enhanced	Vascular anatomy and tissue characterization	3D GRE
MRCP	Biliary and pancreatic ducts	Single-shot fast SE; TE > 500 msec
Balanced SSFP	Vascular anatomy, and fluid	Balanced SSFP

SE, spin echo; STIR, short TI (tau) inversion recovery; FS, fat suppression; GRE, gradient echo; MRCP, magnetic resonance cholangiopancreatography; SSFP, steady-state free precession; CSF, cerebrospinal fluid.

image slice between excitations (TOF effect, as described in Chapter 24). The high signal intensity of blood vessels with or without contrast enhancement reduces the difference in appearance between enhanced and unenhanced 2D single-slice images. On some systems, inversion recovery prepared images (see Chapter 15) can be used for dynamic contrast-enhanced imaging.

For T2-weighted imaging, single-shot techniques have little motion artifact because data for the center of k-space is acquired within milliseconds, but the fine detail is often obscured.

Incorrect timing of image acquisition relative to the bolus of contrast agent is prevented in most cases by using a test dose of gadolinium to determine timing or by using an automated detection method.

Implanted metal (e.g., surgical clips) or undetected external metal on clothing or even in tattoos, is a common source of artifact. Using the shortest possible TE and avoiding fat suppression can minimize the artifact due to metal on gradient echo images. With some instruments, the TE on the 3D-spoiled GRE sequence is minimized by increasing the number of signals averaged from 0.5 to 1.0 and using the maximum allowable sampling bandwidth. The acquisition time is slightly longer if partial Fourier sampling is not used, so adjustments in the number of image slices or the matrix (or both) may be necessary.

Pulse sequences commonly used for body imaging are summarized in Table 27-3.

▼
Essential Points to Remember

Neurological Imaging
1. Spin echo and 3D gradient echo techniques are both acceptable options for obtaining unenhanced images of the brain and spine. They can also be used for contrast-enhanced imaging, although the latter is more suitable for a dynamic technique.

2. For T2-weighted imaging, FSE allows higher spatial resolution and improved definition of CSF spaces with a shorter acquisition time. However, sensitivity to susceptibility contrast is reduced, so T2-weighted SE or T2*-weighted images are preferred for detecting hemorrhage.

3. The FLAIR technique allows depiction of T2 contrast without degradation from high-signal-intensity CSF.

4. Normal brain and cord are characterized by an intact blood-brain or blood-cord barrier, so tumors and damaged brain show greater enhancement on delayed images.

5. On MRI systems with low field strength, the shorter T1 of brain reduces the effects of T1-enhancing contrast agents such as gadolinium chelates. Therefore, the use of a high dose or of magnetization transfer saturation should be considered.

6. MRA and diffusion techniques are commonly included for evaluating suspected cerebrovascular disease and to depict vascular stenoses and cytotoxic edema.

7. Some data suggest that the addition of perfusion imaging can depict ischemic but noninfarcted brain, which is therefore potentially reversible. These images are usually obtained by using dynamic $T2^*$-weighted gradient echo or echo planar imaging after rapid gadolinium chelate injection.

Musculoskeletal Imaging

8. T1-weighted musculoskeletal images should have in-phase TE and sharp edges. For most applications, heavy T1 contrast is not needed, so the TR may be increased to improve coverage.

9. Intermediate-weighted images, with a long TR and a moderate TE, are useful for depicting tendons, ligaments, and fibrocartilage. Tears of these structures are depicted based on T2 contrast.

10. T2-weighted images are useful for depicting fluid, inflammation, and tumor. For most applications, the FSE technique is ideal.

11. STIR imaging is effective for depicting marrow and other soft tissue abnormalities. TE can be increased to add T2 contrast to the inverse T1 contrast that is inherent with STIR.

12. Fat-suppressed T2-weighted images resemble STIR images. If both are obtained, they should be in different planes to maximize their complementary value.

13. The sensitivity of MRI for depicting calcium is improved if gradient echo images with a TE greater than 15 msec ($T2^*$-weighted) are included.

14. Fat-suppressed gradient echo images are ideal for depicting contrast enhancement.

Body Imaging

15. Control of motion artifact, usually through breath holding, is critical for abdominal and thoracic imaging.

16. Imaging at end-expiration is more reproducible, with less unintended motion, than at end-inspiration.

17. Pelvic imaging is less dependent on breath holding than is abdominal and thoracic imaging.

18. Heavily T2-weighted images ($TE_{ef} \geq$ 180 msec), especially with single-shot FSE, are effective for distinguishing solid tissue from simple fluid and static blood, as in hemangiomas.

19. In-phase and opposed-phase images are useful for abdominal imaging and are best obtained as a double-echo gradient echo pulse sequence, where the first echo is used for opposed-phase images and the second echo for in-phase images. There are other alternatives that use a combination of gradient echo or spin echo techniques (or both).

20. Soon after injecting extracellular space gadolinium chelate contrast agents, the images on which veins are first enhanced is similar to a blood-pool image.

21. Several minutes after injecting extracellular space gadolinium chelate contrast agents, enhancement reflects the extracellular space, which is a combination of the vascular and interstitial spaces.

22. Moderately T2-weighted images can help detect solid liver lesions.

These images can be obtained after administering gadolinium chelate contrast agents.

23. Artifact from heterogeneous susceptibility, such as from implanted metal, can be reduced on gradient echo images by using the shortest possible TE and the highest possible bandwidth, as well as by avoiding fat suppression. Using full-Fourier sampling is often necessary to minimize the TE.

Index

Note: Page numbers followed by f refer to figures; page numbers followed by t refer to tables.